Community
Mental Health
for
Older People

Community Mental Health for Older People

Gerard Byrne
BSc(Med) MBBS PhD FRANZCP

Christine Neville
RN RPN BHSc MHSc PhD FACMHN

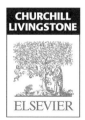

Sydney   Edinburgh   London   New York   Philadelphia   St Louis   Toronto

Churchill Livingstone
is an imprint of Elsevier

Elsevier Australia. ACN 001 002 357
(a division of Reed International Books Australia Pty Ltd)
Tower 1, 475 Victoria Avenue, Chatswood, NSW 2067

© 2010 Elsevier Australia

National Library of Australia Cataloguing-in-Publication Data

---

Byrne, Gerard.

Community mental health for older people / Gerard Byrne, Christine Neville.

9780729538992 (pbk.)

Includes index.
Bibliography.

Mentally ill older people—Care—Australia.
Older people—Health and hygiene—Australia.
Public Health—Australia.

Neville, Christine.

Publisher: Luisa Cecotti
Developmental Editor: Larissa Norrie
Publishing Services Manager: Helena Klijn
Editorial Coordinator: Sarah Botros
Edited by Ruth Matheson
Proofread by Pamela Dunne
Cover and internal design by Lisa Petroff
Cover illustration by Robyn Kennedy
Index by Mei Yen Chua
Typeset by TNQ Books & Journals Pvt Ltd
Printed in Australia by Ligare

PEFC/21-31-17

The book has been printed on paper certified
by the Programme for the Endorsement of
Forest Certification (PEFC). PEFC is
committed to sustainable forest management
through third party forest certification
of responsibly managed forests.

FOREWORD

Currently, 13.3% of the Australian population is aged over 65 and by 2047 this number will rise to 25%. In 2003, mental and neurological disorders accounted for approximately 16% of the disease burden of those aged over 65 (Begg et al 2007). In recognition of this demographic and as a result of strong lobbying by leaders in the fields of psychogeriatric medicine, nursing and other disciplines about the unique needs of the aged, a key direction in the 'National Mental Health Plan 2003–08' was a commitment to improved access to mental health services across the lifespan. This was expressed in 'Key direction 20.2: Ensure older people's mental health services are developed as a key component of the mental health services framework'. In March 2009, while this book was being written, the 'Revised National Mental Health Policy 2008' for Australia was launched. As this book goes to press, the 'Fourth National Mental Health Plan 2009–14' is in development and a 'National Carer Recognition Framework' is to be designed to inform policy development and service delivery for carers, many of whom provide essential support for older mentally ill people.

Necessary and important policy commitment at this level, while a significant step forward, must be made a reality in daily clinical practice. However, it is still questionable if the pace and extent of change has had the intended outcomes, particularly in regard to the care provided to those who are ageing and have a mental illness. For those who have lived with serious and persistent mental illness throughout their adult lives and are now ageing, and for those experiencing mental illness for the first time in late life, the impact of normal ageing processes and events coupled with illness is a daunting experience. It is critical that mental health workers are well trained in ageing-specific psychiatric practice, have an awareness of, and are responsiveness to, the larger context of the healthcare system and have the ability to effectively utilise resources to provide care that is of optimal value. This is a challenging expectation given historic workforce undersupply and retention issues, and the pervasive 'double stigma' of mental illness and ageing in our society, despite the best intentions of policy.

This eminently practical book, aimed at providing information and guidance for multi-disciplinary staff members in mental healthcare teams, creates a context for informed, sensitive and responsive practice. The authors, geriatric psychiatrist Dr Gerard Byrne and geropsychiatric nurse Dr Christine Neville, are seasoned clinicians, teachers and researchers whose collaborative relationship extends over a decade. Their commitment to, and experience with, vulnerable older clients is apparent throughout the book, which uses extensive case exemplars, a DSM–IV framework and current research underpinning best practice to present management strategies. The authors' teaching goal of increasing competence in the complexity of treating older people is certainly consistent with the 'National Mental Health Plan' mandate and is a welcome tool in the preparation of the future mental health workforce. It is comprehensive and accessible enough to serve as a primer for the novice or as a reference text for more experienced mental health workers from all disciplines. For staff needing knowledge of practical geropsychiatric care in long-term care settings, where the overwhelming majority of residents have a diagnosable psychiatric disorder such as dementia, depression or anxiety, this book is invaluable.

Particularly relevant contributions in the book are the chapters on multidisciplinary teamwork, consumer/carer involvement, and rural and cultural/social issues. The contextual tensions and paradoxes that create potential problems for effective teamwork in community mental health teams and limit teamwork to mere rhetoric are highlighted. This approach encourages an awareness of the complexities and dilemmas of policy, models of practice and teamwork patterns in a specialty practice area. Recognition of the unique and essential contribution of consumers and carers to effective treatment and strategies for their meaningful involvement are helpful. The challenges of providing accessible, expert care in rural and remote environments, to Indigenous older people and those from culturally and linguistically diverse (CALD) backgrounds, and to members of minority social groups, are well presented. This reminds mental health workers of the importance of their awareness of, and respect for, difference and how it may be expressed and interpreted in the experiences of ageing and mental illness.

If you are taking the time to read this book, you probably already appreciate what is rewarding about working with older people with mental illness. Your daily work provides dignity and relief from suffering to some of the most vulnerable members of our society. Commitment to this work contributes to improvements in attitudes and expertise that successive generations, including your own, can only benefit from. Congratulations to Gerard Byrne and Christine Neville on an outstanding addition to the field that reflects their expertise, compassion and commitment.

Elizabeth Beattie PhD RN
Professor of Nursing
Queensland University of Technology

Reference

Begg S, Vos T, Barker B et al 2007 The burden of disease and injury in Australia 2003. AIHW Cat. No. PHE 82, AIHW, Canberra

CONTENTS

PREFACE

Community Mental Health for Older People is intended as an introductory text for mental health workers who are interested in the rapidly developing field of older persons' mental health. We hope this book will appeal to both experienced mental health workers as well as those who have just entered the field. Community mental health teams working with older people are usually multidisciplinary and we have written the book with this in mind.

Wherever possible, we have taken an evidence-based approach to our writing. Where evidence has been limited, our approach has been guided by our concern for the humane care of older people with mental health problems. However, we recommend that the reader adopt a critical approach to their clinical work.

The book is divided into seven sections. Section 1 introduces the concepts of population health and burden of disease in relation to the mental health of older people. It then looks at a series of issues integral to evidence-based care in the community, as well as the structure and function of community mental health teams. Section 2 covers several broader background issues that are relevant to all community mental health workers, including sociocultural issues, issues in rural and remote locations, and the role of consumers and carers.

Section 3 addresses the diverse clinical skills that should be acquired by the mental health worker caring for older people, starting with the development of a therapeutic relationship and finishing with risk assessment. Section 4 deals in some detail with the major clinical presentations encountered by community mental health workers dealing with older people, starting with dementia and delirium and finishing with personality disorder. Section 5 canvasses broader management issues from prevention and promotion all the way to electroconvulsive therapy. Section 6 covers legal and ethical issues, including the vexed issue of driving in later life. Finally, Section 7 of the book briefly covers rating scales and outcome evaluation, both of which are now common accompaniments of community mental healthcare of older people. We have provided suggested additional reading at the end of many chapters, as well as a limited number of essential references.

We hope you enjoy reading *Community Mental Health for Older People*.

ABOUT THE AUTHORS

Gerard Byrne is the director of the Older Persons' Mental Health Service at the Royal Brisbane and Women's Hospital and head of the Discipline of Psychiatry within the School of Medicine at the University of Queensland. He has extensive clinical and research experience in the field of old age psychiatry.

Christine Neville is a mental health nurse with a broad experience of community mental healthcare for older people, particularly in regional and rural areas. She received an international award for her work in this clinical area. Christine is the Program Co-ordinator for Mental Health Nursing in the School of Nursing and Midwifery at the University of Queensland.

VERS

RPN BA BSc(Hons)
Addiction and Mental Health Programs, Discipline of Nursing,

Lynn Chenoweth PhD MA(Hons) MAdEd GCert T/L BA RN
Professor of Aged and Extended Care Nursing, Faculty of Nursing, Midwifery and
Health, University of Technology Sydney, Director, Health and Ageing Research Unit,
South Eastern Sydney–Illawarra Area Health Service

Sally Garratt DN(Honaris Causa) MScN BEd DipAppSc(Ned) FRCNA(DLF)
Adjunct Associate Professor ACEBAC, LaTrobe University

David Lie MBBS FRACGP FRANZCP
Senior Lecturer and Clinical Affiliate, Centre for Research in Geriatric Medicine,
University of Queensland; Clinical Director, Older Persons Mental Health Service,
Princess Alexandra Hospital, Brisbane

Bryan McMinn RN MHN BSc MNurs(NP) FACMHN
Clinical Nurse Consultant, Mental Health of Older People, Hunter New England
Mental Health, Conjoint Lecturer, Faculty of Health, University of Newcastle

Rhonda Nay RN BA(UNE) MLitt(UNE) PhD(UNSW) FRCNA FCN FAAG
Professor of Interdisciplinary Aged Care, Director Institute for Social Participation,
Director Australian Centre for Evidence Based Aged Care; Director Australian Institute
for Primary Care; Director TIME for Dementia, La Trobe University/Bundoora
Extended Care Centre

Eileen Petrie PhD MNS PostGradDip CPN RN MRCNA MACMHN
Senior Lecturer, Masters Research Coursework Coordinator, Nursing and Midwifery,
La Trobe University

ACKNOWLEDGMENTS

The writing of *Community Mental Health for Older People* represents many years of work
that has been greatly influenced by professional colleagues and the older people for
whom we have been privileged to provide care. We are grateful to the staff at Elsevier for
their advice and guidance. We would like to express our appreciation to the reviewers
for their insightful feedback during the writing process. Finally, a heartfelt thankyou is
extended to our families for their abiding love, encouragement and support.

Chapter 1

POPULATION HEALTH AND BURDEN OF DISEASE

INTRODUCTION

This chapter introduces the ageing population and its implications for population health and the burden of disease. Special emphasis is given to prevalence data for mental health problems in older people. The chapter also highlights contemporary approaches to epidemiology and health economics as they relate to the mental health of older people. The material presented in this chapter is essential for an understanding of the distribution of mental health problems among older people and is basic knowledge for all mental health workers. More detailed prevalence data are presented in chapters dealing with individual mental health problems.

THE AGEING POPULATION

There is a worldwide trend among developed nations towards population ageing. This trend reflects the combination of steadily rising life expectancy and falling birth rates. Life expectancy is rising due to promotion of healthy lifestyles, prevention of disease and widespread availability of effective medical treatments. Life expectancy in Australia at the age of 65 years is now 82.5 years for males and 86.1 years for females (Australian Institute of Health and Welfare 2007). Falling birth rates are due mainly to improved contraception, later age of marriage, and improved educational and work opportunities for women. The average Australian fertility rate during the period 2000–05 was 1.8 babies per woman. This may be compared with fertility rates for the same period of 2.0 for the United States, 1.3 for Japan and 2.3 for Vietnam (Australian Bureau of Statistics 2007). The replacement fertility rate is the average number of children that each woman needs to have to replace herself and her partner. As the current replacement fertility rate is approximately 2.1, Australia needs an immigration program to maintain or increase its population.

Because women have a longer life expectancy than men, population ageing is associated with population feminisation. Thus, older people are increasingly likely to be women (see Fig 1.1). As a consequence, the prevalence of mental health problems that are more common in women, such as Alzheimer's disease, will increase beyond that predicted by increasing life expectancy alone. Another consequence of the ageing population is that the ratio between older retired people and younger people of working age is rising. In other words, there are increasing numbers of retired people for every

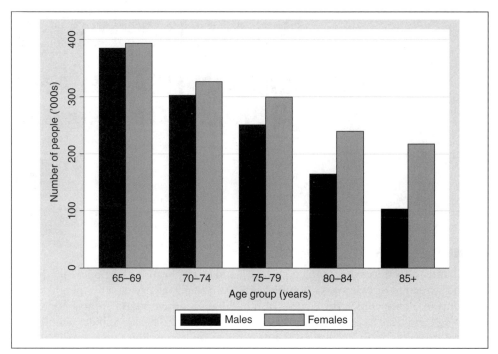

Figure 1.1 Older Australians by age and gender
Source: Australian Bureau of Statistics (2007, Table 3.1, p 82).

working-age person. This so-called elderly dependency ratio is usually calculated as the ratio between the number of people aged 65 years and over and the number of working-age people. At present, the elderly dependency ratio in Australia is approximately 20%. If retired people are dependent upon working-age people for financial and practical support, then it has been argued that this support will be less available in the future. However, the likely significance of this trend is unclear, as more people will have access to superannuation funds in the future, and medical and technological advances might alter caregiving roles.

Australia has one of the highest official marriage rates in the developed world and about 60% of married people can expect to stay married to the same person until one partner dies. However, among people aged 65 years and over, a significant proportion of both men (25.4%) and women (55.6%) no longer have a partner (Australian Bureau of Statistics 2000). As a result, many older people, particularly older women, live alone. Fortunately, 44% of people who live alone own their home without a mortgage (Australian Bureau of Statistics 2004).

Homelessness is a highly politicised issue and accurate data are difficult to obtain. However, in the 2001 national census of Australia, an estimate of the extent of homelessness was made (Chamberlain & MacKenzie 2003). There were estimated to be 99,900 homeless people in Australia, of whom 5995 (6%) were aged 65 years and over. There are also a large number of people living in marginal circumstances, such as caravan parks, who are not counted among the primary homeless in the census. This is an important issue for community mental health services as a high proportion of homeless people have a mental health problem. However, older people are underrepresented among the homeless and are not targeted specifically by programs for the homeless. As an illustration of this, in 2007–08, Australian Supported Accommodation Assistance Program (SAAP) services were accessed by 159 of every 10,000 people aged 15–19 years, but by only 8 of every 10,000 people aged 65 years and over (Australian Institute of Health and Welfare 2009b).

Most of the people seen by older persons' mental health services (OPMHS) are retired from the paid workforce. In Australia in 2007, 84.4% of women and 67.7% of men aged 65–69 years reported that they were retired. In comparison, 97.1% of women and 90.8% of men aged 70 years and over were retired (Australian Bureau of Statistics 2009). Although only 16% of retired people reported that superannuation was their main source of retirement income, this proportion is expected to rise as greater numbers of older people have access to compulsory superannuation funds. About 40% of working-age Australians over the age of 45 plan to cut down their working hours before retiring (Australian Bureau of Statistics 2009).

HOSPITAL CARE

People aged 65 years and over are more likely to be admitted to hospital than younger people and have a higher average length of stay than any other age group, apart from children aged less than one. The term 'hospital separation' refers to the number of people leaving hospital through discharge or death. Hospital separation statistics are complex, but it is instructive to look briefly at how separations for depressive episodes in women vary by age. In 2007–08, 5121 women aged 25–34 years, 7424 women aged 35–44 years, 6472 women aged 45–54 years, 4984 women aged 55–64 years, 2936 women aged 65–74 years, 2611 women aged 75–84 years and 860 women aged 85+ years left hospital after a depressive episode (Australian Institute of Health and Welfare 2009a). Among people aged 65 years and over, Indigenous Australians accounted for 11.5% of hospital separations, whereas non-Indigenous Australians accounted for 37.4% of separations. However, people living in very remote areas have a separation rate 50% higher than the rest of the population (Australian Institute of Health and Welfare 2009a).

RESIDENTIAL AGED CARE

OPMHS deal commonly with people living in residential aged care environments or receiving care at home. In 2008, there were 175,472 Commonwealth-supported residential aged care places in Australia (Australian Institute of Health and Welfare 2009c). In addition, there were 40,280 Community Aged Care Packages (CACP), 4244 Extended Age Care at Home (EACH) packages and 1996 EACH Dementia packages (Australian Institute of Health and Welfare 2009). Current planning targets call for 113 places and packages per 1000 people aged 70 years and over. These targets include 44 high-care places, 44 low-care places, and 25 community-care packages, of which four are for high care (Australian Institute of Health and Welfare 2009c). There has been a steady increase in the proportion of residential aged care facility (RACF) residents who require high care. This currently stands at approximately 70% of all residents. On 30 June 2008, there were 157,087 permanent residents and 3163 respite residents in aged care facilities in Australia (Australian Institute of Health and Welfare 2009c).

EPIDEMIOLOGY

Definitions

'Prevalence' refers to the number of people with a certain disease or disorder per unit of population. Prevalence data are usually expressed as cases per 100,000 of the population. 'Incidence' refers to the number of new cases of a disease or disorder per unit of population. Incidence data are usually expressed as cases per 100,000 of the population per year.

Prevalence and incidence of mental health problems in older people

The *prevalence* of mental health problems in older people is often disputed, mainly because of concern about the methods employed to count people with mental health problems in the community (O'Connor 2006). The standard approach uses fully structured diagnostic interviews administered by trained lay interviewers during systematic doorknock surveys based on census tracts. Such methods are only practicable for counting mental health problems that can be diagnosed by computer algorithm on the basis of respondent self-report. They do not lend themselves to the identification of mental health problems, such as dementia and delirium, which require the respondent to be examined, tested or scanned. Nor do such methods lend themselves to the identification of mental health problems in people who are unable to answer the front door or who decline to participate in the survey. Most diagnostic interviews systematically exclude mental symptoms that are thought to be due to general medical disorders (such as stroke or cancer), although the methods used to determine this are often unsatisfactory. Most population surveys of mental health problems do not include mental state examinations, physical examinations, laboratory investigations or neuroimaging studies, such as computed tomography (CT) or magnetic resonance imaging (MRI) brain scans. Thus, a restricted range of data is obtained at interview and a limited range of mental health problems can be diagnosed.

Despite these limitations, it is instructive to examine the reported prevalence of mental health problems in older people in comparison with the prevalence of mental health problems in young and middle-aged people. Figure 1.2 shows the estimated prevalence of mental health problems by age group for Australians aged between 16 and 85 years based on the 2007 National Survey of Mental Health and Wellbeing (NSMI IW). This survey had a 60% response rate and recruited about 8800 respondents. The NSMHW only counted cases of mood disorder, anxiety disorder and substance-use disorder. The prevalence estimates for older people derived from this survey are associated with high standard errors, and so should be treated with caution. Despite these caveats, it is clear that the estimated rates of so-called 'high prevalence' mental health problems decline sharply with age. However, the mental health problem with the highest prevalence of all, in people aged 65 years and over, dementia, was not counted in this survey. As Figure 1.2 demonstrates, anxiety disorders are the commonest type of mental health problem, other than dementia, at all ages. Anxiety disorders are much more common than mood disorders (mainly depression) and substance-use disorders, although anxiety disorders tend to be the focus of diagnosis and treatment much less often than the other two sets of disorders.

Very little accurate information is known about the true *incidence* of mental health problems in older people. Incidence data are more difficult to obtain than prevalence

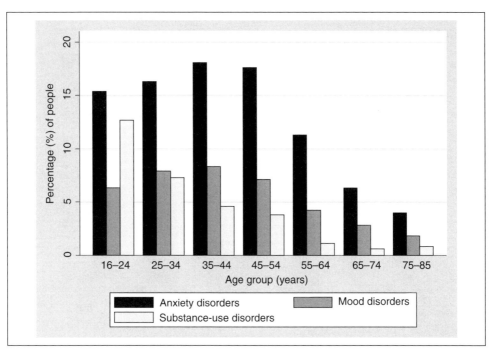

Figure 1.2 Twelve-month prevalence of common mental health problems among community-residing people by age group, Australia 2007
Source: Australian Bureau of Statistics (2008).

data, as the participating individuals must be surveyed twice at a fixed interval (usually 1 year). Attrition in ageing populations adds further to this difficulty.

Although there has been an Australian survey of so-called 'low prevalence' health problems (Jablensky et al 1999), principally schizophrenia and bipolar disorder, this survey specifically excluded older people, and so there are no national data on psychotic disorders in older Australians. However, an epidemiological study from Finland (Perala et al 2007) has provided population-level data on psychotic disorders in older people. These researchers found that the prevalence of psychotic disorders in people aged 65 years and over was 3.6%, much higher than had previously been thought. They found that 2.3% of people aged 65 years and over had a non-affective psychosis, whereas 1.3% of people aged 30–44 years had such a disorder. In other words, schizophrenia and related disorders were found to be more common in older people than in younger adults.

Although no national, population-based prevalence or incidence survey of dementia has been conducted in Australia, various estimates have been made. The prevalence of dementia increases exponentially with age, doubling approximately every 5 years after the age of 65 years (see Fig 1.3). Thus, older people are not at particularly high risk of dementia until the age of 75 years. However, the prevalence of dementia has been shown to be much higher in Indigenous Australians than in the non-Indigenous population (Smith et al 2008). In the Kimberley Region of Western Australia, the estimated prevalence of dementia was 26.8% in Indigenous people aged 65 years and over compared with 6.5% in the non-Indigenous Australian population. Importantly, the prevalence of

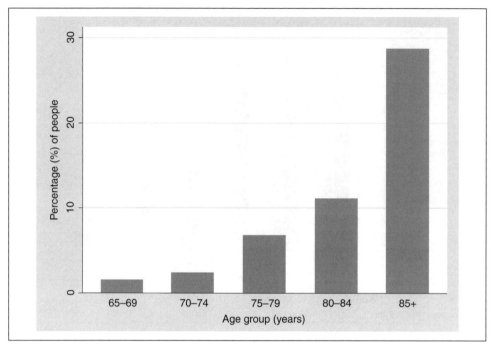

Figure 1.3 Prevalence estimates for dementia
Source: Jorm et al (1987).

dementia was 12.4% in Indigenous people aged 45 years and over, whereas the comparable prevalence in non-Indigenous people was 2.4%.

Although Australian RACFs collect extensive clinical data on their residents, relatively few of these data are published in a readily accessible form. However, independent research has demonstrated very high levels of dementia (Australian Institute of Health and Welfare 2006) and depression (Ames 1993, McSweeney & O'Connor 2008) in Australian aged care facilities. For instance, in 2003 it was estimated from official records that there were 67,650 people with dementia in aged care facilities, representing 48.7% of all residents (Australian Institute of Health and Welfare 2006). This is almost certainly an underestimate. Similarly, McSweeney and O'Connor (2008) found that 24% of newly admitted RACF residents met criteria for a major depressive episode and that a further 20% had subsyndromal depression (minor depression).

Snowdon and colleagues (2006) have studied the pattern of medication prescribing in Sydney RACFs on three occasions—in 1993, 1998 and 2003. Over this 10-year period, they have noted a reduction in the rate of prescribing of regular hypnotic medication (sleeping tablets) from 26.6% to 11.2% and a rise in the rate of prescribing antidepressants from 15.6% to 19.1%. Antipsychotic medication was prescribed to 27.4% of RACF residents in 1993 and to 24.4% of residents in 2003, although in 1998 and 2003 there was increasing use of atypical antipsychotic medication. A significant proportion of this antipsychotic prescribing appeared likely to be 'off label'. The term 'off label' refers to the use of drugs for non-approved indications or in a non-approved manner (e.g. the use of antipsychotics other than risperidone for dementia under the Pharmaceutical Benefits Scheme (PBS)).

BURDEN OF DISEASE

The acronym DALY refers to Disability Adjusted Life Years and is a measure of disease burden based on healthy years lost. The DALY associated with a particular disease or disorder is calculated by summing years of life lost through death (YLL) and years lived with disability (YLD). The use of DALYs allows the disease burden associated with different disorders to be compared on the same scale. DALYs also allow the disease burden associated with the one disorder in different countries to be compared.

The World Health Organization (WHO) sponsored a global burden of disease study using 1990 data that led to a report detailing global patterns of death and disability projected out to 2020 (Murray & Lopez 1996). WHO has more recently published a 2004 update of the report that is freely accessible online (World Health Organization 2008). Using 2003 data, similar methodology was applied to the assessment of disease burden in Australia (Begg et al 2007). Together, mental disorders and neurological disorders accounted for 23% of total Australian burden of disease in 2003 and 43% of non-fatal disease burden. Despite much greater disease burden due to cardiovascular disease and cancer among people aged 65 years and over, mental disorders and neurological disorders, including dementia, still accounted for 15.9% of total disease burden in this group. Mental health DALYs vary considerably by socioeconomic status. In 2003, there was a 53% difference between the mental health DALYs experienced by the lowest quintile of socioeconomic status compared with the highest quintile. These are important findings, as governments now frequently refer to burden of disease figures when allocating funding.

Health economics

The acronym QALY refers to Quality Adjusted Life Years and is a measure of disease burden based on quantity and quality of life following a treatment intervention.

The QALY is critical to the advice provided to health trusts in the United Kingdom by the National Institute for Health and Clinical Excellence (known as NICE) about purchasing health interventions such as new drugs. Considerable controversy arose when NICE initially recommended that the cholinesterase inhibitor medications used to treat the symptoms of Alzheimer's disease were not value for money. However, after a judicial review, NICE issued revised advice indicating that the cholinesterase inhibitors were recommended for people with Alzheimer's disease whose score on the Mini-Mental State Examination (MMSE) was between 10 and 20.

The NICE website is freely accessible at www.nice.org.uk and contains evidence-based advice on a large number of different interventions for a wide range of clinical conditions, including mental health problems. For instance, in relation to generalised anxiety disorder, NICE (2007) recommends that benzodiazepines be used for no longer than 2–4 weeks and that the following treatments (in descending order) should be used instead:
1. psychological treatment using cognitive behaviour therapy (CBT)
2. selective serotonin reuptake inhibitor (SSRI) medication, and
3. self-help with the aid of written material (bibliotherapy).

As another example, NICE (2008) assessed whether transcranial magnetic stimulation (TMS) should be used for treatment-resistant depression. They concluded that there was insufficient evidence of efficacy to recommend TMS in treatment-resistant depression and that TMS should only be used in research studies.

SUMMARY

This chapter has summarised the characteristics of the ageing population and provided an overview of the estimated prevalence of mental health problems in people aged 65 years and over. It has also introduced the acronyms DALY and QALY, which now play an important role in health planning and the allocation of resources by governments.

REFERENCES

Ames D 1993 Depressive disorders among elderly people in long-term institutional care. Australian and New Zealand Journal of Psychiatry 27:379–391

Australian Bureau of Statistics (ABS) 2000 Australian social trends. ABS Cat. No. 4102.0. ABS, Canberra

Australian Bureau of Statistics (ABS) 2004 Marriages, Australia. ABS Cat. No. 3306.0. ABS, Canberra

Australian Bureau of Statistics (ABS) 2007 Australia's welfare. ABS, Canberra

Australian Bureau of Statistics (ABS) 2008 National survey of mental health and wellbeing 2007. ABS Cat. No. 4326. ABS, Canberra

Australian Bureau of Statistics (ABS) 2009 Australian social trends. ABS Cat. No. 4102.0. ABS, Canberra

Australian Institute of Health and Welfare (AIHW) 2006 Dementia in Australia: national data analysis and development. AIHW Cat. No. AGE 53. AIHW, Canberra

Australian Institute of Health and Welfare (AIHW) 2007 Older Australia at a glance 4th edn. AIHW Cat. No. AGE 52. AIHW, Canberra

Australian Institute of Health and Welfare (AIHW) 2009a Australian hospital statistics 2007–08. AIHW Cat. No. HSE 71. AIHW, Canberra

Australian Institute of Health and Welfare (AIHW) 2009b Homeless people in SAAP: SAAP national data collection annual report. SAAP NDC Report Series 13. AIHW Cat. No. HOU 191. AIHW, Canberra

Australian Institute of Health and Welfare (AIHW) 2009c Residential aged care in Australia 2007–08: a statistical overview. Aged Care Statistics Series 28. AIHW Cat. No. AGE 58. AIHW, Canberra

Begg S, Vos T, Barker B et al 2007 The burden of disease and injury in Australia 2003. AIHW Cat. No. PHE 82, AIHW, Canberra

Chamberlain C, MacKenzie D 2003 Counting the homeless 2001. Australian Bureau of Statistics, Canberra

Jablensky A, McGrath J, Herrman H et al 1999 People living with psychotic illness: an Australian study 1997–1998. Commonwealth of Australia, Canberra

Jorm AF, Korten AE, Henderson AS 1987 The prevalence of dementia: a quantitative integration of the literature. Acta Psychiatrica Scandinavica 76:465–479

McSweeney K, O'Connor DW 2008 Depression among newly admitted Australian nursing home residents. International Psychogeriatrics 20:724–737

Murray JL, Lopez AD (eds) 1996 The global burden of disease. Harvard University Press, Cambridge, MA

National Institute for Health and Clinical Excellence (NICE) 2007 Clinical guideline 22. Online. Available: www.nice.org.uk 21 Aug 2009

National Institute for Health and Clinical Excellence (NICE) 2008 Interventional treatment guidance 242. Online. Available: www.nice.org.uk 21 Aug 2009

O'Connor DW 2006 Do older Australians truly have low rates of anxiety and depression? A critique of the 1997 national survey of mental health and wellbeing. Australian and New Zealand Journal of Psychiatry 40:623–631

Perala J, Suvisaari J, Saarni SI et al 2007 Lifetime prevalence of psychotic and bipolar 1 disorders in a general population. Archives of General Psychiatry 64:19–28

Smith K, Flicker L, Lautenschlager NT et al 2008 High prevalence of dementia and cognitive impairment in Indigenous Australians. Neurology 71:1470–1473

Snowdon J, Day S, Baker W 2006 Current use of psychotropic medication in nursing homes. International Psychogeriatrics 18:241–250

World Health Organization (WHO) 2008 The global burden of disease: 2004 update. WHO, Geneva. Online. Available: www.who.int/healthinfo/global_burden_disease/2004_report_update/en/index.html 27 May 2009

Chapter 2

NORMAL, HEALTHY AND SUCCESSFUL AGEING

INTRODUCTION

This chapter introduces the concept of normal ageing and contrasts it with healthy ageing and successful ageing. Mental health workers regularly encounter unhealthy ageing, so it is useful to have a clear idea of normal ageing and successful ageing. The concepts of brain reserve and the clinician's illusion are also described.

NORMAL AGEING

Normative or normal ageing involves adapting to declining physical health, dealing with life transitions and coping with loss and grief. Many older people do this without difficulty. The Australian Institute of Health and Welfare (AIHW) produces regular statistical overviews of the characteristics of older Australians (Australian Institute of Health and Welfare 2007) and many of the statistics in this chapter are derived from this source. Approximately two-thirds (67.3%) of older Australians rate their general health as good or better, whereas one-third (32.7%) rate their health as fair or poor (Australian Institute of Health and Welfare 2007). Despite these optimistic self-ratings, the majority of older Australians do have one or more chronic health problems. These include high blood pressure (71.8%), high cholesterol (61.8%), impaired glucose tolerance (22.1%) and obesity (20.1%). Other big health issues in normal ageing include osteoarthritis, impaired eyesight due to cataracts and macular degeneration, impaired hearing, and poor dental health due to lack of universal access to dental care.

Not surprisingly, older people have more than twice the rate of visits to their general practitioners as younger adults (Australian Institute of Health and Welfare 2007). In 2005–06, this amounted to 8.6 visits per year for people aged 65 years and over compared with about 4 per year for people under 65 years of age. While the majority of older people do not have cognitive impairment or a serious mental health problem, anxiety and depressive symptoms are quite common. In 2004–05, 3.2% of people aged 65 years and over reported very high levels of psychological distress and 7.7% reported high levels of psychological distress on a standardised self-report measure.

Life transitions are common in later life. Some older people are fortunate to be able to continue working beyond the normal retirement age in an occupation that they find enjoyable and fulfilling. More commonly, however, retirement comes at the usual time, if not earlier than expected, due to poor health or prevailing economic conditions. The majority of older people have had children and by the time of their retirement from the paid workforce also have grandchildren. In well-functioning families, grandparents are likely to be happily involved in helping their adult children care for their children. In less fortunate families, grandparents will need to substitute for absent or dysfunctional parents. Some older couples might be able to coordinate their other roles sufficiently to become what are termed 'grey nomads' in Australia or 'snow birds' in Canada and the United States (Higgs & Quirk 2007). Grey nomads travel around the country, often congregating in camping grounds and caravan parks in picturesque locations. They commonly drive campervans or tow caravans. Some older couples do this for part of the year, whereas others have no permanent residence and travel for the whole year. There is often a preference for warmer climates and outdoor activities.

Loss and grief are normal accompaniments of the human condition, but are more commonly experienced in later life. Among Australians aged 65 years and over, 71.3% of men and 44.6% of women are married, whereas 12.3% of men and 42.1% of women are widowed. Largely as a consequence of spousal bereavement, 29% of older Australians live alone (Australian Institute of Health and Welfare 2007). Spousal bereavement is associated with a temporary rise in symptoms of anxiety and depression, and occasionally with mental health problems requiring treatment.

Regular physical activity is undertaken by 49% of older Australians. Walking is most popular, with 29.1% of those aged 65 years and over walking on a regular basis. Other popular types of physical activity include lawn bowls (5.6%), golf (5.4%), aerobics or similar classes (5.4%), swimming (4.2%) and cycling (1.7%) (Australian Institute of Health and Welfare 2007). Reported physical activity varies by self-rated general health status. Over 60% of older people who rated their health as excellent participate in sport or physical activity, while only about 20% of older people who rate their health as poor do so (Australian Bureau of Statistics 2006).

There is clearly some room for increased participation in regular physical activity by older people. Importantly, there is now evidence that regular physical exercise is not only good for physical health and longevity, but also for cognitive function. Epidemiological evidence indicates that men who walk at least 3 kilometres per day reduce their risk of dementia by almost one-half compared with sedentary men (Abbott et al 2004), and experimental evidence indicates that walking for 50 minutes three times a week significantly improves cognition (Lautenschlager et al 2008). In laboratory studies on rodents, voluntary physical exercise has been found to be associated with increased neurogenesis (production of new brain cells) and it is possible that the same might be true in humans.

The availability of good social support and social networks seems to improve the resilience of older people, just as it does young and middle-aged people. Older people tend to prune their social networks so that they are smaller and more focused on supplying their needs. However, normal older people generally perceive their social networks to be adequate. Perhaps surprisingly, social networks seem also to modify the effect of brain pathology on the risk of cognitive decline (Bennett et al 2006). In other words, older people with good social networks seem somehow able to tolerate more brain pathology before developing clinical signs of cognitive impairment or dementia. Older people are increasingly using the internet to stay in touch with friends and relatives. In 2004–05, 20% of older people used a computer at home, with the majority having internet access. This will rise dramatically over the next few years, as 51% of those aged 55–64 used a computer at home in 2004–05 (Australian Institute of Health and Welfare 2007).

Access to transport is a key requirement in later life. Of older people residing in the major Australian cities in 2006, 84.4% of men and 52.2% of women had access to a motor vehicle they could drive (Australian Institute of Health and Welfare 2007). The proportions were even higher in provincial cities and rural areas. Older people without cognitive impairment and those with insight into mild cognitive impairment generally modify their driving behaviour as their driving skill changes (Pachana & Petriwskyj 2006). For instance, older people often restrict their driving to good conditions and daylight hours. Despite these self-imposed changes in driving behaviour, older people are overrepresented in motor vehicle accident statistics. This may be because many older people tend to drive short distances and most accidents occur close to home.

Two factors that are commonly associated with unhealthy ageing are features of normal ageing for some people. Although modest regular alcohol consumption might be associated with reduced risk for some cardiovascular outcomes, 8.1% of older Australians engage in a risky level of alcohol intake. In addition, 7.9% of older people smoked cigarettes in 2004–05 (Australian Institute of Health and Welfare 2007). Smoking is one of the most important modifiable risk factors for cardiovascular disease, stroke and cancer.

Falls occur commonly among older people and risk-reduction measures include regular weight-bearing exercise like walking, balance exercises, avoidance of unnecessary psychotropic medications, and avoidance of risky alcohol intake. In some older people, cerebrovascular disease is an important additional risk factor for gait abnormalities and falls.

Dental health is another component of normal ageing. One consequence of improved conservation of teeth is that today's older people have more teeth than previous generations and thus are at greater risk of tooth decay and gum disease than previously. However, older people are still generally at lower risk of tooth decay than middle-aged and younger people. In the absence of a universal system of dental care, limited access to affordable dental care is an issue for some older people.

The role of work in later life is coming under greater scrutiny as an increasing proportion of the workforce is over the age of 55 years. These trends are affecting health workers also. In 2006, 20.6% of male health workers and 14.6% of female health workers were aged 55 years or over (Australian Institute of Health and Welfare 2009). In recognition of better health and increased longevity, governments in developed nations around the world are pushing back the conventional retirement age to beyond 65 years. People in jobs that are not physically demanding and in jobs where excellent health is not a requirement may elect to work beyond the conventional retirement age, particularly if the public contribution to pensions declines, as seems inevitable. Workers in physically demanding jobs (e.g. the building trades and underground mining) and workers in jobs that demand excellent health (e.g. airline pilots and professional athletes) may need to seek employment in less physically demanding fields in later life. Unless birth or immigration rates increase dramatically, there will be relatively fewer working-age people to support older people, and one consequence of this is that older people will need to continue working longer.

One issue that is related to healthy and successful ageing is whether employers will be prepared to allow older workers to work reduced hours so that they can manage their transition to retirement in a graduated fashion. In the 2006 Australian census, 48% of full-time workers indicated that they intended to work part time before retiring from the workforce. Interestingly, 24% of employed people indicated that they intended to retire at 70 years or over.

Superannuation will become increasingly important for a happy retirement. However, at present, only 44% of Australians aged 65–69 years have any superannuation. Those older people without superannuation and who do not own their own homes are likely to suffer significant financial strain and potential psychological distress unless they obtain support from their children.

These work-related changes are likely to have a major impact on the lives of older people. Some older people see work as a phase through which one moves to retirement, and as a means of generating income so as to live comfortably. In other words, they work to live. Others see work as an integral component of their lives and an expression of their personality, and not something to be set aside prematurely. In other words, they live to work. Personal choices and sociocultural factors are likely to be key determinants of which of these approaches to work is taken by the older person. However, it is possible to age successfully while adopting either approach.

HEALTHY AGEING AND SUCCESSFUL AGEING

The terms healthy ageing and successful ageing are often used interchangeably and both suggest something better than normal ageing. In healthy ageing, serious morbidity is compressed so that it occurs as close as possible to the moment of death. In successful ageing there is an emphasis on happiness and fulfilment, as well as physical health.

Peel and colleagues (2005) reviewed behavioural determinants of healthy ageing. Modifiable risk factors included smoking status, physical activity level, body mass index, diet, alcohol use and certain health practices. The Australian Longitudinal Study of Women's Health (ALSWH) (Lee & ALSWH team 2003) has studied predictors of poor mental health in very large cohorts of young, middle-aged and older women, and found the following risk factors:
- having many physical symptoms
- making frequent visits to the general practitioner
- being unmarried
- having financial problems
- smoking tobacco
- not being physically active
- being overweight or obese, and
- using illicit drugs.

Similarly, predictors of successful mental health ageing have been studied in 601 octogenarian men from the Health In Men Study (HIMS) (Almeida et al 2006). Successful mental health ageing was defined as the absence of depression or cognitive impairment. Those men with high school or university education, and who undertook regular physical activity, were more likely to have good mental health at 5-year follow-up. Older age, non-English-speaking background, and, curiously, regular consumption of full cream milk were associated with poor mental health outcome (Almeida et al 2006). Just why the consumption of full cream milk should be associated with poor mental health outcome is unknown, but it might relate to risk of cerebrovascular disease or to possible associations with other unmeasured risk factors.

Vaillant and Mukamal (2002) have studied predictors of successful ageing in several cohorts, including in male Harvard University graduates who were enrolled in the Grant Study of Adult Development starting in 1938. Six factors identified before 50 years of age predicted good health and happiness between 75 and 80 years of age. These were: never being a smoker, or stopping smoking when young; the absence of alcohol abuse;

having a stable marriage; doing some exercise; not being overweight; and using mature psychological defences. Six factors that did not predict good health and happiness in later life were also identified. These were: ancestral longevity; cholesterol level; stress; parental characteristics; childhood temperament; and positive affect and ease in social relationships.

BRAIN RESERVE

So far in this chapter we have been considering healthy ageing as a holistic concept and one that can be applied to the overall health of the individual. However, cognitive ageing is worthy of special consideration. Approximately 6.5% of people aged 65 years and over have dementia (Australian Institute of Health and Welfare 2007; see Ch 19), so there is considerable interest in how to prevent this common disorder. The concept of 'brain reserve' relates to individual differences in life experience that are linked prospectively to a reduced risk of cognitive impairment or dementia (Valenzuela & Sachdev 2006). Thus, in this model, the clinical symptoms of dementia emerge when brain pathology exceeds brain reserve. Brain reserve factors include high childhood intelligence, high educational achievement, high occupational work complexity, effortful cognitive lifestyle activities and possibly also physical activity (Fratiglioni & Wang 2007). Overall, these factors when present are capable of reducing the risk of dementia by about 50% (Valenzuela 2008). These findings are in keeping with earlier work from the 'Nun Study' which found that young recruits who wrote reflective essays in their early twenties with high idea density and high grammatical complexity were less likely to develop dementia in their eighties (Snowdon et al 1996). These are important findings and suggest that early life factors have an enduring influence on later life cognitive function. It seems that the presence of brain pathology such as that due to Alzheimer's disease is, in many cases, insufficient on its own to cause cognitive impairment or dementia.

THE CLINICIAN'S ILLUSION

Mental health workers generally work with highly symptomatic and often very disabled older people. While it is quite appropriate for this to be the case, the experience can bias the clinician's view of the severity and chronicity of mental illness. Older people with mental health problems of long duration are more likely to appear in the caseload because the usual caseload is strongly biased towards prevalent (i.e. existing) cases, rather than incident (i.e. new) cases, and the overall prognosis often looks much worse than it usually is. This is the clinician's illusion (Cohen & Cohen 1984). Knowledge of normal ageing and successful ageing might be a partial antidote to this illusion.

SUMMARY

In this chapter, we have introduced the concept of normal ageing and outlined its characteristics for older Australians. We have also described the concepts of healthy and successful ageing and looked at predictors of successful ageing from US and Australian research. We have looked briefly at work in later life, and the concepts of brain reserve and the clinician's illusion.

FURTHER READING

Australian Institute of Health and Welfare (AIHW) 2007 Older Australia at a glance, 4th edn. AIHW Cat. No. AGE 52. AIHW, Canberra

Slater H 1995 The psychology of growing old. Open University Press, Buckingham

Vaillant GE 2002 Aging well. Little, Brown, Boston, MA

REFERENCES

Abbott RD, White LR, Ross GW et al 2004 Walking and dementia in physically capable elderly men. Journal of the American Medical Association 292:1447–1452

Almeida OP, Norman P, Hankey G et al 2006 Successful mental health aging: results from a longitudinal study of older Australian men. American Journal of Geriatric Psychiatry 14:27–35

Australian Bureau of Statistics (ABS) 2006 Sport and social capital, Australia, 2006. ABS Cat. No. 4917. ABS, Canberra

Australian Institute of Health and Welfare (AIHW) 2007 Older Australia at a glance, 4th edn. AIHW Cat. No. AGE 52. AIHW, Canberra

Australian Institute of Health and Welfare (AIHW) 2009 Health and community services labour force 2006. AIHW Cat. No. HWL 43. AIHW, Canberra

Bennett DA, Schneider JA, Tang Y et al 2006 The effect of social networks on the relation between Alzheimer's disease pathology and level of cognitive function in old people: a longitudinal cohort study. Lancet Neurology 5:406–412

Cohen P, Cohen J 1984 The clinician's illusion. Archives of General Psychiatry 41(12):1178–1182

Fratiglioni L, Wang H-X 2007 Brain reserve hypothesis in dementia. Journal of Alzheimer's Disease 12:11–22

Higgs PF, Quirk F 2007 'Grey nomads' in Australia: are they a good model for successful aging and health? Annals of the New York Academy of Sciences 1114:251–257

Lautenschlager NT, Cox KL, Flicker L et al 2008 Effect of physical activity on cognitive function in older adults at risk for Alzheimer disease. Journal of the American Medical Association 300:1027–1037

Lee C, ALSWH team 2003 Women and mental health in Australia. Summary report prepared for the Australian Commonwealth Department of Health and Ageing. Australian Longitudinal Study on Women's Health, University of Newcastle and University of Queensland, Report No. 78. Online. Available: www.alswh.org.au/Reports/SynthesesPDF/mentalhealth_summary.pdf 12 Apr 2009

Pachana NA, Petriwskyj AG 2006 Assessment of insight and self-awareness in older drivers. The Clinical Geropsychologist 30:23–38

Peel NM, McClure RJ, Bartlett HP 2005 Behavioral determinants of healthy aging. American Journal of Preventive Medicine 28:298–304

Snowdon D, Kemper S, Mortimer J et al 1996 Linguistic ability in early life and cognitive function and Alzheimer's disease in late life: findings from the Nun Study. Journal of the American Medical Association 275:528–532

Vaillant GE, Mukamal K 2001 Successful aging. American Journal of Psychiatry 158:839–847

Valenzuela MJ 2008 Brain reserve and the prevention of dementia. Current Opinion in Psychiatry 21:296–302

Valenzuela MJ, Sachdev P 2006 Brain reserve and dementia: a systematic review. Psychological Medicine 36:441–454

Chapter 3

EVIDENCE-BASED CARE IN THE COMMUNITY

INTRODUCTION

The community mental health worker caring for older people will develop over time a certain pattern to their clinical work. It is likely that this pattern will have been influenced by their general professional education and training (e.g. as a nurse or social worker), by their previous experience in the workplace (e.g. in an adult mental health service) and by their exposure to the older persons' mental health services (OPMHS) team in which they currently work. They are likely to have had professional supervision as well as direction from line managers. In addition, their OPMHS team may have clinical pathways or protocols that guide the clinical approach to older people with particular problems. Some mental health workers might even have encountered pharmaceutical company representatives seeking to promote their products. Finally, the worker is likely also to bring their patterns of behaviour to their work. These patterns have been informed by their personal experiences with the healthcare system, and those of their family and friends. So the knowledge, skills and attitudes brought by the worker to the clinical situation are likely to have been moulded over time by a variety of influences. As only some of these influences are likely to be reliable and valid sources of evidence, it is worth examining more formally the types of evidence that might inform clinical behaviour.

This chapter provides a detailed outline of the evidence-based approach to healthcare. However, much of standard care in older persons' mental health is still based on historical practice and humane principles, rather than evidence. In the absence of satisfactory evidence, a scientific approach should be taken to practice by the individual mental health worker and by the mental health team of which they are a member. Standard practices that are not yet based on evidence should be subject to critical scrutiny by the health worker.

QUANTITATIVE VERSUS QUALITATIVE METHODS

Before considering the scientific method and the types of empirical evidence that underpin evidence-based clinical practice, it is worth outlining the differences between quantitative and qualitative methods. Quantitative methods involve the collection of observations using numbers. For example, change in the average score on the Hamilton Depression Rating Scale is commonly used to establish the extent of improvement in older people with major depressive disorder in clinical trials of new psychological or pharmacological treatments. By contrast, qualitative methods involve the collection of observations without using numbers. For example, a focus group might be used to find out which aspects of a respite care service are most helpful to the carers of people with dementia. In clinical research, qualitative data are sometimes used to complement quantitative data.

Both quantitative and qualitative approaches involve the collection of data. However, the collection of data alone does not constitute evidence unless the data are analysed within a model or in relation to a hypothesis. This principle is as true for quantitative data as it is for qualitative data. Quantitative methods usually involve deductive reasoning, whereas qualitative methods usually involve inductive reasoning. Many research papers use deductive reasoning based on quantitative methods to arrive at their main finding and then inductive reasoning to generalise from the particular circumstances of their study to the broader case.

Although quantitative methods such as randomised controlled trials and quantitative meta-analyses (see below) are strongly preferred to other types of evidence by the Cochrane Collaboration and other groups promoting evidence-based medicine, qualitative methods can add considerably to knowledge in a number of fields relevant to mental health, including phenomenology, sociology and anthropology. Qualitative methods can generate types of data that provide clinically relevant nuances to quantitative data.

THE SCIENTIFIC METHOD

The scientific method refers to the gathering of empirical evidence through observation and experiment to enable hypotheses to be tested. An alternative term for the modern version of the scientific method is the hypothetico-deductive method. This method is generally considered to be the only reliable approach to obtaining unbiased evidence about the world around us. A hypothesis is considered scientific if it is falsifiable—that is, if it is possible, at least in principle, to prove it wrong. This does not mean that all human wisdom is to be found via the scientific method, just that this is the only *reliable* way to gather *unbiased* evidence. Other, non-scientific approaches to the world around us might include such fields of inquiry as astrology and psychoanalysis. These latter endeavours are considered non-scientific because they do not lead to falsifiable hypotheses.

Scientific inquiry traditionally begins with observations from which potential explanations, or hypotheses, are generated. These hypotheses lead to predictions, which can be tested by further observation or through experiment. This process is often followed iteratively until stable findings provide a reliable explanation for the observations. Findings from scientific inquiry are usually subjected to peer review before publication.

TYPES OF EVIDENCE

Much of the 'evidence' that we use in clinical practice is quite informal and would not pass close scrutiny. This includes clinical anecdotes provided by co-workers, editorials in clinical journals and opinion pieces written by leading exponents of a particular theory or treatment. Much of this 'evidence' is not reliable or unbiased, cannot be falsified, has not been subject to independent peer review, and is often best disregarded.

Scientific approaches to clinical evidence include peer-reviewed case studies, case series, case-control studies, cohort studies, randomised controlled trials, secondary analyses, systematic reviews and meta-analyses. Each of these will now be briefly outlined.

Case study

There are two broad types of single case studies: descriptive and analytic. In a descriptive case study, a single informative clinical case is presented in written or oral form, usually to a specialised audience. Many descriptive case studies are examples of qualitative research. Some clinical journals have regular or occasional case studies that illustrate the work-up and management of cases. These are useful for the presentation of rare or unusual examples of mental health problems that the average mental health worker is unlikely to encounter often. Of course, it is difficult to generalise from a single case study but they often alert clinicians to illness manifestations that they might not have been aware of or complications that they had not previously considered. However, descriptive single case studies generally require replication before too many clinical implications can be drawn.

In analytic case studies (often termed 'N = 1' studies), an intervention is trialled in a clinical setting. For instance, a new or experimental approach might be applied in a novel clinical situation. Often these N = 1 studies use an A–B–A design where a conventional approach, or treatment as usual, is given in the first phase (A), followed by the experimental treatment in the second phase (B), followed by a third phase where the first phase treatment (A) is repeated.

Case series

In a case series, a small collection of informative clinical cases is presented, either using the descriptive approach or an analytic approach, as described for single case studies. Often these will be consecutively seen cases that have been accumulated over several years. This is a particularly useful approach to the presentation of uncommon combinations of mental health problems. A case series has the potential to drive clinicians to examine their own practices and researchers to generate testable hypotheses about the aetiology and management of particular presentations of clinical disorders. Descriptive case series may be considered a type of qualitative research.

Case-control study

Case-control studies are sometimes known as controlled comparison studies. Although this type of cross-sectional observational study is generally considered weaker than cohort studies (which are longitudinal observational studies) and experimental studies, it is sometimes the only feasible type of study that can be done when researchers are interested in studying uncommon conditions. In the case-control study, cases (people with the condition of interest) are compared with controls (people who do not have the condition of interest). It is important that the controls are in all other important respects similar to the cases, except that they do not have the condition of interest. Because case-control studies are cross-sectional in design, they do not lend themselves readily to causal thinking.

Cohort study

Cohort studies are observational studies that employ a longitudinal perspective. They lend themselves to causal thinking. In the typical cohort study, a population sample (the cohort) is followed over time (often years) to see what happens to them. For instance, a cohort study might be used to investigate predictors of depression as people grow older. Information on potential predictors is obtained at baseline, and so is not confounded by knowledge of which participants will ultimately develop depression. The main limitations of cohort studies are the length of time they take to run and the associated expense of mounting them, the difficulty of keeping the cohort intact during a lengthy period of follow-up (people move house, get fed up with the study, or die), and the problem of trying to predict at the beginning of the study which potential predictor variables are likely to be relevant.

Despite these limitations, cohort studies are a good way of generating lists of possible risk factors or protective factors for clinical conditions, including mental health problems. However, these risk factors or protective factors still need to be rigorously tested in randomised controlled trials before they can usefully be introduced into clinical practice. Quite often, when randomised control trials are used in an attempt to modify risk factors that have previously been identified in cohort studies, the interventions turn out not to have any impact on disease incidence or prevalence. For example, oestrogen and non-steroidal anti-inflammatory drugs (NSAIDs) were demonstrated in cohort studies to be protective against the future development of Alzheimer's disease, but in subsequent randomised controlled trials seemed to have little, if any, protective effect.

Randomised controlled trials

Well-conducted randomised controlled trials (RCTs) generate much stronger evidence for the efficacy of treatments or preventive interventions than observational studies such as case-control studies and cohort studies. As a consequence, most regulatory authorities such as the US Food and Drug Administration (FDA) and the Australian Therapeutic Goods Administration (TGA) require at least two rigorous RCTs before considering a new drug for licensing.

The critical feature of an RCT is an intervention (or treatment) that is randomly assigned to some of the participants, while other participants receive the control intervention (in drug trials, this is commonly a placebo drug or a comparison drug). Random assignment is not the same thing as giving every second person the intervention and the others the placebo. It involves the use of some formal method of generating random numbers (often a computer program) and then using these numbers to assign participants to treatment arms of the study.

The RCT approach may be used for drug trials and for non-pharmacological trials. Thus, the development of a new drug for the treatment of Alzheimer's disease and the development of a new type of cognitive behaviour therapy (CBT) for depression in older people would both usually involve several RCTs conducted by different researchers. However, human drug trials are further subdivided according to a classification scheme, as follows:

- The Phase 0 study is a newly described category for 'first in human' clinical trials.
- Phase I studies involve the use of a drug in a small group of normal healthy volunteers, usually young men. Phase I studies are conducted to assess the safety of the drug in healthy people, but do not usually have a sufficient number of participants to determine the efficacy of the drug.
- Phase II studies are conducted on larger numbers of volunteers who suffer from the condition that the drug has been designed to treat. Phase II studies aim to establish the correct dose of the drug (Phase IIA studies) and how well the drug works (Phase IIB studies). Many Phase II studies use the RCT approach and include a placebo group.

- Phase III studies are usually multisite RCTs designed to compare the efficacy and toxicity of the new drug with an existing treatment.
- Phase IV studies are surveillance studies conducted after a drug has been marketed. Phase IV studies are usually designed to study the adverse effect profile of the drug in treated populations.

Because of the critical importance of RCTs, most medical journals now require the authors of papers describing the results of RCTs to have registered their RCT on a public access website prior to any people being recruited to the study. The US National Institutes of Health (NIH) clinical trials website (www.clinicaltrials.gov) and the Australian New Zealand Clinical Trials Registry website (www.anzctr.org.au) record information about all clinical trials regardless of whether they involve pharmaceutical agents or non-pharmacological interventions such as CBT. Scientific journals that publish the findings from clinical trials usually now require researchers to describe their research according to the CONSORT guidelines (Altman et al 2001).

Measures of statistical and clinical significance

As previously outlined, the scientific method requires the collection of data and the testing of hypotheses through either observational or experimental studies. Various numerical measures are used to report the results of hypothesis testing. These include p-values, the effect size, odds ratios, confidence intervals and the number needed to treat. The p-value conventionally represents the probability that the finding of an experiment could have happened by chance alone. For example, a p-value of less than 0.05 indicates that if the experiment were to be conducted in a similar manner 100 times over, it would produce a similar result at least 95 times.

Importantly, a p-value does not indicate the magnitude of the difference between an experimental intervention and a control condition. For this, we need an effect size, often shortened to ES and often represented by Cohen's d. When using Cohen's d to measure ES, around 0.3 is said to be a small effect, around 0.5 is said to be a medium effect and 0.8 or greater is said to be a large effect. A variety of other statistics may be used to represent the ES, but these will not be discussed here. Another way of representing the difference between two groups is to use the odds ratio (OR). As its name suggests, the OR is the ratio between two sets of odds. If the odds of a person aged 75 having depression is five in 100 (0.05) and the odds of a person aged 40 having depression is 20 in 100 (0.2) then the OR is 0.05/0.2 or 0.25. That is, the 75-year-old has one-quarter the odds of having depression as the 40-year-old.

The confidence interval (CI) is used to estimate the uncertainty in a numerical finding. The wider a CI, the less certain the finding. In health and medical research, a CI of 95% is commonly used, indicating that if the experiment were to be conducted 100 times, 95 times out of 100 you would get a result within the limits of the CI. Thus, an odds ratio of 0.25 might have a 95% CI of 0.2–0.3 or a 95% CI of 0.01–2.5. The first CI is narrow, so one can be confident that the OR is likely to be accurate. The second CI is wide, so one can have little confidence that the OR is accurate.

Another metric that is useful in human clinical trials is the 'number needed to treat' (NNT). The NNT can be defined as the number of people who need to be treated with an intervention for one person to respond who would not have responded to a placebo. Treatments with better efficacy have smaller NNTs. A related concept is the number needed to harm (NNH).

Measures of statistical significance often provide little information about the likely clinical significance of research findings. For this, we need to use a different approach. In determining clinical significance it is useful to have data also from normal people—so-called normative data. If a research finding is statistically significant and the intervention brings people with a particular clinical condition (e.g. a major depressive episode) back into the normal range on a clinical scale (e.g. the Hamilton Depression Rating Scale), then the findings are likely also to be clinically significant. Thus, moving a person from a pathological score to a normal score on a scale might suggest clinical significance. Paradoxically, statistical approaches have also been taken to estimate the clinical significance of change scores using a metric called the Reliable Change Index (RCI) (Jacobson & Truax 1991). Alternatively, if a person satisfies diagnostic criteria (e.g. DSM–IV or ICD–10) for a major depressive episode before the intervention and does not meet these criteria after the intervention, it could be argued that they have achieved clinically significant change in their diagnostic status.

Secondary analyses

In secondary analyses the researcher uses data already collected by others. For instance, a government agency may have collected data on self-reported mental health during a survey in a defined geographic area or in a population census. These data might later be available in a de-identified form to researchers who might be interested in looking at the relationship between mental health and, say, age and income.

Systematic reviews and meta-analyses

Review articles summarise a large amount of material and make it available to the reader in a more easily assimilated form. Most clinicians are not going to have the time or inclination to search the original research literature on a particular subject unless they are planning to conduct some original research themselves. However, many clinicians look for summaries of published research to guide their own clinical practice. This has become much more important within the context of evidence-based clinical practice. Review articles are often written like opinion pieces in which the author says what they think about a topic and provides evidence in support of their view. Unfortunately, such review articles are unlikely to provide a sound basis for clinical practice. Clinical practice should be based on an unbiased appraisal of the available evidence. To achieve this, the modern clinician will generally integrate their own clinical experience with the findings from systematic reviews and meta-analyses.

The systematic review is fundamental to the development of evidence-based clinical practice. In this type of literature review, the authors identify and synthesise all the high-quality research that is available on a particular clinical question. Some, but not all, systematic reviews include a quantitative meta-analysis, which is a statistical technique for summarising the findings from a series of similar studies.

Cochrane reviews

The Cochrane Collaboration publishes health-related systematic reviews and meta-analyses and provides the results of these without charge on their website (www.cochrane.org). For instance, if one searches the Cochrane database on the topic of antipsychotic drug treatment for late-onset schizophrenia, one finds a single systematic review (Arunpongpaisal et al 2003) reporting that there is 'no trial-based evidence upon which to base guidelines for the treatment of late-onset schizophrenia'. Similarly, if one searches on the topic of antipsychotic drug treatment for older people with schizophrenia, there is one systematic review (Marriott et al 2006) reporting that 'there are little robust data available to guide the clinician with respect to the most appropriate drug to prescribe'. The Cochrane Collaboration uses quantitative data and eschews qualitative data.

Joanna Briggs Institute

The Joanna Briggs Institute (JBI), based in Adelaide, also undertakes systematic reviews and provides the results to its subscribers (www.joannabriggs.edu.au). It takes a somewhat different approach to that taken by the Cochrane Collaboration and includes both quantitative and qualitative evidence in its summaries and reviews. It focuses particularly on nursing and midwifery topics. The open-access JBI 'Best Practice' series covers several topics of relevance to community mental health of older people. These include the 'Management of constipation in older adults', 'Strategies to reduce medication errors with reference to older adults' and 'Strategies to manage sleep in residents of aged care facilities'. These clinical management reviews are relatively brief, are easy to read and identify the quality of evidence for each recommendation.

Clinical practice guidelines

The AGREE Collaboration (2001) has defined clinical practice guidelines (CPGs) as 'systematically developed statements to assist practitioner and patient decisions about appropriate health care for specific clinical circumstances'. However, CPGs are only as good as the evidence on which they are based. To assist healthcare workers 'to undertake their own assessment before adopting the recommendations' found in a set of guidelines, the AGREE Collaboration developed an Appraisal Instrument (AGREE Collaboration 2001). The Appraisal Instrument covers six domains: scope and purpose; stakeholder involvement; rigour of development; clarity and presentation; applicability; and editorial independence.

OTHER ISSUES IN RELATION TO EVIDENCE
Levels of evidence

Levels of evidence (or quality of evidence) have been described by several research organisations, including the Australian National Health and Medical Research Council (NHMRC), the Oxford Centre for Evidence-Based Medicine (OCEBM) and the Joanna Briggs Institute (JBI). Although levels of evidence are commonly described for studies of treatment interventions (see below), there are also published tables of levels of evidence for aetiology, screening, diagnosis and prognosis.

The NHMRC levels for treatment interventions are:

I	Systematic review of level II studies
II	Randomised controlled trial
III–1	A pseudo-randomised controlled trial
III–2	A comparative study with concurrent controls
III–3	A comparative study without concurrent controls
IV	Case series (with post-test data or pre-test and post-test data)

Efficacy versus effectiveness

A distinction is normally made between efficacy and effectiveness of any treatment intervention. Efficacy refers to whether the intervention works under ideal experimental conditions. Effectiveness refers to whether the intervention works under 'real world' circumstances. The difference in meaning between these two terms is important because sometimes treatment interventions that work quite well in the model participants often recruited to clinical trials do not work nearly as well in the usual type of people seen by mental health services. For instance, a treatment for psychosis might work quite well in people who do not have any comorbid general medical problems. However, when the same treatment is used in people with common general medical problems such as type 2 diabetes and Parkinson's disease, serious adverse effects emerge that limit the dose that can be used and, as a consequence, the effectiveness of the drug.

Generalisability

The issue of generalisability of research findings follows on from the previous discussion of efficacy and effectiveness. When the clinician seeks to apply findings from the research literature to their own practice, how should they judge the published research? This is a particularly important issue in relation to the mental health of older people. Relatively little research has been done into treatment interventions for older people with mental health problems. Thus, one is left with trying to generalise to older people from studies based mainly on younger people without significant comorbidity. The clinician should establish the age range of the study sample and whether the study included 'real world' cases or only ideal cases. If older people were recruited to the study, was a significant proportion of the participants aged 80 years and over? If not, then the study is not likely to generalise well to the 'old old'.

Next, the clinician must ask whether many potential participants were excluded from enrolment in the study and whether many actual participants dropped out of the study during the treatment intervention. Clinical trials in which more than 20% of the participants dropped out during treatment are usually judged to be of inferior quality and are unlikely to generalise well to the general population of people being treated. The next issue is whether comorbidity was permitted. In other words, were people with more than one mental health problem (e.g. major depression and generalised anxiety disorder) or a mental health problem plus a general medical condition (e.g. schizophrenia plus type 2 diabetes) enrolled in the study? In practice, many older people with mental health problems have additional comorbid mental or physical disorders, and research studies that do not reflect this might have limited generalisability.

Another important question is whether the study was conducted on community-residing people, on residential aged care facility (RACF) residents or on hospital inpatients. Findings might not transfer well between these settings. Other important questions might include whether people from culturally and linguistically diverse backgrounds and people with diverse educational and occupational backgrounds were enrolled in the study. The answers to these and related questions should help the clinician determine whether study findings will generalise well to the people they treat.

Types of qualitative evidence

The techniques of qualitative research include face-to-face interviewing, focus groups, written descriptions by participants, and observations of verbal and non-verbal behaviour. Sometimes, observers are also involved in the action, so-called participant observers. Qualitative research often generates large amounts of textual data that can be a challenge to interpret. To assist with this task, several computer software programs have been developed, including the evocatively named NVivo and Nud*ist.

HOW TO LOCATE THE EVIDENCE

It has never been easier to locate the evidence that supports clinical practice. Although textbooks on old-age psychiatry and shorter books on particular mental health problems are likely to be found in any good health service library, they are generally too detailed for a quick introduction to the field and too out of date to consult for the latest evidence. Electronic databases are the most powerful and flexible method of locating the evidence, particularly as the evidence is mainly to be found in journal articles. Most modern mental health services have ready access to electronic library resources, including web-based databases such as MEDLINE, PsycINFO and CINAHL. Most hospital and university libraries offer short instructional courses on the use of these databases.

Although these databases cover the fields of medicine, psychology and nursing respectively, in practice there is considerable overlap between them in terms of journal coverage. Articles of relevance to mental health practice, including the mental health of older people, are to be found in all three databases. However, even if the mental health service does not have access to these databases, there is free public access to MEDLINE via PubMed (www.ncbi.nlm.nih.gov/pubmed). As previously noted, the Cochrane library is easily accessible (www.cochrane.org).

While MEDLINE and the other online databases allow thousands of journals to be searched for relevant articles, several journals focus specifically on mental health problems in older people. These include *International Psychogeriatrics*, the *International Journal of Geriatric Psychiatry*, the *American Journal of Geriatric Psychiatry* and *Aging and Mental Health*. Mental health workers specialising in the care of older people are advised to regularly browse the table of contents of one or more of these journals.

A recent publication phenomenon is the development of electronic open access journals. Such journals offer free public access to all. In psychiatry there are now more than 30 open access journals, although none yet that specialise in the mental health of older people. Open access journals can be identified through the Directory of Open Access Journals (see www.doaj.org).

EXAMPLES OF EVIDENCE

Community outreach services

Although there is a long-cherished view that mental health services to older people should be delivered in the community, what is the evidence that such outreach services are effective? To help answer this question, Van Citters and Bartels (2004) undertook a systematic review of the published evidence on the effectiveness of community-based mental health outreach services for older adults. They discovered 14 studies including five RCTs. Two of the 14 studies were actually studies of gate-keeping programs. Of the remaining 12 studies, eight involved participants living in their own homes or in public housing, two involved residents of aged care facilities and two involved mixed cohorts. Although the complex results of this systematic review are difficult to summarise briefly, the five RCTs demonstrated that the interventions provided by community outreach services led to significantly reduced depressive symptoms (four studies) and significantly reduced overall psychiatric symptoms (one study). A quantitative meta-analysis was not possible due to widely varying study designs. The authors concluded that their systematic review provided 'qualified support for the effectiveness of multidisciplinary psychogeriatric outreach services' (Van Citters & Bartels 2004).

Psychological interventions for caregivers of people with dementia

Selwood et al (2007) undertook a systematic review of psychological interventions for the family caregivers of people with dementia. They found 10 good-quality studies. These studies provided clear evidence that six or more sessions of *individual* behavioural management therapy focused on the care recipient's behaviour improved caregiver psychological health, both immediately and in the longer term. However, they found that *group* behavioural management therapy, with the exception of one Australian inpatient study (Brodaty & Gresham 1989), was ineffective. Selwood et al (2007) also found that individual and group caregiver support interventions are effective in alleviating depression and distress both immediately and for some months.

Management of constipation in older adults

A Joanna Briggs Institute (JBI) systematic review of the management of constipation was summarised in a JBI Best Practice article (Joanna Briggs Institute 2008). This review found grade A evidence (strong support that merits application) for prevention of constipation using education about hydration and a high-fibre diet, and for screening of older adults for polypharmacy, laxative use and cognitive impairment. It found grade B evidence (moderate support that warrants consideration) for monitoring bowel movements, using osmotic agents (e.g. lactulose) and bulking agents (e.g. bran), and for bed exercises in people unable to walk.

Treatment of late-onset psychosis

A Cochrane systematic review (Arunpongpaisal et al 2003) reported that there was no methodologically sound RCT evidence on the use of currently available antipsychotic medication in people with late-onset schizophrenia (LOS) (age of onset >40 and <59) or with very late onset schizophrenia-like psychosis (VLOSLP) (age of onset >60). There is an urgent need for RCTs of antipsychotic medication in people with LOS and VLOSLP. Thus, clinicians treating people with these types of LOS with antipsychotic medication must rely on efficacy evidence obtained in younger people, together with their own clinical experience.

Treatment of anxiety

A quantitative meta-analysis (Pinquart & Duberstein 2007) investigated the comparative efficacy of behavioural and pharmacological treatments for anxiety disorders in 32 studies that enrolled a total of 2484 participants aged 60 years and over. Most of the participants were suffering from generalised anxiety disorder or panic disorder. There was a wide range of pharmacological agents used, although antidepressants were the predominant class used. Most of the behavioural interventions employed CBT. Although the uncontrolled ES of pharmacological interventions ($d = 1.76$) was much greater than the uncontrolled ES of behavioural interventions ($d = 0.81$), when non-specific changes in the control groups were taken into account, the comparative ESs ($d = 0.83$ for pharmacological interventions and $d = 0.80$ for behavioural interventions) were not significantly different. However, interpretation of the comparative efficacy of behavioural and pharmacological interventions was difficult because the pill placebos used in the pharmacological studies were associated with much greater improvement ($d = 1.06$) than the control conditions used in the behavioural studies ($d = 0.10$). Nevertheless, both pharmacological and behavioural interventions for anxiety disorders in older adults showed large ESs. Thus, the evidence suggests that both pharmacological treatments and behavioural treatments have good efficacy in older adults with anxiety disorders.

A subsequent meta-analysis (Thorp et al 2009) has investigated the efficacy of different behavioural treatments for late-life anxiety in 19 published studies. Unlike the previously described meta-analysis, this review included adults aged 55 years and over. These reviewers also used studies that included participants with anxiety symptoms as well as participants with anxiety disorders. This review compared CBT without relaxation training (CBT – RT) with CBT plus relaxation training (CBT + RT) and with relaxation training (RT) alone. Interestingly, CBT alone and CBT + RT were no better than RT alone. Thus, the available evidence indicates that RT is an evidence-based treatment for anxiety in later life. This information is likely to be very useful to clinicians working in OPMHS, as RT is relatively simple and inexpensive to administer.

Treatment of depression

A Cochrane review (Wilson et al 2008) has investigated psychological treatments for depression in older people and found that there was limited evidence on which to base conclusions. However, they found seven clinical trials that compared CBT with a control condition. In five clinical trials (N = 141) in which CBT was compared with a control condition and the outcome assessed by a clinician on the Hamilton Depression Rating Scale (HDRS), CBT was superior to control with a mean advantage of 9.85 points on the HDRS. All of the people were outpatients. One potential threat to the generalisability of these findings is that some of the studies included in this review used people aged 55 years and over, which is rather young by contemporary standards of later life.

A recent meta-analysis (Thompson et al 2007) found five RCTs (N = 165) in which antidepressant medication was compared with placebo for the treatment of depression in people with Alzheimer's disease. Most of the participants (134 or 81.2%) were outpatients and the remainder were RACF residents. Antidepressants were superior to placebo in terms of both treatment response (OR 2.32; 95% CI 1.04–5.16) and remission of depression (OR 2.75; 95% CI 1.13–6.65). The number needed to treat (NNT) for both response and remission was five. However, the astute reader will note that the confidence intervals around these odds ratios are rather wide, and disturbingly close to one at the bottom end.

SUMMARY

Contemporary evidence-based approaches have particular relevance to treatment interventions in community mental health, and several examples of this have been provided. Although these approaches usually employ quantitative methods and deductive reasoning, there is an important place also for qualitative methods and inductive reasoning, particularly in the social sciences that are relevant to mental health.

REFERENCES

AGREE Collaboration 2001 Appraisal of guidelines for research and evaluation (AGREE) instrument. Online. Available: www.agreecollaboration.org 14 June 2009

Altman DG, Schulz KF, Moher D et al (for the CONSORT Group) 2001 The revised CONSORT statement for reporting randomized trials: explanation and elaboration. Annals of Internal Medicine 134:663–694

Arunpongpaisal S, Ahmed I, Aqeel N, Paholpak S 2003 Antipsychotic drug treatment for elderly people with late-onset schizophrenia. Cochrane Database of Systematic Reviews, Issue 2. Art. No.: CD004162. DOI:10.1002/14651858.CD004162

Brodaty H, Gresham M 1989 Effect of a training programme to reduce stress in carers of patients with dementia. British Medical Journal 299(6712):1375–1379

Jacobson NS, Truax P 1991 Clinical significance: a statistical approach to defining meaningful change in psychotherapy research. Journal of Consulting and Clinical Psychology 59:12–19

Joanna Briggs Institute 2008 Management of constipation in older adults. JBI Best Practice 12(7):1–4

Marriott R, Neil W, Waddingham S 2006 Antipsychotic medication for elderly people with schizophrenia. Cochrane Database of Systematic Reviews, Issue 1. Art. No.: CD005580. DOI:10.1002/14651858.CD005580

Pinquart M, Duberstein PR 2007 Treatment of anxiety disorders in older adults: a meta-analytic comparison of behavioral and pharmacological interventions. American Journal of Geriatric Psychiatry 15:639–651

Selwood A, Johnston K, Katona C et al 2007 Systematic review of the effect of psychological interventions on family caregivers of people with dementia. Journal of Affective Disorders 101:75–89

Thompson S, Herrmann N, Rapoport MJ, Lanctot KL 2007 Efficacy and safety of antidepressants for treatment of depression in Alzheimer's disease: a meta-analysis. Canadian Journal of Psychiatry 52(4):248–255

Thorp SR, Ayers CR, Nuevo R et al 2009 Meta-analysis comparing different behavioral treatments for late-life anxiety. American Journal of Geriatric Psychiatry 17:105–115

Van Citters AD, Bartels SJ 2004 A systematic review of the effectiveness of community-based mental health outreach services for older adults. Psychiatric Services 55:1237–1249

Wilson KCM, Mottram PG, Vassilas CA 2008 Psychotherapeutic treatments for older depressed people. Cochrane Database of Systematic Reviews, Issue 1. Art. No.: CD004853. DOI:10.1002/14651858.CD004853.pub2

Chapter 4

MODELS OF MENTAL HEALTHCARE AND ORGANISATIONAL ISSUES

INTRODUCTION

Although there is evidence for the effectiveness of older persons' mental health services (OPMHS) (Draper 2000), the most effective components of such services have not yet been clearly identified. There are many different ways to deliver community mental health services to older people. This chapter covers models of care delivery and associated organisational issues. It assumes the presence of a national health service with universal access.

AREA-BASED SERVICES

In countries with national health systems, such as Australia, New Zealand and the United Kingdom, most public sector mental health services are organised and delivered within a defined geographical area or district. Inpatient beds and mental health teams are generally provided on an historical basis with forward planning of both bed numbers and community teams determined by population data. Subspecialty mental health services such as OPMHS teams are a more recent phenomenon and in many places have been grafted on to adult mental health services.

The OPMHS is likely to see people with a wide variety of mental health problems. However, in comparison with adult mental health services, the older persons' service is likely to see a higher proportion of women and more people with mood disorders and cognitive disorders.

In more fortunate districts, acute inpatient mental health facilities for older people have been purpose-built and are co-located with geriatric medical services. More commonly, however, older people with mental health problems are admitted to general adult inpatient wards. This is often a rather unsatisfactory situation because the needs of younger people with, for example, acute psychosis are quite different from the needs of older people with, for example, severe depression. Because of their physical frailty, older people are vulnerable to falls. Some older people with cognitive impairment are prone to wander into other people's rooms, precipitating retaliatory assaults. In addition, older inpatients often require substantially more physical nursing care and more medical interventions, mandating a quite different staffing mix. Wards with mixed groups of younger and older people often have difficulty providing for the needs of each group.

Because community mental health services for older people are a relatively new phenomenon in most places, their implementation has generally been planned. However, some districts have autonomous community-based services and others have integrated hospital and community services. This particular issue is dealt with in more detail in Chapter 5.

While larger provincial towns often have their own OPMHS, in rural and remote regions, mental health services for older people are generally provided by a lone mental health worker who must cover a vast geographic area, usually in an off-road vehicle. In some rural locations, there are fly-in fly-out mental health teams that augment the work of the local worker.

INTEGRATED HOSPITAL AND COMMUNITY SERVICES

An integrated model of hospital and community care is useful for the management of complex problems in older people with serious mental health problems such as major depression with psychotic features, bipolar disorder with comorbid physical problems such as Parkinson's disease, and very late onset schizophrenia-like psychoses complicated by dementia. In each example, the combination of complexity and severity mandates access to hospital beds, but chronicity mandates assertive community follow-up. In such cases, the integrated hospital and community model allows essential continuity of care.

In integrated hospital and community care, the inpatient and community parts of the service share personnel, have common team meetings and share case notes. In an integrated service, the hospital team knows well the strengths and limitations of the community team and can better judge when it is appropriate to discharge a person. Similarly, the community team knows well the strengths and limitations of the inpatient team and can better judge which people are likely to benefit from inpatient care. The community team might also be better able to judge when an illness has reached the stage where inpatient care is needed. In addition, access to certain types of treatment, including electroconvulsive therapy (ECT), is often restricted to inpatient units.

For practical reasons, not all personnel can be shared. For instance, the requirement of shiftwork for most inpatient nursing personnel means that they are less likely to be able to participate much in community care. However, most allied health workers such as social workers, occupational therapists and clinical psychologists are able to work across the inpatient and community parts of the service. Similarly, most medical personnel, including psychiatrists and trainee psychiatrists (registrars), are able to work across both sectors. It is also often feasible to rotate nursing and junior medical staff between community and inpatient roles so that they are familiar with both.

In integrated services, team meetings (including ward rounds) are attended by representatives from the inpatient unit and from the community team. In some services, completely integrated meetings are held in which inpatients and those people in the community are discussed, although these can be rather lengthy. In other integrated services, separate team meetings are held with the inpatient and community teams, with representatives from the other team in attendance. There are great advantages in having cross-representation at team meetings or ward rounds. These include both teams having advance notice of impending admissions and discharges, and a larger group of health workers to share the responsibility of providing care for challenging people.

One major advantage of integrated services is the early involvement of community case managers in the care of inpatients who have not previously been case managed and the continuing involvement of community case managers where the person has been admitted from their care. Early engagement of case managers during the inpatient phase of clinical care can greatly facilitate discharge planning and allow this to begin at the time of admission.

Community case managers bring with them a wealth of knowledge about individuals and this can be used to facilitate an early commencement of inpatient treatment, as work-up time can be minimised. Community case managers can often introduce the person to the inpatient unit and the inpatient staff. They can also introduce the person's family to the inpatient team. Each of these steps has the potential to make the transition to inpatient care less traumatic for the person and their family. It might also make the whole inpatient treatment phase more efficient, with reduced length of stay.

There is nothing more irritating to busy mental health workers than missing clinical files. These are a common occurrence when hospital and community mental health services within the same geographical area insist on having separate and independent clinical files. One essential feature of an integrated hospital and community mental health service for older people is a single integrated clinical file. Ideally, this would be an electronic file but, at the time of writing, in most jurisdictions this will still be a physical chart. Preferably, this clinical file should be the same file used by district medical and surgical services, so that a holistic approach can be taken to mental and general healthcare.

One perennial question is: Who covers the after-hours roster? In many mental health services, the OPMHS team is too small to cover nights and weekends in its own right, so this task is covered by a shared roster to which all teams contribute.

Australian experts (Snowdon 1993, Snowdon et al 1995) have recommended the provision of eight acute inpatient beds per 100,000 of the total population for older people with mental health problems, and British experts (Royal College of Physicians and Royal College of Psychiatrists 1989) have recommended the provision of 15 beds per 100,000 total population. However, planning documents in Australia generally specify the provision of approximately four acute inpatient beds per 100,000 of the total population for older people with functional mental health problems. They usually make no allowance for inpatient mental health beds for older people with dementia associated with severe behavioural and psychological symptoms. The net effect is that districts often have too few acute inpatient beds for older people with mental health problems, including dementia. Similarly, planning documents often specify approximately four full-time equivalent (FTE) older persons' community mental health staff per 100,000 of the total population, rather than a number based on the number of older people and the likely prevalence of mental health problems.

PRIVATE SECTOR SERVICES

In most countries with well-developed public mental health systems, there are also private practitioners providing fee-for-service mental healthcare. In Australia, there is a flourishing private sector involving mainly psychiatrists and clinical psychologists, with smaller numbers of social workers and occupational therapists in independent private practice. There is also a relatively large number of private psychiatric hospitals, many of which are now providing community outreach services to people with private health insurance. Public sector and private sector services often need to work together to provide optimal care for people. In Australia, people with private health insurance cover have the option to be admitted to a private psychiatric hospital and have private community follow-up or to be admitted to a public hospital and have public or private community follow-up.

Contemporary private psychiatric hospitals generally have a multidisciplinary staff consisting of mental health nurses, clinical psychologists and occupational therapists. Although some private hospitals employ psychiatrists or psychiatric registrars (trainee psychiatrists), others rely on visiting psychiatrists for their medical input. Many also have visiting general practitioners and general physicians. Care arrangements can sometimes be complex and it is important for mental health services to avoid a silo mentality in which it is difficult for people to move between public and private healthcare providers.

WHO CARES FOR THE 'GRADUATES'?

The term 'graduates' has been used to describe those people with early-onset psychotic disorders, particularly chronic schizophrenia, who make it into old age. Because of higher mortality rates among young and middle-aged people with chronic psychoses, it is a select group who live through to later life. These individuals often have complex care needs and longstanding relationships with adult mental health teams. Thus, the question which arises is whether they should continue to be cared for by their adult mental health team or transfer to the care of an OPMHS team when they reach 65 years, or whatever age of transition is used locally.

The principle of continuity of care would argue in favour of their staying with their adult team, as they are likely to know them well. However, older people with early-onset psychotic disorders often have significant general medical problems due to risk factors such as smoking and obesity, and poor access to general practitioners. OPMHS are often more used to addressing the physical health needs of older people and often have better links with general practitioners and geriatricians. As the older person with an early-onset psychotic disorder ages, they may develop increasing frailty associated with gait disorder and dementia. They may need to have access to community aged care services, including home-delivered meals, home help and in-home respite services. Some will ultimately need residential care. All of these services are likely to be very familiar to the older persons' team, and so this is an argument in favour of transferring the care of the older person with an early-onset psychotic disorder to an OPMHS team.

WHO CARES FOR PEOPLE WITH DEMENTIA?

As the population ages, the number of people with dementia will increase significantly. Some of these people will have clinically significant problems with their mental state or behaviour. These problems are known collectively as the behavioural and psychological symptoms of dementia (BPSD) (see Ch 28). An important issue for any OPMHS is the extent to which it will be responsible for the assessment of older people with BPSD. Most OPMHS take the view that BPSD is core business for their service and spend much of their time on the assessment and management of such people. However, many people with dementia do not have clinically significant BPSD and it is debatable whether those with uncomplicated dementia should be dealt with by mental health services. There is a good argument for people with uncomplicated dementia to be managed by their general practitioners with the assistance of a memory clinic. Specialised driving assessment clinics, often run by occupational therapists, are generally beyond the scope of the OPMHS.

Younger people with dementia should be assessed by clinicians with specialised knowledge of this area. If there is a local memory clinic or some other type of specialised dementia assessment service, then this should be used to undertake the work-up and confirm the diagnosis. Later on in the clinical course of early-onset dementia, there are often issues with BPSD, and the OPMHS is likely to be in a good position to offer advice and support.

TRANSCULTURAL ISSUES

In larger OPMHS teams it may be possible to employ some workers with a similar ethnic or language background to the main minority groups in the local community. However, in smaller teams this is often not possible. In such cases, it is essential to have access to transcultural mental health workers who can conduct specialised mental health assessments in the person's own language. If such transcultural mental health workers are not available, it is useful to have access to professional interpreter services, either in person or on the telephone.

SOURCES OF REFERRALS

From whom should community OPMHS teams accept referrals? Although specialist medical services traditionally accept referrals only from other doctors, this model is not appropriate for OPMHS. Legitimate referrals may come from a host of different sources, including the older person themselves, their family members, their local doctor, a community health worker, staff from an adult mental health service, nursing personnel from a local residential aged care facility (RACF), and the local police station. Many OPMHS require that the person's general practitioner is aware of the referral to minimise frivolous referrals and to allow for easy handover to the general practitioner when the OPMHS has completed their episode of care.

DOMICILIARY OR CLINIC-BASED CONSULTATIONS

Although many adult mental health teams conduct most of their consultations in hospital outpatient departments or centralised clinics, domiciliary consultations (home visits) seem to come naturally to OPMHS community teams. In most instances, more clinically relevant information is obtained from a home visit than from a clinic visit. On home visits, the person's partner or adult child is often present and able to provide collateral information. On home visits, the OPMHS clinician can observe the living environment and see if any delusion-based modifications have been made (e.g. to exclude poison gas from getting in through the cracks around the front door). The kitchen can be checked for the adequacy of food supplies and the back veranda can be checked for empty alcohol bottles. On a home visit, the older person should have ready access to their spectacles and hearing aids. The clinician should be able to directly examine the Webster Pak® or Dosette® box, or look at the medication containers. The clinician can also look for hazards in the home, such as loose runner carpets or dangers in the kitchen.

Occasionally, the clinician will not be able to enter the house or apartment because of the extent of hoarding or because the person has frank persecutory delusions. However, clinic or hospital visits should generally be reserved for those, usually younger, older people who are particularly concerned about their privacy or have serious dependency issues.

CASE MANAGEMENT MODEL

The traditional case management model involves the use of mental health workers (usually registered nurses, social workers, occupational therapists and clinical psychologists) to conduct community-based assessments, devise management plans and implement time-limited case management. In this model, most contact with the person is made by the case manager, who obtains the assistance of other personnel as needed. Under such a model, the medical staff is used in the initial work-up of the person and in regular reviews at 3-month intervals. The case manager visits the person at home and makes regular telephone contact between home visits. The case manager reports back at regular intervals to team meetings about the person's progress. In OPMHS teams, the case managers also provide education and support to carers and family members of the person.

CONSULTATION–LIAISON MODEL

In the community-based consultation–liaison model, mental health workers are consulted by general practitioners, by community health workers or by RACF personnel to assess a person under their care and make recommendations for future management. In some places, particularly where no inpatient mental health service exists, a community mental health service might provide consultation–liaison services to hospital medical and surgical wards. Occasionally, an OPMHS would be engaged in this role. In all of these versions of the consultation–liaison model, the person remains under the care of the referrer. Quite often, the problems raised by consultative requests are common to more than one of the people referred by an individual referrer and allow the possibility of providing more general clinical advice to the referrer. This might take the form of impromptu educational sessions or planned training workshops for staff.

THE DAY HOSPITAL

Day hospitals were once widely used in mental health services, although they are no longer considered to be an essential component of adult mental health services. Day hospitals are still used by geriatric medicine services, as they allow older people access to a wide range of nursing and allied health interventions without requiring a hospital admission. Although still popular in the United Kingdom (Hoe et al 2005), there is limited evidence for the efficacy of day hospitals in the OPMHS context. In Australia, community mental health teams have largely replaced day hospitals for the ongoing management of people with functional mental health problems. Similarly, various forms of respite care, including centre-based day respite, have replaced day hospitals for the care of people with dementia.

THE MEMORY CLINIC

Memory clinics assess and manage people with cognitive complaints, including people with subjective memory complaints, mild cognitive impairment and dementia. Older people attending memory clinics tend to be a little younger (mid-70s) than older people seen by an OPMHS (late 70s). Memory clinics are generally run on a multi-disciplinary and multispecialty basis. They are often staffed by geriatricians, psycho-geriatricians, neurologists, neuropsychologists, nurses and social workers. The availability of a local memory clinic is likely to reduce the workload of geriatric medical services and OPMHS. However, the memory clinic will be a source of referrals to the OPMHS, as some people with dementia will go on to develop clinically significant BPSD. Similarly, when older people with uncomplicated dementia are referred to the OPMHS, they can be referred on to the memory clinic, which is likely to have better resources for the assessment and management of such people.

RESIDENTIAL AGED CARE FACILITIES

Residential aged care facilities (RACFs) provide care for older people with dementia and other chronic disabilities. In the Australian setting, they may provide either high care (nursing home care) or low care (hostel care), or both. They are often locked to prevent the egress of confused older people. Community mental health teams work closely with the staff of RACFs, as many older people with challenging behaviours and other mental health problems reside in aged care facilities. Residents of aged care facilities commonly have mental health problems (McSweeney & O'Connor 2008) and are often prescribed psychotropic medications (Snowdon et al 2006). In some places, specialised psychogeri-atric RACFs are managed by the OPMHS. This arrangement has the potential to allow greater flexibility in managing acute inpatient beds and the longer term management of older people with severe mental health problems, including BPSD.

INVOLUNTARY CARE IN THE COMMUNITY

Involuntary care in the community is a well-established part of community mental health-care and at first glance seems to be a sensible practice. It is designed to maintain a least restrictive approach to involuntary treatment and to minimise frequent readmissions to hospital of people with serious mental health problems. However, the available evidence suggests that it actually reduces neither admissions nor bed days (Kisely et al 2007). Nevertheless, involuntary treatment in the community is a normal part of the role of the OPMHS team. Thus, the model of care adopted by OPMHS teams needs to take into account the requirements of the local Mental Health Act in relation to involuntary care in the community. In practice, this means that all clinical staff will need to understand the involuntary provisions of the Mental Health Act and sufficient staff will need to be authorised under the Act to carry out the procedures required by the Act. Similarly, many people being cared for by the OPMHS team are likely to be under guardianship and administration orders. Such orders may dictate where they can live and their access to money. Thus, OPMHS personnel will need to develop good working relationships with personnel from the local office of the Adult Guardian (or equivalent).

THE POLICE SERVICE

The police service comes into frequent contact with older people with mental health problems. The police are asked to assist when older people are found wandering in the street and when older people assault others. Older people often call the police to complain about their neighbours and many of these complaints turn out to be due to persecutory delusions. OPMHS teams often need to call the police for assistance in transporting people who are being taken involuntarily to hospital and in gaining entry to houses and apartments when it is suspected that an older person may have come to harm.

SOCIAL AND COMMUNITY SERVICES

The well-functioning OPMHS will need to have collaborative relationships with income support services and with accommodation services. The latter might include providers of private hostel accommodation, providers of emergency accommodation as well as the local public housing provider. Similarly, the OPMHS will have collaborations with community health providers, including those providing domiciliary nursing care, and providers of respite care. Thus, it is clear that the health and welfare milieu in which the OPMHS team operates is a complex one.

SUMMARY

Older people with mental health problems are seen in a wide variety of clinical and non-clinical settings, each with its own model of care. The complexity of these arrangements is magnified by differences in funding models between the public and private sectors. In the ideal situation, a district will have a public sector, integrated hospital and community mental health service for older people. In some locations, there will also be private sector mental health services.

FURTHER READING

Melding P, Draper B 2001 Geriatric consultation–liaison psychiatry. Oxford University Press, Oxford

REFERENCES

Draper B 2000 The effectiveness of old age psychiatry services. International Journal of Geriatric Psychiatry 15:687–703

Hoe J, Ashaye K, Orrell M 2005 Don't seize the day hospital! Recent research on the effectiveness of day hospitals for older people with mental health problems. International Journal of Geriatric Psychiatry 20:694–698

Kisely S, Campbell LA, Scott A et al 2007 Randomized and non-randomized evidence for the effect of compulsory community and involuntary out-patient treatment on health service use: systematic review and meta-analysis. Psychological Medicine 37:3–14

McSweeney K, O'Connor DW 2008 Depression among newly admitted Australian nursing home residents. International Psychogeriatrics 20:724–737

Royal College of Physicians and Royal College of Psychiatrists 1989 Care of elderly people with mental illness. Royal College of Physicians, London

Snowdon J 1993 How many bed-days for an area's psychogeriatric patients? Australian and New Zealand Journal of Psychiatry 27:42–48

Snowdon J, Ames D, Chiu E, Wattis J 1995 A survey of psychiatric services for elderly people in Australia. Australian and New Zealand Journal of Psychiatry 29:207–214

Snowdon J, Day S, Baker W 2006 Current use of psychotropic medication in nursing homes. International Psychogeriatrics 18:241–250

Chapter 5

COMMUNITY MENTAL HEALTH TEAMS

INTRODUCTION

This chapter considers community mental health teams for older people. It examines their composition and function. In those places with universal health systems, such as Australia, New Zealand and the United Kingdom, assessment and care of older people with mental health problems is usually carried out by community-based multidisciplinary teams. In urban centres, there are often multidisciplinary teams devoted to the care of older people. As the scientific literature on this topic is sparse, this chapter is based mainly on our own experiences over many years working in dedicated community mental health teams for older people.

TEAM SIZE

Community mental health teams for older people usually consist of 6 to 12 health workers, together with one or more administrative personnel. Smaller teams can be more difficult to sustain, as members are often the only representatives of their professional groups, there is less intraprofessional support available and it is difficult to arrange leave cover. Larger teams are usually broken into subunits because when teams have greater than 12 members their team meetings become lengthy and difficult to manage. Teams with 6 to 12 members can tolerate periods of absence for sick leave, recreation leave and parental leave without an unacceptable load falling to other team members.

TEAM COMPOSITION

The core professions needed by a community mental health team for older people include medicine, nursing, social work, occupational therapy and psychology. There are advantages in also having input from pharmacy, speech pathology, dietetics and physiotherapy, although such personnel are likely to be used solely for their profession-specific knowledge and skills, rather than for generic mental health tasks, such as initial assessment and case management. Even with the advent of mobile communications technology, community teams cannot work well without competent support from administrative personnel.

LEADERSHIP

In many places, including Australia, there are statutory requirements for people to be admitted to mental health services, including community mental health teams, under a specialist psychiatrist. As a result, in many community mental health teams for older people, a psychiatrist is likely to have ultimate clinical decision-making responsibility. The local Mental Health Act is also likely to require a psychiatrist to take responsibility for people managed under its involuntary treatment provisions. Depending upon the psychiatrist's personality and inclination, the psychiatrist might also take on service development and innovation roles.

There is another leadership role needed in all but the smallest community mental health teams. Team leaders, often drawn from the ranks of senior nurses, have important administrative responsibilities as teams grow beyond about six members.

TEAMWORK

Teamwork often comes naturally to people attracted to working in community mental health teams for older people. The specific knowledge and skills of the various health professions are essential to the day-to-day work of such teams. Thus, there are plenty of opportunities for health workers to practise their own professions, as well as more generic mental health worker roles such as case management. As a result, personnel are more likely to derive satisfaction from their working lives and staff turnover is often quite low.

Sometimes, however, personnel are drafted in from adult mental health teams and do not have a strong inclination towards working with older people. In such circumstances, it will be incumbent upon existing members of the team to introduce the new worker to the quite different philosophy of the community mental health team for older people. It is often invaluable for new workers to work alongside enthusiastic and experienced workers to gain familiarity with the work style and philosophy.

WORKLOAD

Clinicians working in community mental health teams for older people can expect to be busy. Typical tasks include individual counselling and behaviour therapy, family meetings, and liaison work with general practitioners, community health workers and residential aged care facilities. They will need to work with local retail pharmacies to provide people with medication-dispensing systems. They will need to assist people to access local health and welfare services, as well as income maintenance and accommodation services. They will need to negotiate through the various parts of the local Mental Health Act. They may need to transport people to various appointments, including the local pathology provider to have blood tests done.

Caseload allocations are likely to be based on the number of cases, case complexity and local issues, including sociodemographic factors, living arrangements, geographic location and traffic patterns. The work model adopted by the team might also influence workload allocation.

GENERIC CLINICAL ROLES

Despite ample opportunities to practise specific professional roles in most community mental health teams for older people, there are generic clinical roles that most members of such teams will need to gain familiarity with. All team members will need to be competent at doing initial clinical assessments, including mental state examinations, and all team members will need to understand case management as it is applied to older people with mental health problems. Teams vary in the extent to which they mix the application of generic and profession-specific roles. However, as a broad generalisation, mental health teams for older people probably use profession-specific skills more frequently than adult mental health teams.

THE VALUE OF DIFFERENT PERSONALITY TYPES

In his excellent book on community mental health teams, Burns (2004, pp 23–24) recommends a mix of personality types in a community mental health team. He recognises that 'a core of unflappable staff' is necessary for people to feel 'contained and safe'. But he also indicates that it is useful to have personnel who 'thrive on crises or who can communicate excitement and enthusiasm'.

THREATS TO TEAM COHESION

There are some common threats to team cohesion. These include lack of agreed roles for team members, lack of clear reporting structures and lines of responsibility, inequitable workload distribution, and lack of adequate professional supervision. It is essential that team members understand the balance between generic case management roles and profession-specific roles that they are required to undertake. This may sometimes require careful negotiation between the worker and the team leader, and is best established at the beginning of employment with the team. Effective teams need effective team leaders, and personnel need to be quite clear about lines of clinical responsibility. The local Mental Health Act will define some of these responsibilities, and team protocols need to take these requirements into consideration. The team leader must meet very regularly with team members so that issues can be identified and resolved at the earliest opportunity.

Perceptions of inequitable workload distribution are common sources of dissatisfaction within mental health teams. Distribution of workload should generally be on a numerical basis—that is, each worker should be allocated approximately the same number of older people. Some consideration needs to be made for case complexity, although much mental health work with older people involves considerable complexity. Professional supervision is critical to professional development and risk management, and is dealt with in more detail below.

Some conflict is inevitable, even in well-functioning teams. In itself, conflict is not necessarily a bad thing, as it often precipitates an examination of a practice. However, conflict that does not have a forum or is not allowed to surface is likely to fester and could destabilise a team. Mental healthcare in the community is difficult enough without destructive forces within a team using up everyone's emotional energy.

TOLERANCE AND HUMOUR

In any community mental health team for older people, there is likely to be a mix of personality styles and a mix of motivations for working in this challenging field. Sometimes, these differences will cause friction among team members. Tolerance is an essential ingredient for working with the mentally ill and an essential ingredient for working in a well-functioning team. Humour is often useful in defusing a difficult situation that has arisen within a team, although it does take some time to know just how far to take certain types of humour.

PROFESSIONAL SUPERVISION

All mental health workers should have access to professional supervision. The worker should meet regularly with their professional supervisor, who may or may not be their line manager. In multidisciplinary teams, the line manager is often someone from a different professional discipline who is responsible for day-to-day decision making, including workload allocation, approving leave applications, and for arranging back-up. These tasks should be differentiated from professional supervision, which should provide the worker with a supportive forum in which they can discuss clinical issues that have arisen in their work and can focus on knowledge acquisition, skills training and professional development more generally. Professional supervision may be provided on a one-to-one basis or in a group setting, according to local requirements and supervisor availability. In some professions, professional supervision is augmented by a formal requirement for continuing professional development (CPD). Health professional registration boards and local health districts are increasingly moving towards each worker meeting annual formal requirements for CPD and accreditation.

OPERATIONAL MODELS

The term 'medical model' is now obsolete and is rarely used. However, the role of medical personnel in teams is still often discussed. In some teams (e.g. single-member or dual-member rural or remote teams), there may be no medical personnel, so referral to outside medical personnel is regularly needed. In other teams (e.g. well-resourced urban teams), there may be several medical personnel. In the latter case, the team will need a clear understanding of how the medical input is to be used. Teams often differ as to whether a medical practitioner (e.g. a psychiatrist or training registrar) should be involved in every assessment interview. Some teams take the view that the investment of medical time during the initial contact with the older person will save time later on, as experienced medical personnel are likely to be able to decide rapidly whether the referral is appropriate to the service and whether it is appropriate to manage the person in the community. Other teams take the view that it is more efficient for initial assessments to be undertaken by non-medical personnel, with later review by medical staff at a clinic. There is no one correct approach to this issue.

DOMICILIARY ASSESSMENT AND CARE

A critical feature of community mental health teams for older people is their capacity to undertake domiciliary assessments and to provide domiciliary care. Most older people are seen in their own homes or in other residential environments, including aged care facilities such as nursing homes. In this way, the mental health worker can make a more accurate assessment of the fit between the person, their carer and their usual environment. The mental health worker can also assess threats to safety in the person's usual environment. Many frail older people find it difficult to get to outpatient clinics, particularly if they have gait disorders or impaired vision.

In contrast, when older people are seen in the clinic, they often present differently and much useful data are unavailable. Taking a routine domiciliary approach to assessment and care allows the community mental health team the opportunity to provide assertive outreach if resources permit.

Mental health teams for older people usually develop protocols that cover domiciliary visits. In most instances, initial domiciliary visits are undertaken in pairs to minimise risk to the workers involved. In cases where the risk to the worker is considered low, a single worker may undertake subsequent visits.

AGE POLICY

Most community mental health teams for older people have a flexible age policy. They usually take people aged 65 years and over presenting for the first time with symptoms that suggest mental illness. They may also take older people with longstanding mental health problems who have more recently developed comorbid conditions associated with ageing, such as dementia or Parkinson's disease, or people who are now living in an aged care facility. They often also take younger people with health problems, such as dementia, which normally present in later life.

ADMINISTRATIVE SUPPORT

All mental health teams for older people require competent administrative support. There is usually a clear division of labour between clinical personnel and administrative officers. Clinical personnel usually do rostered shifts as the duty intake officer, during which they handle inquiries from the people in their care, as well as carers and referrers. If there are no inquiries, the mental health worker can update their clinical files, make telephone calls or study areas of clinical interest. In contrast, administrative officers should staff the base office, undertake clerical duties including typing, make appointments, and monitor the field visit log to assist with maintaining the safety of workers on domiciliary visits.

TEACHING AND TRAINING ROLES

Mental health teams for older people are often highly sought after student placements because of the challenging mix of people with comorbid mental health problems and physical disorders, and the often highly competent staff of such teams. Student placements from all disciplines should be encouraged and students should be made to feel welcome.

Mental health teams for older people are also highly sought after as higher level placements for many types of established clinical personnel, including registrars undertaking advanced training in the psychiatry of old age. There is a great need for clinical psychologists with specific training in the psychology of old age; therefore, clinical students should be encouraged to do placements within mental health teams for older people.

Although teaching roles are sometimes seen as an additional burden for an already overstretched community team, the presence of enthusiastic students can revitalise a jaded clinician. Teaching is essential for the long-term survival of specialised mental health teams for older people.

PERSONNEL TRAINING

Newly employed health workers will need to undergo induction procedures to obtain payroll numbers and name badges. They will also be given standardised training in fire safety and in cardiopulmonary resuscitation. In mental health services, there will also be mandatory training in aggression management and in the use of the local Mental Health Act. There may also be required training modules in computer skills and in the documentation of mental health outcomes. All of this might well take a week or more to complete, so managers of community mental health teams need to factor in this down time when taking on new personnel.

In the course of employment in a community mental health team, there should be in-service training opportunities in community services, Indigenous mental health, transcultural mental health, forensic mental health and in the latest advances in mental health for older people. There will be further requirements in terms of maintenance of standards in relation to the local Mental Health Act. In some jurisdictions, there will be mandatory training requirements in child safety. Some of these requirements may be able to be met via online courses of instruction.

COMMUNICATIONS

Modern community teams require mobile communications systems, including mobile telephones and paging devices. Personnel need to be able to call the office from the field. It is often necessary to call people who are hearing impaired by telephone to ask them to open the front door. It is sometimes necessary to call the police for the safety of the mental health worker or because of concerns about the safety of the person.

As most routine record keeping is now done online, it is essential for mental health workers to have access to an office with a desktop computer connected to the health services network. Such a network is likely also to have electronic reference texts and databases of value to busy health workers. The modern mental health worker needs keyboard and computer skills to enable them to work efficiently. With increasing emphasis on electronic record keeping, all mental health workers should learn to touch-type.

TRANSPORT

Motor vehicles are not an optional extra for community teams; they are an essential component of their work. The vehicles must be fit for purpose, which usually means that they must be safe and easy to drive. They will generally have automatic transmissions, doors that allow easy access for older people, and boots into which a collapsible walking frame can readily fit. In certain rural and remote settings, four-wheel drive vehicles will be essential, but in most urban environments medium-size sedans will suffice. Small sedans are often inappropriate for older people. In harsh climates, such as those encountered in much of Australia, it will be necessary to obtain vehicles fitted with air conditioning. Consideration will need to be given also to fitting out the vehicles with communications gear, which will vary in type according to the setting. In some urban settings it will be necessary for vehicles to have automatic toll devices to allow tollway access. If medications are to be transported in vehicles, it will be necessary to have a suitable, secure container for such medications. If laboratory samples (e.g. blood and urine) are to be transported in vehicles, it may be necessary to consider insulated or even refrigerated containers.

RECORD-KEEPING ISSUES

Most community teams use standardised assessment protocols to ensure that a uniform minimum data set is obtained on each person. While such protocols are a useful aide memoire, they do not substitute for the well-informed clinical judgment of an experienced mental health worker. When using standardised assessment protocols, whether paper-based or computerised, the clinician must be careful not to inappropriately truncate their clinical note taking to conform to the protocol.

AUDIT ACTIVITIES

Audit activities are often seen as tedious and of dubious benefit. However, they elucidate systematic difficulties with compulsory record keeping that prompt a review of documentation. If all personnel are involved in audit activities, it allows everyone 'ownership' of the data and minimises the individual burden involved.

RESEARCH ACTIVITIES

Research is not for everyone, as it requires considerable perseverance and the pervasive curiosity to look beyond the obvious and continually ask questions. Funding can be challenging to obtain and there are many obstacles between the initial good idea and the final paper for publication. However, mental health workers who have conducted research projects leading to published papers can derive enormous satisfaction from their endeavours. There are few things as reinforcing as conducting research that advances knowledge that is likely to be of benefit to people. It is important that clinical research be translated into action at the coalface or else the effort may have been wasted. Routine clinical data collections can be used as a basis for research activities. Research into mental health for older people often involves important issues of informed consent and substitute decision making. It will sometimes involve the local Guardianship Tribunal.

TEAM MEETINGS

The team meeting is one of the fundamental activities of a community mental health team and it is difficult to conceive of a well-functioning team for older people without such a meeting. Team meetings are almost always conducted weekly. However, their tasks differ from team to team. Some teams use the weekly team meeting to discuss all incoming referrals, whereas other teams delegate this task to a team leader. Most teams use the team meeting as a forum for the presentation and discussion of all newly assessed people. Team meetings are the usual forum for routine case reviews—brief presentations every 3 months or so. Such review presentations will often involve discussion of requirements for reports under the relevant Mental Health Act. Importantly, the team meeting allows the discussion of people who are to be discharged from the team, as well as those to be admitted to the care of the team. The team meeting is not a substitute for a daily handover or for individual supervision.

Generally speaking, the team meeting will be attended by all of the clinical personnel from the team and their students and trainees. The team meeting is often also a convenient forum for visits from representatives from other service providers, such as case managers from adult teams hoping to transfer people, and domiciliary nurses from community health teams wishing to discuss mental health issues.

In some teams, the team meeting is also a forum for discussion of business matters, including leave, workload, students, training and research. In other teams, a separate business meeting is run on a monthly basis to deal with these issues.

Team meetings require an agenda and minutes, and a member of staff should be allocated to this task. The agenda is a useful prompt to team members about what needs to be discussed during the meeting. The minutes provide a useful audit trail for later reference.

BURNOUT

Staff burnout is an ever-present threat in busy community mental health teams. The burden of increasingly onerous record-keeping requirements adds to the natural strains of caring for seriously mentally ill people. Mental health workers are often highly dedicated individuals who empathise strongly with the people in their care. However, things do occasionally go wrong and mental health workers have a tendency to blame themselves. Sometimes, the system unfairly blames the mental health worker for something beyond their control.

Burnout has many different manifestations, depending upon the personality of those involved. Quite commonly, work performance declines and the mental health worker is reluctant to carry out their usual home visits. Their number of sick days might increase and dysphoria and anergia might be evident. Sometimes, burnout is manifested by irritability and intolerance. Prevention of burnout includes ensuring that mental health workers do not work excessive hours and that everyone is required to take regular recreation leave. If overnight or on-call work is required, then rostered fatigue leave will be needed. Team-building activities, including social events during the working week, may also assist with preventing burnout. Small prizes to reward good work also tend to boost morale. Team leaders need to be vigilant for early signs of burnout and should take pre-emptive action. Burnout and its prevention are also issues for discussion during professional supervision. Sometimes, burnout is merely a euphemism for mental health problems, including depression and anxiety. In such instances, the staff member should be referred promptly for professional assistance.

SUMMARY

This chapter has provided a detailed overview of the structure and function of the community mental health team for older people. It has canvassed many of the organisational and operational issues that are relevant to such teams. It has touched on supervision, conflict and burnout.

FURTHER READING

Burns T 2004 Community mental health teams: a guide to current practices. Oxford University Press, Oxford

Cummings SM 2009 Treating older persons with severe mental illness in the community: impact of an interdisciplinary geriatric mental health team. Journal of Gerontological Social Work 52(1):17–31

REFERENCE

Burns T 2004 Community mental health teams: a guide to current practices. Oxford University Press, Oxford

Chapter 6

CULTURAL ISSUES

INTRODUCTION

An older person's cultural background has a great influence on many aspects of their mental health. When considering treatment options, it is imperative to consider a person's cultural background. Australia like many other countries is culturally diverse, but its Anglo-Saxon or Western population is dominant. The culturally and linguistically diverse (CALD) section of the population is chronically underserviced and their health needs are not clearly articulated. This chapter provides an introduction to and an overview of issues important to understanding the complex relationship between cultural issues and mental healthcare. It highlights some of the cultural factors that influence seeking of mental healthcare, access to and utilisation of mental health services, and the quality of mental healthcare received by older people from CALD backgrounds.

The structure of this chapter follows the premise of delivering culturally congruent care. The four basic constructs for culturally congruent care are:

1. cultural diversity
2. cultural awareness
3. cultural sensitivity, and
4. cultural competence.

Cultural diversity is referred to in terms of race and ethnicity. Cultural awareness is a cognitive construct that requires knowledge of major between-group differences, such as food preferences and religious practices. Cultural sensitivity lies in the affective domain and relates to a person's attitude about themselves and others, and their openness to learn along cultural dimensions. Finally, cultural competence is a behavioural construct that encompasses the actions that are in response to cultural diversity, awareness and sensitivity. Some behaviours constituting cultural competence have been identified as workforce diversity and training, interventions addressing barriers, transcultural communication practices and adapting care based on the assessment of individual needs (Schim et al 2007).

CULTURAL DIVERSITY

There is diversity, not often recognised, found with the original Australian peoples—the Aboriginal and Torres Strait Islanders. The tribal groups alone have up to 300 different languages (Harkins 1994). Based on the 2006 Australian census, Aboriginal and Torres Strait Islander people make up just over half a million (2.5%) of the total Australian population. The structure of the population is relatively young, with very small numbers of older people. Only 2.8% of the total Indigenous population are aged 65 years and over (approximately 16,000 people altogether) and 0.8% are aged 75 years and over. Overall, people aged 65 years and over constitute less than 3% of the Indigenous population, whereas people aged 65 years and over make up 13% of the non-Indigenous population (Australian Bureau of Statistics 2008).

The reason for this disparity is Indigenous people have a lower life expectancy based on poorer living standards due to systemic discriminatory practices since white settlement over 200 years ago. As these issues are addressed, the life expectancy of Indigenous Australians is increasing, albeit very slowly. Indigenous people mainly live in metropolitan (30%) and regional (43%) areas, with the remaining 27% residing in remote areas. In remote areas they make up 12% of the population and 45% in very remote areas. Some of these people continue to speak their traditional languages and do not have English as their second language or read English (Australian Institute of Health and Welfare 2007). The mental health status of Indigenous Australians is very poor as well. This can be attributed to chronic feelings of dislocation due to repeated losses that have occurred for many generations. These losses have been related to relocation from tribal lands, disruption of cultural practices and language, forced removal of children and the breakup of extended families, and high mortality and morbidity rates (McKendrick & Ryan 2007).

Nearly 54% of Australia's population aged 65 years and older were born overseas, representing more than 200 different ethnic communities. About 39% of these older people are from English-speaking countries, with the vast majority (61%) from non-English-speaking countries. It is the latter that is continuing to grow faster than other segments of Australia's population, so much so that population projections indicate that in the next 10 years one in every four people over the age of 80 will be from a CALD background (Australian Institute of Health and Welfare 2007).

Clearly, English language proficiency is a major issue in older people's capacity to find and use services that suit their needs. Therefore, this chapter focuses on older people from non-English-speaking countries. Currently, the commonest ethnic groups in the upper end of the older population (older old) are Italians and Greeks who migrated to Australia during the post-World War II period. However, since the early 1970s, with the dismantling of the White Australia policy, the migration patterns have changed, with the primary immigrant groups being from Lebanon, Vietnam, Malaysia and the Philippines. These people make up a significant part of the lower end of the older population (younger old). This pattern of immigration has implications for the future delivery of culturally specific mental health services for older people.

CULTURAL AWARENESS

According to the statistical evidence (Australian Institute of Health and Welfare 2008), most migrants are very healthy because this is a criterion set down in government immigration policies. However, the act of migration and resettling in another country puts people under a lot of stress, because it usually means they no longer have family and friends close by for support. The value of established networks, such as health and welfare services, should not be underestimated in maintaining good mental health. The experience of 'culture shock' is very real and this can have detrimental effects on a person's overall wellbeing (Minas & Silove 2007). There is a difference between people who have migrated voluntarily and those who have been forced to migrate as refugees, or asylum seekers. Many people who have arrived in Australia in the last few years have come from countries that have been devastated by political unrest and wars, and not surprisingly often have a mental health problem that can range from chronic mental health problems to trauma and distress. These extreme symptoms are particularly prominent in people who have been detained, tortured or fled persecution, and they are therefore very susceptible to mental health problems (Silove 2002).

Some ethnic groups with a long history of migration to Australia are very well established and because of their sizeable concentrations have, over the years, lobbied for and built up services that meet their specific ethnocultural needs. But the commonalities between the ethnic groups are fewer than their differences. The groups most at risk with regard to mental health are smaller ethnic groups who are very disadvantaged, not only from extreme social isolation, but also from many health, economic and political perspectives. The major issue is lack of knowledge about health services and entitlements due to poor reading and conversational ability in the English language. This issue is followed by more enduring negative influences, such as poor childhood nutritional and healthcare standards, leading to a poorer overall health status. Not having the benefit of being educated to at least the minimal education standards of a country such as Australia can mean employment is limited to intermittent, low-paid, unskilled jobs. In some cases, a person could have qualifications but they are not recognised by Australian standards. Additionally, not having complete employment means a lack of insurance and superannuation contributions that may support a person upon retirement (Minas 1990).

An older person trying to cope with the accumulative stresses associated with the immigration experience and ongoing racial or cultural discrimination could be vulnerable to mental health problems. Added to this vulnerability is how the older person's cultural background influences their interpretation, response and ability to cope with a mental health problem, their perception of mental healthcare providers, and how they are likely to utilise and respond to mental health treatment.

If health matters are viewed as a family affair with multiple family members involved with the care of the older person, then the family has a great influence on an individual's health-seeking behaviour and pathway to formal mental healthcare treatment (O'Brien & Jackson 2007). There are likely to be highly contrasting family household structures among the various ethnic groups. While some will have living arrangements similar to what is known as the 'nuclear family', there remains a high propensity for living with children in multigenerational households. According to the Australian Institute of Health and Welfare (2007), family care remains an important source of support for older people from non-English-speaking backgrounds who were born overseas, with 70% living with their families compared with 58% of Australian-born older people. Additionally, they have lower usage of residential aged care facilities, but a higher use of community aged care packages.

However, it would not be prudent to assume these older people live in supported, extended families. The situation could be the exact opposite, with all the younger adults out working long hours and the older people expected to be at home caring for children. Such circumstances could create significant stresses. For example, for some older Aboriginal and Torres Strait Islander people, such an arrangement may prevent them from participating in important kinship responsibilities, such as a death ceremony which can take place over a number of weeks (McGrath & Phillips 2008). Additionally, even when an extended family network exists, caring may still be shouldered by one person, so the assumption should not be made that the need for professional care is reduced because of an 'extended family' living situation.

Another reason the older person may live with their family is dependency due to the inability to speak English and handle money. Some older Italian women in North Queensland, for example, although they have lived in Australia for 50 years or more, have very poor English proficiency due to living in isolated, predominantly Italian farming communities, and not being involved in outside workforce or business dealings. Such circumstances create an environment where the needs of the individual are attempted to be managed within the family and community. Seeking help outside of such protective environments is also challenging, particularly if one has faced difficulties or prejudices in the past. It is not surprising that people would hold unconventional health beliefs and practices, and look to family for decision making and care, rather than the formal service agencies, or that they would have a degree of caution in interacting with and using them (Dare 2006).

Older people in many cultures are traditionally held in high esteem and viewed as leaders and teachers. It is expected that families will care for their older members. However, despite these close family bonds, as the younger generations become assimilated to Western ways, they can become critical of older people's traditional practices which are not seen as relevant. This diminishes the role and status of the older person. As the younger generations become involved in the work and school culture of their new country, a divergence in cultural values will invariably arise and the older person will begin to feel more lonely, isolated and alienated because they are not involved and lack understanding of many things. Additionally, if the person is an older member of a poorer, less-established, marginalised group, they may have fewer peers close to their age, thereby exacerbating the feelings of alienation and loneliness (Abrahamson et al 2002, Dare 2006, Dein & Huline-Dickens 1997).

The family dynamics in many cultures involve extremely complex processes with intricate protocols. Within Aboriginal and Torres Strait Islander families, for example, the concept of family has a collective approach in which there is much ascribed status to family members, the needs of the family outweigh the needs of the individual, mutual goals exceed individual goals and there are strong bonds of mutual obligation (O'Brien & Jackson 2007). In these circumstances, health matters become family decisions and it is important for the whole family to be involved in the decision. This is usually done with family meetings where everyone with a right and responsibility attends. Issues discussed might include the disease, current and potential symptoms, treatment options and caring issues. All the family members like to be well informed about progress and need to know what to expect (McGrath et al 2005, McGrath et al 2007).

Sometimes, a lot of consultation can take place and the family may advise the older person, but the older person is not obliged to listen to younger family members. If such a dilemma occurs, it may turn out that another approach is needed, such as the involvement of an Aboriginal health worker. This person may be more successful in having a positive impact on the healthcare issue that needs to be addressed (McGrath et al 2005, McGrath et al 2007, McGrath & Phillips 2008, O'Brien & Jackson 2007, Stein-Parbury 2009).

The stigma of mental illness permeates many cultures, causing feelings of shame and embarrassment for all involved. Stigma can be so powerful in some cultures that it can ruin a family's public image and respect within the community. Not only is the whole family marginalised because they are seen as having 'bad breeding', but the individual is also subjected to fear, rejection and ridicule (Cloutterbuck & Zhan 2005, Minas 1990). The effect of these negative attitudes and beliefs on the individual can range from denial of the mental health problem and expression of psychological distress through the body rather than in the mind, lack of disclosure of problems to family members and health-care professionals, serious delay in seeking help, and irreparable damage to family relationships and consequently support (Cloutterbuck & Zhan 2005, Dare 2006, Minas 1990). Stigma is a strong barrier in the utilisation of mental health services to the extent that, in some Asian families, the acceptance of formal support services can be seen as moral failure (Minas 1990).

CULTURAL SENSITIVITY

Ethnocultural factors contribute to and influence how a person interprets the nature of their problem, its cause and severity, how symptoms are manifested and communicated, treatment preference, how the mental health problem is managed within the family and community context, pathways taken towards the utilisation of formal mental health services and subsequent satisfaction with care. To provide effective mental healthcare, the worldview in which the mental health problem is occurring must be understood. This is achieved by taking into consideration social, historical and ethnocultural factors (Stein-Parbury 2009).

Generally, in Western culture the cause of mental health problems is attributed to psychological stress and/or chemical imbalances. The entire process of managing a mental health problem is within a biomedical framework based on scientific reductionism where the mind, body and soul are often separated. Some non-Western cultures conceptualise mental health problems as having wider social, religious and metaphysical causes, such as spirit possession, punishment for evil acts committed by themselves or others, and general disharmony in many realms (McKendrick & Ryan 2007). Aboriginal and Torres Strait Islander people and Maori view mental health, social and emotional well-being as part of a holistic understanding of life that encompasses the individual, their family and the community (McKendrick & Ryan 2007, Swan & Raphael 1995). Therefore, cultural orientation influences how an individual explains, organises and manages a mental health problem.

It is imperative that any symptoms of a mental health problem are viewed in their cultural context. For example, if a person believes they are distressed because of spirit visitation, this could be interpreted as a psychotic episode and lead to a misdiagnosis (McKendrick & Ryan 2007). An affected person may reject modern science altogether and subscribe to traditional health practitioners, remedies and spiritual rituals. In this case, an older person could be particularly vulnerable if culturally unsafe health professionals interpret this as a sign of incapability and use the Mental Health Act to force 'standard' treatment (Stein-Parbury 2009).

A significant reason why people from CALD backgrounds are suspicious and reluctant to utilise mental health services is that they fear and mistrust the services and their providers (McGrath et al 2007). Such attitudes regarding the use of formal health services may have been shaped by past experiences where there is a history of health services being difficult to access, and where staff may have been generally hostile and used discriminatory and racist practices. Under such difficult circumstances, it is not surprising that people would hesitate to seek needed help and, when they do, care may be sub-standard and sought too late. As a result, people are less likely to seek mental healthcare services, and this leads to the underrepresentation and underutilisation of mental health services (Cloutterbuck & Zhan 2005, Minas 1990, Stein-Parbury 2009).

Other difficulties have stemmed from key social and ethnocultural factors, such as low English literacy levels which make people from CALD backgrounds prime candidates for misdiagnosis, experiencing fear of dying or being hospitalised involuntarily, and lacking knowledge about forms of treatment, medications and the mental health-care system generally. This lack of knowledge means people may be ambivalent about accepting assistance and are unable to determine whether they have received quality care, or not, in regard to what constitutes routine care and good outcomes (Cloutterbuck & Zhan 2005, Harkins 1994, McGrath et al 2007, Minas 1990, Stein-Parbury 2009).

CULTURAL COMPETENCE

Consultation is vital to the process of achieving cultural competence. Older people from CALD backgrounds are aware of their health problems and should be consulted about their health needs, including the best means by which to tackle the problems (Kleiman 2006). Such information may not be forthcoming, but being with, talking with and making observations can provide insight into the unique characteristics of specific ethnic groups and an understanding of the values that they hold (O'Brien & Jackson 2007). Other ways of dealing with some of these issues include developing partnerships with consumers and carers from culturally diverse backgrounds so that knowledge can be shared and processes put into place that are culturally inclusive (McGrath et al 2007). Such practices can be achieved by arranging and/or attending forums or community activities to learn, share ideas and opinions, and establish networks (Brach & Fraserirector 2000, McGrath et al 2007). Learning some of the language such as basic phrases and having available translated material on mental health issues can make a real difference with older people (McGrath et al 2007, O'Brien & Jackson 2007).

To appreciate cultural differences it is important to know normative cultural values and to conform with specific cultural expectations (Cloutterbuck & Zhan 2005). This goes a long way in establishing a meaningful rapport with the individual and their family. The process starts with finding out information from family members and health workers on how to conduct a successful interaction. Questions to be asked could be:

- What are the right channels?
- Who are the right people to speak with? (This person has to have the right relationship to the older person; otherwise, information may not be shared or communicated as openly.)
- Who has to be involved so that the right information is passed on?

With Aboriginal and Torres Strait Islander people, there is women's business and men's business. When a female health professional asks an Indigenous male a question about their health, a response may not be forthcoming. This may not be because the man is unconcerned about his health, but rather that it is men's business and it will not be shared with a woman. Also within this culture, nurturing and caring for the sick is seen as women's business (McGrath et al 2005, Maher 1999, Stein-Parbury 2009).

Having contact with elders or leaders from different groups is helpful, so advice can be sought and information obtained as to who should be spoken to about a particular person or issue. It may also be appropriate to ask them to pass on information. There is a need to be careful with how information is delivered because, if it is taken literally, it may have unfortunate consequences. For example, if it is bad news, this may have to be explained as the illness is nobody's fault; otherwise, an individual may be 'blamed' for the illness. Simple questions such as 'What is the best way to do this?' and not charging in, or talking down to people, will go a long way to ensure any encounters are successful and good-quality outcomes are achieved. Asking permission to do things fosters respect and trust, as does being involved in the community. Face-to-face contact, mutual familiarity and going out and talking to families in the communities also builds trust and rapport, as well as gaining some insight into the community's strengths and vulnerabilities, obstacles and resources that may either positively or negatively affect the care of the older person (McGrath et al 2005, O'Brien & Jackson 2007).

At an individual level, if the mental health worker is unfamiliar with certain cultural values, they run the risk of offending the person, which could result in a poor outcome and it may take an enormous effort to make up any ground that has been lost. Typical assessment techniques of probing questions may be seen as disrespectful and inappropriate (Minas 1990). Therefore, establishing an effective therapeutic relationship requires consideration of use of proper titles and names, knowing the appropriate degree of personal and physical interaction, and understanding cultural nuances. For example, in some Asian cultures, remaining silent, calm, non-challenging, controlled and containing personal feelings, even in the most difficult circumstances, is the defined behaviour (Parsons 1990). Superficially, it may appear that no problems exist. However, to get the correct information in order to make accurate judgments, the mental health worker may have to be very tactful and specific in their questioning style.

On the other hand, Aboriginal and Torres Strait Islander elders may be reluctant to engage in discussions about their mental health because they are shy and frightened. This may be because the health professional is seen as an authority figure, a sense of a class difference is felt, or that poor English proficiency is a cause for embarrassment because they feel they are presenting as being unintelligent (McGrath et al 2007). In these circumstances, the older person may feel more comfortable with an Aboriginal health worker present or an interpreter. In some communities where there is a concentration of a particular ethnic group, health services that focus on the specific needs of the group have been established. These health services are even more effective if staff are from the same ethnic background (Cloutterbuck & Zhan 2005, McGrath et al 2007, O'Brien & Jackson 2007, Stein-Parbury 2009).

Aboriginal health workers and health workers from across the different CALD communities have an important role to play in the delivery of healthcare (McGrath et al 2007, O'Brien & Jackson 2007). Health workers occupy positions in health services, community organisations or other government agencies (McKendrick & Ryan 2007). They are usually known and respected members of the community who have received mental health education for their role. Therefore, they guide other community members through the health system and provide entry into the communities for health staff. Health workers can assist the older person to explain their health problem to the staff and, conversely, explain Western medicine in a more comprehensible manner to the older person. Overall, the role of the health worker has improved access to healthcare by being seen as giving greater community participation and control in healthcare (Brach & Fraserirector 2000, McGrath et al 2007, O'Brien & Jackson 2007).

Interpreters are very important from a number of perspectives. Even if the older person is proficient in English, stress or cognitive impairment can cause people to revert to their native language. Interpreters can overcome barriers produced by the use of different terminology. They may understand how the perceptions and explanation of mental illness differ between cultures and may be able to broker some common understanding. Ideally, an interpreter would have expertise in the area of mental health and not have any conflict of interest. It would be vitally important that they are acceptable to the older person from age, gender and status perspectives. Generally, because they are able to relate to people from their own culture, this makes enormous inroads in expediting successful outcomes for all involved (Brach & Fraserirector 2000, McGrath et al 2005).

It is prudent clinical practice to be familiar with the mental health beliefs and practices commonly held by the CALD population being served and to determine whether or not the individual prescribes to these beliefs and practices (Campinha-Bacote 2002). Eliciting what the older person believes is causing their distress, or mental health problem, helps in assessment, negotiating treatment and setting mutual goals (Kleiman 2006). Even though the cultural group may have been exposed to Western medicine and have the necessary information about it, some people, particularly older people, will revert to traditional medicines, practitioners, folklore and beliefs to varying degrees (Campinha-Bacote 2002). This choice should be respected and if necessary negotiated on how to safely incorporate traditional healers and practices and Western medicine into the healthcare plan (Brach & Fraserirector 2000, O'Brien & Jackson 2007). Sometimes, culture-bound syndromes may explain an older person's behaviour (American Psychiatric Association 2000). In Maori, for example, *Mate Maori* (Maori Sickness) results from:

> *... exposure to spiritual forces engendered by transgression of cultural prohibitions. These states can be precipitated by the sufferer's own egregious actions or by those members of his whanau, particularly ancestors; spiritual forces therefore are considered pertinent to the 'sickness' (McKendrick & Ryan 2007, p 452).*

Presenting symptoms may be bizarre thoughts, hearing voices, disconnected speech and behavioural changes, which could all be misdiagnosed as a serious mental health problem. Treatment with cultural and spiritual interventions has better response (Plunkett 2003).

The use of assessment scales is encouraged to support and augment clinical decision making. However, before using scales, it is necessary to check if it has been validated for use with the population it is intended to be used upon. Some scales have been developed with universal characctristics that are easily transferable across many different ethnocultural groups. The Rowland Universal Dementia Assessment Scale (RUDAS) (Storey et al 2004) is one such example. Some other scales that are commonly used, such as the Mini-Mental State Examination (MMSE) (Folstein et al 1975), have been tested with many different groups of people. A rudimentary database search using the terms 'MMSE' and 'translation' revealed the MMSE has recently been validated and translated into Arabic and Sinhalese.

SUMMARY

Culture directly affects mental health, not only as a personal experience for the older person, but also in the understanding and acceptance of mental health problems. Many older people and their families from CALD backgrounds do not seek treatment for mental health problems. The barriers that have been identified in this chapter include beliefs of what mental illness arises from, poor access to mental health services due to lack of knowledge about what is available, available services being culturally inappropriate, language and cultural barriers, and stigma associated with mental illness. By employing strategies to strengthen culturally congruent care, some of these barriers may be overcome to ensure good-quality outcomes for the older person.

TIPS FOR CULTURALLY CONGRUENT MENTAL HEALTHCARE

The following tips for culturally congruent mental healthcare have been adapted from the World Federation for Mental Health (2007):

1. Get to know the culture you are interacting with and develop an understanding of how values, practices and beliefs influence human behaviour.
2. Talk with and listen to community members about their needs in regard to advocacy and service delivery.
3. Be respectful by getting to know the community leaders and their role.
4. Spend time clarifying issues and addressing doubts.
5. Approach non-government organisations, mental health groups, and religious and ethnic leaders, to gain support for your role.
6. Understand and respect communication processes and be inclusive.
7. Support actions with the use of evidence-based data and credible sources/ information.
8. Use a scientific approach, as this defuses emotions and makes acceptance of issues easier.
9. Avoid making value judgments about other people's behaviour.
10. Be cautious with the use of language, as some words may be offensive. Explain issues in a broader context of health.
11. Do not dictate knowledge; listen and behave in a neutral way.
12. Try and determine areas of common interest.
13. Look for and emphasise the positives. Every society has positive and negative features.
14. Appreciate that things may move very slowly, but small changes are significant and can be enduring over time.

USEFUL WEBSITES

Multicultural Mental Health Australia (MMHA): www.mmha.org.au
World Federation for Mental Health: www.wfmh.org

REFERENCES

Abrahamson TA, Trejo L, Lai DWL 2002 Culture and mental health: providing appropriate services for a diverse older population. Mental Health and Mental Illness in Later Life Spring:21–27

American Psychiatric Association 2000 Diagnostic and statistical manual of mental disorders, 4th edn. American Psychiatric Publishing, Arlington, VA

Australian Bureau of Statistics (ABS) 2008 Australian demographic statistics, December quarter 2008. ABS Cat. No. 3101.0.0. ABS, Canberra

Australian Institute of Health and Welfare (AIHW) 2007 Older Australia at a glance, 4th edn. Cat. No. AGE 52. AIHW, Canberra

Australian Institute of Health and Welfare (AIHW) 2008 Australia's health 2008. Cat. No. AUS 99. AIHW, Canberra

Brach C, Fraserirector I 2000 Can cultural competence reduce racial and ethnic health disparities? A review and conceptual model. Medical Care Research and Review 57(1):181–217

Campinha-Bacote J 2002 Cultural competence in psychiatric nursing: have you 'asked' the right questions? Journal of the American Psychiatric Nurses Association 8:183–187

Cloutterbuck J, Zhan L 2005 Ethnic elders. In: Melillo KD, Houde SC (eds) Geropsychiatric and mental health nursing. Jones and Bartlett, Boston, MA

Dare K 2006 Addressing elder abuse and impaired capacity in CALD. Paper presented at the forum on 'Addressing elder abuse and impaired capacity in CALD'. Online. Available: www.justice.qld. gov.au/files/Guardianship/diversity0906.rtf 30 June 2009

Dein S, Huline-Dickens S 1997 Cultural aspects of ageing and psychopathology. Aging and Mental Health 1(2):112–120

Folstein MF, Folstein SE, McHugh PR 1975 'Mini-Mental State': a practical method for grading the cognitive status of patients for the clinician. Journal of Psychiatric Research 12:189–198

Harkins J 1994 Bridging two worlds: Aboriginal English and cross-cultural understanding. University of Queensland Press, Brisbane

Kleiman S 2006 Discovering cultural aspects of nurse–patient relationships. Journal of Cultural Diversity 13(2):83–86

Maher P 1999 A review of 'traditional' Aboriginal health beliefs. Australian Journal of Rural Health 3:229–236

McGrath P, Ogilvie KF, Rayner RD et al 2005 The 'right story' to the 'right person': communication issues in end-of-life care for Indigenous peoples. Australian Health Review 29:306–316

McGrath P, Patton MAS, Ogilvie KF et al 2007 The case for Aboriginal health workers in palliative care. Australian Health Review 31(3):430–439

McGrath P, Phillips E 2008 Insights on end-of-life ceremonial practices of Australian Aboriginal peoples. Collegian 15:125–133

McKendrick J, Ryan E 2007 Indigenous mental health. In Bloch S, Singh BS (eds) Foundations of clinical psychiatry. Melbourne University Press, Melbourne

Minas IH 1990 Mental health in a culturally diverse society. In Reid J, Trompf P (eds) The health of immigrant Australia: a social perspective. Harcourt Brace Jovanovich, Sydney

Minas IH, Silove D 2007 Transcultural and refugee psychiatry. In: Bloch S, Singh BS (eds) Foundations of clinical psychiatry. Melbourne University Press, Melbourne

O'Brien LM, Jackson D 2007 It's a long way from the office to the creek bed: remote area mental health nursing in Australia. Journal of Transcultural Nursing 18(2):135–141

Parsons C 1990 Cross-cultural issues in health care. In: Reid J, Trompf P (eds.) The health of immigrant Australia: a social perspective. Harcourt Brace Jovanovich, Sydney

Plunkett F 2003 Epidemiology: Maori mental health. Online. Available: www.teiho.org/Epidemiology/ DisparitiesInMaoriMentalHealth.aspx 1 July 2009

Schim SM, Doorenbos A, Benkert R, Miller J 2007 Culturally congruent care: putting the puzzle together. Journal of Transcultural Nursing 18(2):103–110

Silove D 2002 The asylum debacle in Australia: a challenge for psychiatry. Australian and New Zealand Journal of Psychiatry 36:290–296

Stein-Parbury J 2009 Patient and person: interpersonal skills in nursing. Elsevier, Sydney

Storey JE, Rowland JTJ, Conforti DA, Dickson HG 2004 The Rowland Universal Dementia Assessment Scale (RUDAS): a multicultural cognitive assessment scale. International Psychogeriatrics 16(1):13–31

Swan P, Raphael B 1995 Ways forward: national consultancy report on Aboriginal and Torres Strait Islander mental health. AGPS, Canberra

World Federation for Mental Health 2007 Mental health in a changing world. World Federation for Mental Health, Woodbridge, VA

Chapter 7

SOCIAL ISSUES

INTRODUCTION

When exploring the mental health problems of older people, the extent to which they are exacerbated by social issues is as important as what results from biological factors. The opening section of this chapter concentrates on ageism and how this affects an older person's self-esteem. This negative attitude directed at older people adds another layer of stress in an already stressful period of life. Women have a greater life expectancy than men, although the downside of this fact is having a greater propensity for the less desirable aspects of ageing, such as poor health and social isolation. Marital status also influences mental health outcomes for older people in relation to social and supportive relationships and how these interact. The chapter concludes with a discussion on mental health issues for non-heterosexual older people, an often-overlooked topic.

AGEISM

Understanding the concept of ageism and how it affects older people is one of the fundamental issues of working with older people. Butler (2009, p 211) describes ageism as 'age prejudice', which relates to the prejudice and stereotypes that are applied to older people solely on the basis of their age. This type of discrimination, where older people are seen as somehow inferior to others, is very prevalent and pervades all aspects of daily life. It includes disparaging remarks that dismiss and belittle older people, adverse media portrayals, the poor design of goods and services, and broader political agendas.

A good example of ageism was found in recent research conducted into mental health services by the UK Healthcare Commission (2009). This study revealed that older people have less access to psychological therapies, out-of-hours and crisis mental health services, and alcohol services. More damning were the findings that there was an 'unjustified reluctance' to take referrals for older people and particularly those with dementia. Ageism affects people personally, socially, culturally and economically. It prevents people from receiving adequate healthcare and reduces their opportunity to fully participate in their communities. This attitude is particularly prevalent in Western societies, and people from other cultural backgrounds are often surprised at the limited degree of respect afforded to older people in countries such as Australia.

Ageist attitudes are formed through stereotyping. A stereotype is:

... an exaggerated, superimposed and generalised portrayal of a group. It involves the adoption of an oversimplified, narrow and standardised image to explain the behaviour or characteristics of individuals and groups (Germov 1998, p 353).

Stereotypes can be positive or negative, and they can be damaging. Positive stereo-typing can take the form of older people always being seen as wise and trustworthy with many life experiences to call upon in times of need. Negative stereotyping occurs when older people are seen as old fashioned, slow, demented, unproductive and incap-able of making important decisions. Both positive and negative stereotyping can create problems when caring for older people. As a mental health worker, it is necessary to examine one's own values and beliefs in relation to this topic. This can be done through professional supervision or undertaking value clarification exercises, which are available on the internet or in textbooks (Stein-Parbury 2009).

Identifying, not accepting, and challenging ageism should be the cornerstone for community-based care. Other strategies include valuing and respecting individuality, being mindful of older people's dignity, being committed to equality and diversity, showing kindness and compassion about any abnormal behaviours, communicating effectively and respectfully, and promoting a healthy lifestyle for older people (Nursing and Midwifery Council 2009).

GENDER

With regard to social issues, the differences between older men and older women are quite marked. First, women have a longer life expectancy than men. For the age group 65–85 years of age, women outnumber men by three to one, and this ratio increases in the 85+ age group where women outnumber men by six to one. The life expectancy for women is 86.1 years of age, whereas it is 82.5 years for men (Australian Institute of Health and Welfare 2007). A longer life expectancy can mean greater exposure to losses associated with health, family and friends, and living a significant period of life with some form of chronic disability or illness. For a man, living longer could mean finding himself in a world surrounded by women, which may not concern some men, but finding someone to share confidences may be difficult, thereby increasing a sense of isolation.

A significant number of older women have poor socioeconomic circumstances and often live below the poverty line (Butler 2009). This is usually a reflection of an absent work history or one characterised by low wages, interrupted careers for the purposes of childbearing and rearing, and lower superannuation entitlements. Widowhood, living alone and inadequate income are all predictors of poorer psychological outcomes in later life.

An overrepresentation of women will be particularly noticeable in the 'old old' age group (>80 years of age). It is predicted that this group will double in size over the next two decades and triple during the next 50 years to comprise more than 9% of the Australian population or 2.3 million people in 2051. In 2008, there were 3400 people aged 100 years and over, and this figure alone is projected to grow to 40,000 people by 2051 (Australian Bureau of Statistics 2008). This group of very old people will have special needs in relation to physical and mental health.

In regard to their mental health, older people commonly underreport their symp-toms or express distress through somatic symptoms like headache or tiredness, and therefore often do not receive an appropriate diagnosis. Although women are more likely than men to seek help in relation to difficulties created by mental health prob-lems, when compared with their younger counterparts (24–65-year-olds), older women are less likely to seek treatment and, when they do get treatment, it is often given at a lesser level. Treatment is usually sought in the general healthcare sector, rather than the specialised mental health services (Australian Institute of Health and Welfare 2008).

This difference between men and women is also reflected in specific disorders, such as anxiety and depression, where prevalence rates are twice as high for women as for men (Australian Bureau of Statistics 1997, Bergdahl et al 2007). In relation to dementia, it is thought the higher prevalence in women can be explained by the fact that many more women live to the age when dementia is more prevalent and women with dementia tend to live longer as well (Australian Institute of Health and Welfare 2006). One area where men feature more predominantly is with suicide rates. For many years, older men had the highest rates of suicide, which has only recently been surpassed by 15–34-year-old males (De Leo et al 2001).

Older women are also more prone to late-onset schizophrenia than older men (Castle 2005). This gender disparity has not yet been fully explained, but it usually occurs in socially isolated women who have remained undiagnosed for a considerable period of time. The symptom profile is generally mild. These older women usually only come to the attention of mental health services when neighbours become worried or the police are called on a regular basis because, for example, the older woman believes she has an 'intruder', which is really symptomatic of a persecutory delusion. Although the symptoms are usually distressing, they can be treated pharmacologically with good outcomes. However, this should be done cautiously and with some form of social support. Hassett (1998) gave a classic example of such a situation in her paper about an older lady who believed she had a plumber in her roof. Hassett warned against being too aggressive in treatment. Dealing with the 'delusion' often occupies a lot of time for the older person and, once this is removed, they can lose a sense of purpose and become vulnerable to depression.

Just as important as diagnosed disorders are the underdiagnosed disorders. For example, older women are often undiagnosed in the areas of alcohol abuse, and prescription (especially benzodiazepines) and over-the-counter medication abuse. The Australian National Drug Strategy Household Survey (Australian Bureau of Statistics 2001) found that on a daily basis, 40% of older women consumed over-the-counter medications. Such medications could easily be taken for psychological distress as well as physical problems. For men, on the other hand, excess alcohol consumption remains a major form of substance abuse, which often occurs with a mood disorder.

Women are the primary users of mental health services. They have twice the rate of anxiety and depression and are more willing to seek treatment. Traditionally, men negate concerns about their health and therefore their usage of health services is much lower than women. This not only happens when they are acutely ill, but they are also less likely to take preventive health actions or comply with health regimes. Reasons for this are embedded in how a society constructs the notion of masculinity (e.g. men should be in control of their emotions and not succumb to sickness). A depressive illness can be particularly damaging for the male psyche because the symptoms of the illness make a presentation that is in opposition to the stereotypical image of a 'male' (Emslie et al 2006).

MARITAL STATUS

Emotional and economic wellbeing is linked to marital status. Older men are more likely to be married (71.3%) than older women (44.6%), whereas widowhood affects 12.3% of men and 42.1% of women (Australian Institute of Health and Welfare 2007).

Widowed men are more likely to remarry than widowed women. In most marriages, the woman tends to be younger than the man (Australian Bureau of Statistics 2009). The implication of these social factors is that if an older man becomes ill and needs assistance, the primary caregiver is likely to be his wife, whereas if an older woman becomes ill she will probably be living alone and the likely carer will be a child or some other person.

Since the 1960s there has been an increase in divorce rates and remarriages (Australian Bureau of Statistics 2009). As a consequence, characteristics of people who are now entering old age include greater age discrepancies between spouses, with the man being considerably older than the woman. Step-relationships have become more common. This could mean the inclination to care for an older parent who is not a 'blood relative' may not be as strong. Having a strong relationship with one's offspring is important for old age, as children are a major source of social support.

A marriage can be a supportive function for mental wellbeing or it can be an undermining factor. Conflict or difficulties in a marriage can be particularly distressing for an older person, especially if it is a relatively new phenomenon brought about by a recent change (e.g. in physical health or perhaps retirement where two people may find themselves spending more time with each other). Widowhood, particularly if it has occurred more than once, is a predictor of depression and also suicide. Older men are at an increased risk for suicide in the year following the death of their spouse.

SEXUAL ORIENTATION AND GENDER IDENTITY

Old age does not change one's sexual identity. It is hard to judge the number of older people of gay, lesbian, bisexual, transgender or intersex (GLBTI) orientation or identity. Since 1999 the Australian Bureau of Statistics (Australian Bureau of Statistics 2009) has been gathering data on same-sex couples and, in the 2006 census, 0.4% of adults (around 50,000) said they were living with a same-sex partner. It is thought this figure is an undercount of the true number of people living in same-sex relationships, with some people being reluctant to identify as being in a same-sex relationship, or others may have not identified because they did not know that same-sex relationships would be counted in the census (Australian Bureau of Statistics 2009). Additionally, this may not be a good reflection of the size of this population group, as it may not have included people of transgender, intersex or bisexual orientation, and those GLBTI people who are not in a 'couple' relationship. In 2007, Callan and Mitchell estimated there were 390,000 older GLBTI people living in Australia.

As heterosexuality is the dominant social process in Australia, GLBTI people can be marginalised and excluded socially, resulting in feelings of disconnectedness and invisibility, which in turn has negative effects on their health and wellbeing (Callan & Mitchell 2007). Being a minority group, it is easy to direct attention away from their specific needs and health issues. These actions are exacerbated for older GLBTI people when ageist attitudes that also exist in the wider GLBTI community are thrown into the mix. Chamberlain and Robinson (2002) give a particularly poignant example in their research where older gay men from working-class backgrounds suffer not only exclusion from mainstream society, but also the gay subculture with its strong propensity to honour youth and beauty.

There are a number of reasons why the health status of GLBTI people is poorer than their heterosexual counterparts. Underutilisation of health services occurs because the GLBTI person may be unsure if staff attitudes will make them feel accepted or rejected (Peate 2008). Having to hide one's sexual orientation or gender identity can lead to social isolation, anxiety and psychological distress, and in some cases may provoke serious and chronic mental health problems, such as altered body image and drug and alcohol abuse. GLBTI people are often subjected to verbal and physical attacks because of their sexual orientation or gender identity (Victorian Gay and Lesbian Rights Lobby 2000).

Harrison (2005) has written extensively on this topic and is critical of the Australian aged care policy and system which does not take into account a GLBTI person's family and household composition, who is involved in the caring relationship and what the financial arrangements may be. The prospect of being placed in an aged care facility can be a major concern from real or anticipated homophobia and heterosexist attitudes by staff (Cohen et al 2008). These concerns extend to fear of exposure to abuse (emotionally and physically), hostile reception, poorer standard of care because of staff prejudices, or negative reactions to anatomical differences for intersex people. Expression of sexuality and sexual needs is a topical issue in the aged care literature, with very little consideration of same-sex affection.

SUMMARY

Impacts certain demographics can have on prevalence of MH problems.

Ageist community attitudes can have far-reaching and damaging effects on older people. Such attitudes prevent full participation in community activities and can leave older people susceptible to social isolation, poor self-image and feelings of uselessness. Another important social issue for the mental health worker to consider is gender and what impact this difference has on the ageing experience. Women tend to live longer than men, but in these extra years they often have to cope with significant losses such as partners and children, declining physical health and inadequate incomes. All of these losses increase social marginalisation and the likelihood of mental health problems.

There are some commonalities between men and women when treating them for mental health problems, but there may be some circumstances where differences have to be acknowledged and a gender-specific focus in regard to treatment may have to be put in place. This chapter ended with a discussion on the mental health needs of GLBTI people. This group of people do require special consideration, as they often have to contend with a counterproductive social environment, as well as the perils of ageing and ageist attitudes.

FURTHER READING

Kimmel D, Rose T, David S 2006 Lesbian, gay, bisexual, and transgender aging: research and clinical perspectives. Columbia University Press, New York

USEFUL WEBSITES

Gay and Lesbian Health Victoria runs a clearinghouse of health-related information: www.glhv.org.au
Lesbian and Gay Alzheimer's Society Carer's Network: www.alzheimers.org.uk/Gay_Carers/ residentialcare.htm

REFERENCES

Australian Bureau of Statistics (ABS) 1997 Mental health and wellbeing: profile of adults, Australia. ABS, Canberra

Australian Bureau of Statistics (ABS) 2001 National drug strategy and household survey. ABS, Canberra

Australian Bureau of Statistics (ABS) 2008 Population by age and sex, Australian states and territories. ABS Cat. No. 3201.0. ABS, Canberra

Australian Bureau of Statistics (ABS) 2009 Australian social trends. ABS, Canberra

Australian Institute of Health and Welfare (AIHW) 2006 Dementia in Australia: national data analysis and development. AIHW Cat. No. AGE 53. AIHW, Canberra

Australian Institute of Health and Welfare (AIHW) 2007 Older Australia at a glance, 4th edn. AIHW Cat. No. AGE 52 AIHW, Canberra.

Australian Institute of Health and Welfare (AIHW) 2008 Mental health services in Australia 2005–06. Mental Health Series No. 10. AIHW Cat. No. HSE 56. AIHW, Canberra

Bergdahl E, Allard P, Lundman B, Gustafson Y 2007 Depression in the oldest old in urban and rural municipalities. Aging and Mental Health 11(5):570–578

Butler RN 2009 Combating ageism. International Psychogeriatrics 21(2):211

Callan M, Mitchell A 2007 'It's none of my business': gay and lesbian clients seeking aged care services. Geriaction 25(3):31–33

Castle DJ 2005 Epidemiology of late-onset schizophrenia. In: Hassett A, Ames D, Chiu E (eds) Psychosis in the elderly. Taylor & Francis, London and New York

Chamberlain C, Robinson P 2002 The needs of older gay, lesbian and transgender people. ALSO Foundation, Melbourne

Cohen HL, Curry LC, Jenkins D et al 2008 Older lesbians and gay men: long-term care issues. Annals of Long Term Care 16(2):33–38

De Leo D, Hickey PA, Neulinger K, Cantor CH 2001 Ageing and suicide. Commonwealth Department of Health and Aged Care, Canberra

Emslie C, Ridge D, Ziebland S, Hunt K 2006 Men's accounts of depression: reconstructing or resisting hegemonic masculinity? Social Science and Medicine 62(9):2246–2257

Germov J 1998 Glossary. In: Germov J (ed) Second opinion: an introduction to health sociology. Oxford University Press, Melbourne

Harrison J 2005 Pink, lavender and grey: gay, lesbian, bisexual, transgender and intersex ageing in Australian gerontology. Gay and Lesbian Issues and Psychology Review 1(1):11–16

Hassett A 1998 A patient who changed my practice: the lady with a plumber in her roof. International Journal of Psychiatric Clinical Practice 2:309–311

Healthcare Commission 2009 Equality in laterlife: a national study of older people's mental health services. Healthcare Commission, London

Nursing and Midwifery Council 2009 Care and respect every time: new guidance for the care of older people. Online. Available: www.nmc-uk.org/aArticle.aspx?ArticleID=3607 7 June 2009

Peate I 2008 The older gay, lesbian and bisexual population. Nursing and Residential Care 10(4):192–194

Stein-Parbury J 2009 Patient and person: interpersonal skills in nursing. Elsevier, Sydney

Victorian Gay and Lesbian Rights Lobby 2000 Enough is enough: a report on the discrimination and abuse experienced by lesbians, gay men, bisexuals and transgender people in Victoria. Victorian Gay and Lesbian Rights Lobby, Melbourne

Chapter 8
ISSUES IN RURAL AND REMOTE LOCATIONS

INTRODUCTION

Australia has always taken pride in its rural heritage, and much of its modern-day nationhood grew from the values that emanated from this agricultural background. One-third of Australia's population is spread throughout rural and remote regions. The population in these regions also includes a significant number of Aboriginal and Torres Strait Islander people, and although specific cultural issues are addressed in Chapter 6, problems within rural and remote regions are magnified for these people because their health levels and socioeconomic status are markedly lower than that of other Australians.

Many rural and remote communities suffer isolation, socioeconomic disadvantage and limited services. Providing mental healthcare for older people in these circumstances is compounded by these issues and presents many unique challenges for all involved. These challenges are in relation to steadfast rural values, access to mental health services and overcoming social isolation. This chapter finishes with some innovative practices, such as telehealth and mental health first aid, which assist in dealing with some of the challenges associated with providing effective mental healthcare for older people in rural and remote areas.

Remoteness

DEMOGRAPHICS

A significant proportion of Australia's older population lives in areas classified as regional, rural and remote. This means all those areas outside major cities, such as regional towns, coastal settlements, small inland towns, farming communities and what is referred to as 'the bush' or 'the outback'. The Australian Standard Geographical Classification (ASGC) remoteness areas classification (Australian Bureau of Statistics 2001) gives one of five remoteness categories to areas depending on their distance from different sized urban centres, where the population size of the urban centre governs the range and types of services available (see Fig 8.1). The Accessibility and Remoteness Index of Australia (ARIA) (Department of Health and Family Services 1994) classifies rurality and considers settlement at five levels. At level 1 there are populations between 200 and 5000, at level 2 there are populations between 5000 and 17,999, at level 3 there are populations between 18,000 and 49,999, at level 4 there are populations between 49,999 and 250,000, and at level 5 there are populations over 250,000.

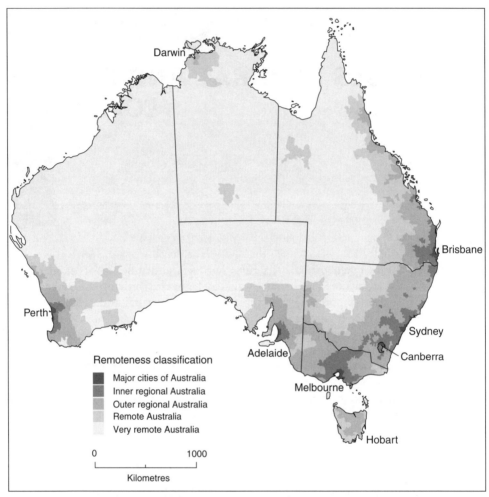

Figure 8.1 The Australian Standard Geographical Classification (ASGC) remoteness areas of Australia
Source: Australian Bureau of Statistics (2001).

The 2006 census (Australian Institute of Health and Welfare 2007) established that 24% of older people live in inner regional areas, 11% in outer regional areas, 1.2% in remote areas and 0.5% in very remote areas. Generally, 36% of older people live outside of the metropolitan cities, whereas 33% of people under 65 years of age live in the same areas. The figures for Indigenous Australians add an important perspective when discussing the mental health needs in rural and remote locations. Although, overall, Indigenous people only constitute 2.5% of the total Australian population, they make up 12% of the population in remote areas and 45% of the population in very remote areas. Another factor to consider is the expanding number of retirees moving from the cities to coastal and rural locations. They usually retire to these areas because of the attractive features of rural communities, such as a slower pace of life, friendliness and cheaper accommodation, so their retirement funds go further. However, these communities often do not have the infrastructure to cope with the perils of ageing on a large scale.

THE MENTAL HEALTH OF OLDER PEOPLE IN RURAL AND REMOTE LOCATIONS

maybe not in UK

Generally, people in rural and remote areas have poorer health outcomes when compared to their urban counterparts. The reasons for this disparity are: lower incomes; lower levels of education; riskier occupations; poor access to goods and services; limited access to health services; shortage of healthcare providers; higher levels of personal risk factors, such as drug and alcohol abuse, smoking and domestic violence; and, in some very remote areas, the lack of basic necessities such as clean water, fresh food, and safe and habitable accommodation. All of these factors make rural and remote locations challenging for older people, particularly when they need mental healthcare.

In regard to mental health, the Australian Institute of Health and Welfare (2008b) reported that there are no statistically significant interregional differences in the prevalence of major psychiatric disorders such as depression and anxiety. In fact, men aged 65 years and over were significantly less likely to experience depression than their urban counterparts. However, the National Health Survey (Australian Bureau of Statistics 2006) collected information on psychological distress by asking 10 questions about emotional state in the four weeks prior to interview. People with very high levels of psychological distress potentially have the need for help from a health professional. Men in rural and remote areas were 1.2 times more likely than men in metropolitan areas to show high to very high levels of psychological distress. Men aged 46–64 years scored the most distress, closely followed by men 65 years of age and over. Older women scored the highest amount of psychological distress for women. When the scores of men and women were combined, the 65 years and older cohort had the most psychological distress overall.

The provision of mental healthcare to older people in rural and remote areas has its own set of difficulties. The social characteristics of the rural communities are likely to exacerbate an illness. Limited resources, coupled with embedded social problems such as higher rates of alcohol abuse, prescribed and non-prescribed substances and domestic violence, all may contribute to pervasive and serious symptoms of anxiety and depression.

RURAL VALUES

Rural people do perceive themselves as being different from city people. The personal characteristics of being conservative, strong, stoic, independent, self-sufficient and self-reliant are embedded in the stereotype of how to make a success of living in harsh, isolated and deprived environments. Unfortunately, when one has to deal with a mental health problem, these values are maintained and are a reason why country people are less likely to seek help for any distress they are experiencing. This could be such a sensitive issue that even to mention that they may require 'counselling' could be taken as an insult and they may cut off any further contact. Mental health issues are a topic not readily discussed.

ACCESS TO MENTAL HEALTH SERVICES

Australians in rural and remote areas do not have the same level of access to quality health services as their urban counterparts. This situation is compounded for mental health services (Perkins 2008). There is a dire shortage of specialist mental health professionals and often a high turnover of staff. Additionally, knowledge and interest regarding mental health issues among generalist healthcare staff is often limited. For example, they may not be up to date with current, effective treatments. When the responsibility for the management of an acutely ill person falls onto primary care providers, such as general practitioners (GPs), ambulance/retrieval officers, hospital emergency staff, Aboriginal health workers and in some circumstances police, the likelihood of ideal outcomes for the older person may be greatly reduced, despite the best intentions of the people involved. In the primary care setting, mental health problems are usually complicated by associated chronic physical conditions and/or drug and alcohol abuse, making the situation even more difficult for underresourced health services. However, with mental healthcare, there may be some advantage in rural and remote areas including closer integration between the GP, hospital care and community care, and easier access to some community services and residential aged care facilities (RACFs) (Australian Institute of Health and Welfare 2000).

Nowadays, some rural and remote areas have visiting specialist mental health teams. There are some disadvantages to this concept. These teams can lack specific expertise due to recruitment issues. High staff turnovers mean that there could be new staff every visit, and so no rapport or continuity of care is established. The team may not have the capacity to make home visits, which are often necessary when caring for older people. In addition, it may not be economically viable for the team to visit unless there is a certain number of older people waiting to be seen. In this situation, assessment and treatment would be delayed and follow-up for older people inconsistent.

If a rural community is fortunate enough to have a local mental health worker, then the expectations of what this person can realistically do must be given careful consideration. A mental health worker can play a role in all or part of the following areas: health promotion, and preventive, curative and rehabilitative services. To ensure that they are effective in their role, it is important that the barriers of working in a rural area are addressed. To prevent professional isolation, the mental health worker needs to know where they can seek advice. This can be achieved through having well-developed communication channels with specialist services, developing valuable networks so there is support from other health professionals to share concerns, obtaining support for decisions and sourcing the right information. Such networks are essential to prevent burnout and to provide continuity of care for the older person. Ideally, there should be a mental health specialist or a specialist mental health service available for consultation and backup.

Local mental health workers are in the unique position of having sensitivity towards local issues and being able to raise awareness of such issues to help in breaking down any prejudices. Activities such as writing articles for the local newspaper, doing radio interviews, providing information stalls at community events, guest speaking at local schools, club meetings and council meetings, and setting up support groups, will have positive benefits. A lot of consistent work can also be done to improve collaboration between mental health services, GPs, aged care assessment teams, police, ambulance officers and emergency room staff.

Due to the lack of specialised services in rural and remote areas and inability of general health services to take on older people with serious mental health problems, a large proportion of the burden of care falls onto families and other informal caregivers. Even when services do exist, there can be a reluctance to use them due to the previously described stoicism, privacy and confidentiality reasons. Support groups can be set up, but if travel time and transportation difficulties prevent involvement in this type of activity, carers can be referred to online services or websites that mental health organisations have set up (Dow et al 2008). These provide excellent information and support for older people and their carers. Crisis lines also have an important role to play in assisting people in emergency situations.

Greater difficulties in accessing healthcare due to distance, time, cost and transport availability, and longer delays in accessing services, can make mental health problems more serious, resulting in admission to hospital. People in rural and remote areas have higher rates of hospitalisation (Australian Institute of Health and Welfare 2008a). Admission to the local hospital or a RACF for a mental health problem may not be an ideal option if it is not resourced to meet the older person's needs. However, due to lack of availability of and inability to gain access to mental health beds in the larger centres, older people who are acutely ill with primary psychiatric diagnoses are sometimes treated in general beds of the local hospital with staff who may not have the knowledge of how to treat a mental health problem. The older person and their family may be very uncomfortable with this outcome. Concern could be about privacy and confidentiality issues.

Through lack of understanding, prejudices against an individual and their family can easily develop, with long-term consequences. In a small community, anonymity is difficult. People may be very sensitive to the stigma attached to mental health problems and experience feelings of shame, humiliation and embarrassment. In such circumstances, it may be prudent to use services in other areas if appropriate or available. Another issue that may arise in a small community is there could be conflicting roles and boundaries between the healthcare workers and the older people—they may be related or socially connected. In such situations, the health professional needs to explain to the older person and their relatives what their professional role is and how they are legally and ethically bound in regard to privacy and confidentiality (Hungerford 2006).

If the situation is an emergency or dangerous, the hospital may not be able to admit the person, and in these situations police cells are sometimes used. Although this might only occur in extreme circumstances, it could be very traumatic and humiliating for the older person. Another option is to be admitted to distant city facilities. Specialist care may be received, but the disadvantage could be separation from families, communities and social networks whose support is needed in times of mental health problems (Hungerford 2006).

SOCIAL ISOLATION

Older people with mental health problems who live in a rural and remote area may be further disadvantaged by social isolation. Substantial evidence exists that lack of social integration and emotional support has a negative effect on mortality through poorer physical and mental health outcomes, including decreased cognitive functioning (Bennett et al 2006).

Rural and remote areas have a higher rate of suicide, mainly on account of the devastating actions of younger men and the high number of Indigenous people residing in these areas, but older people also appear on the registers (Australian Bureau of Statistics 2005). Easier access to very lethal means such as guns, driving recklessly on poor roads and the lack of emergency services for quick responses all feed into the high rates of completed suicides. Prevention and risk assessment for suicide is an essential clinical skill for any health worker in rural and remote areas (see Ch 21).

THE POSITIVES OF RURAL AND REMOTE AREA WORK

The challenges to the provision of mental healthcare to older people have been discussed at length, but what is happening on the positive side of the equation? Mental health workers often work closely with other health and social services, and people get to know each other well on a professional and personal basis. People enjoy living and working in rural and remote areas and the people invest a lot of time, energy and money into their communities. People in these regions are keen to use available technologies and to try out innovations that will improve health outcomes. Over the last decade there have been such practices as telehealth and mental health first aid, which are making an impact.

Telehealth

Telehealth involves the use of telecommunications such as videoconferencing, telephone services and online health to diagnose, treat and evaluate health at a distance (Jones 2001). These are useful systems that allow greater access to specialised information so that care is improved. These forms of communication can be used for meetings, consultations, supervision, educational sessions and clinical work. This is an area that has not reached its potential, although advances such as tools to assist in screening older people have been made. The Telephone Interview for Cognitive Status (Brandt et al 1988) and the Structured Telephone Interview for Dementia Assessment (STIDA) (Go et al 1997) are two examples. There may be some conditions or presentations for which this type of service is not appropriate, but, overall, the research indicates that this type of service is as feasible and clinically acceptable as face-to-face contact. Mental health workers, older people and family carers can access such programs as the following:
- general information services
- psychoeducational programs
- automated programs to distract people with Alzheimer's disease as a tool for behavioural symptoms
- support services for staff, family caregivers and older people, and
- health maintenance programs.

Mental health first aid

Mental health first aid (MHFA) (Sartore 2008) is a recent development, particularly in light of the devastating social and economic consequences of drought. An MHFA program aims to equip non-health professionals with basic skills to identify when a person has some psychological distress and how to encourage them to seek professional help. These non-health professionals are chosen because they are respected, local people who belong to front-line agencies that have close and ongoing links to farmers and their families, particularly in times of considerable stress. They come from backgrounds such as drought support workers, financial counsellors, stock and station agents, and government department staff.

Traditionally, these types of occupations have always made up part of the community's social network and have played an important role as albeit very informal 'front-line' counsellors. However, in times of great pressure, this is not enough because even though they are aware of the enormous difficulties people are facing, they also feel helpless.

By applying MHFA, they can recognise when people are in serious difficulty, such as an acute psychosis or clinical depression, and feel confident in linking these people with services for mental health advice and support. Having awareness and understanding of mental health issues and being comfortable and empathetic in talking about them goes a long way to breaking down the barriers produced by stigma.

SUMMARY

Rural and remote life is characterised by extreme fluctuations in environmental conditions, limited resources, lack of formal social support systems and isolation, with many people living hours from their nearest neighbour or town. People in these areas, including older people, make less use of GPs and mental health services than their urban counterparts, despite a similar prevalence of mental health problems. The provision of effective mental healthcare is stymied by the lack of qualified mental health staff, the fear of stigma and the attitude of rural stoicism.

To improve outcomes for older people, there needs to be greater community access to mental healthcare. Mental health workers and other key members of the community who have direct contact with people in stressful situations need to be able to identify when a person is unwell, apply early intervention techniques and know how to refer for appropriate treatment. It is vital to put in strategies to engage with local communities to raise awareness of mental health problems so that the older people who suffer from these conditions can recover and live without stigma.

USEFUL WEBSITE

Mental Health First Aid: www.mhfa.com.au

REFERENCES

Australian Bureau of Statistics (ABS) 2001 Australian standard geographical classification. ABS Cat. No. 1216.0. ABS, Canberra

Australian Bureau of Statistics (ABS) 2005 Suicides Australia. ABS, Canberra

Australian Bureau of Statistics (ABS) 2006 National health survey. ABS, Canberra

Australian Institute of Health and Welfare (AIHW) 2000 Health in rural and remote Australia. AIHW, Canberra

Australian Institute of Health and Welfare (AIHW) 2007 Older Australia at a glance, 4th edn. Cat. No. AGE 52. AIHW, Canberra

Australian Institute of Health and Welfare (AIHW) 2008a Australia's health 2008. AIHW Cat. No. AUS 99. AIHW, Canberra

Australian Institute of Health and Welfare (AIHW) 2008b Rural, regional and remote health: indicators of health status and determinants of health. Rural Health Series No. 9. AIHW Cat. No. PHE 97. AIHW, Canberra

Bennett DA, Schneider JA, Tang Y et al 2006 The effect of social networks on the relation between Alzheimer's disease pathology and level of cognitive function in old people: a longitudinal cohort study. Lancet Neurology 5:406–412

Brandt J, Spencer M, Folstein M 1988 The Telephone Interview for Cognitive Status. Neuropsychiatry, Neuropsychology and Behavioural Neurology 1(2):111–117

Department of Health and Family Services (DHFS) 1994 National rural health strategy. DHFS, Canberra

Dow B, Moore K, Scott P et al 2008 Rural carers online: a feasibility study. Australian Journal of Rural Health 16:221–225

Go RC, Duke LW, Harrell LE et al 1997 Development and validation of a Structured Telephone Interview for Dementia Assessment (STIDA): the NIHM genetics initiative. Journal of Geriatric Psychiatry and Neurology 10:161–167

Hungerford C 2006 Treating acute mental illness in rural general hospitals: necessity or choice. Australian Journal of Rural Health 14:139–143

Jones 2001 Telepsychiatry and geriatric care. Current Psychiatric Reports 3:29–36

Perkins D 2008 Mental health academics in the university departments of rural health: roles and contributions. Australian Journal of Rural Health 16:325–326

Sartore G-M, Kelly B, Stain HJ et al 2008 Improving mental health capacity in rural communities: mental health first aid delivery in drought-affected rural New South Wales. Australian Journal of Rural Health 16:313–318

Chapter 9
CONSUMERS AND CARERS

INTRODUCTION

Older people experience a broad range of mental health problems and contact with specialist mental health services is increasing. This contact brings a desire on the part of consumers and carers to have greater participation in the management of these services so their unique needs are better addressed. The population served by older persons' mental health services (OPMHS) is different from other mental health services. One of these points of difference is the greater presence of other people involved with the care of the older person, be that a spouse, a child or a neighbour. Many people derive a lot of satisfaction from being a carer and they are a very valuable resource, but recognition needs to be given to this role, and also the issue of carer burden and ways to reduce burden.

CONSUMER AND CARER PARTICIPATION IN MENTAL HEALTH SERVICES

Since the early 1990s, beginning with the National Inquiry into Human Rights of People with Mental Illness (Human Rights and Equal Opportunity Commission 1993), there has been a considerable shift in philosophical thinking about consumer and carer participation in mental health services. No longer is their presence a neglected, unsupported and almost invisible group of family members struggling to deal with the impact of mental illness on their lives (Mental Health Council of Australia and Carers Association of Australia 2000). Consumer and carer groups have developed into highly structured, funded organisations to achieve their purpose of support and advocacy for consumers and carers.

All the current government policy documents have a consistent and strong reference to the importance of consumer and carer involvement in the management of mental health services to the extent that it is listed as a quality indicator (Australian Health Ministers 2003, Australian Health Ministers Advisory Council 1996). The input of consumers and carers extends from direct involvement in the mentally ill person's treatment and care plan through to the broader areas of service planning, delivery and evaluation. Beyond being a major stakeholder, another reason why consumer and carer input is important is because their perceptions of what is important in a mental health service can differ significantly from that of the service providers. Lelliott et al (2001), for example, found that consumers placed greater value on social and staff relationships as well as purposeful daytime activities, rather than having all attention focused on controlling their symptoms.

How 'participation' is defined and implemented will determine the feasibility of participation. Indeed, barriers to consumer and carer participation do exist, and these have to be dealt with on an ongoing basis. Some consumers and carers do not want to be involved as they have other priorities in their lives. There may be a considerable amount of family conflict and ill-feeling where the carers may not want involvement, or the consumer may not want their carer involved. Geographical distance, not speaking the dominant language or having compromised health status themselves could be other barriers for carers. Additionally, some mental health service staff may resent consumer and carer participation or have issues with privacy and confidentiality. Knowing the barriers and working out strategies to overcome these will empower consumers and carers so their participation is maximised.

Integration of consumer and carer input for mental health service delivery needs to be facilitated. This is essential so that tokenism is avoided and the benefits realised. Facilitation involves delineating the participation role and educating staff and other carers and consumers about the role and how it articulates with the service. The consumers and carers themselves need to have training and support on how to participate effectively as well. Lloyd and King (2003) have provided ideas for a broad approach to maintain the momentum for consumer and carer participation. The ideas include multidisciplinary and service discussions about strategies to continually improve partnership, creating links between government and non-government sectors, distributing promotional material, incorporating consumer and carer participation into service plans and policy and procedure documents, conducting joint research and evaluation, encouraging working party and committee membership, conducting multidisciplinary and service forums, and involvement in staff education and training. The paid employment of carer and consumer consultants in mental health services has been a successful strategy. These consultants draw on their experience and that of other consumers and carers. They can have an array of roles in areas such as advocacy, education, management and research.

SUPPORT

It is well known that recovery from mental illness is enhanced with support from family and friends. For family and friends to maintain these roles, they in turn need support. Support can come from the mental health services, which can provide information and ready communication. Support also comes from consumer and carer organisations, which to their credit have become very effective organisations in a relatively short period of time. This effectiveness has been achieved through their being able to identify and assist with the specific needs of carers, and lobbying and representing on behalf of carers. Below are listed some of the consumer and carer groups that function at a national level, with many local branches throughout the country.

Mental Health Council of Australia

The Mental Health Council of Australia (MHCA) is a registered charity that was established in 1997 (see www.mhca.org.au). It is a non-government organisation (NGO) that represents and promotes the interests of the Australian mental health sector to achieve better mental health outcomes for all Australians. Membership consists of national organisations representing consumers, carers, special needs groups, clinical service providers, public and private mental health service providers, researchers and state/territory community mental health peak bodies. Its activities are centred around health promotion, education and research, and contributing to the reform agenda for Australia's mental health system.

Carers Australia

Carers Australia is the national NGO made up of a network of carers' associations in each state and territory (see www.carersaustralia.com.au). Its purpose is to improve the lives of carers through the provision of services such as counselling, advice, advocacy, education and training. Carers Australia also represents and promotes the recognition of carers to governments, businesses and the wider public.

Mental Health Carers Arafmi Australia

Mental Health Carers Arafmi Australia (ARAFMI) is an NGO that provides support for families, carers and friends of people with mental health issues (see www.arafmiaustralia.asn.au). The first ARAFMI group was formed in Sydney in 1975 by a group of carers who identified the need for a service that would specifically address the concerns of carers, relatives and friends. The movement quickly spread to other Australian states and to the Northern Territory, and it became the primary provider of services for carers of people with a mental illness in Australia. Its support services provide counselling, mutual support groups, telephone support, and information and referral services.

Mental Illness Fellowship of Australia

The Mental Illness Fellowship of Australia (MIFA) began in 1986 as the Schizophrenia Fellowship and in 2001 became what it is known as today (see http://esvc000144.wic027u.server-web.com). The MIFA is an NGO and describes itself as a not-for-profit, grassroots, self-help, support and advocacy organisation of people with serious mental illnesses, their families and friends.

Alzheimer's Australia

Alzheimer's Australia is the peak NGO representing people living with dementia, their families and carers (see www.alzheimers.org.au). Alzheimer's Australia provides leadership in policy and service development. Each state and territory has an office that is responsible for providing information, support, advocacy and education services.

Consumer Advisory Groups

Consumer Advisory Groups (CAGS) for mental health are found in many health services in most Australian states. These groups are non-government bodies, but are funded by government and their purpose is to represent the views of consumers to government for the development of legislation and policy. These views are formulated by information that is gathered from committees, consumer groups and forums, and by undertaking research about consumer experiences with the mental health system.

SPECIAL CHARACTERISTICS OF OLDER CONSUMERS

The consumers of community mental health services for older people have a different profile from consumers of other adult mental health services. Foremost are the physical changes and medical comorbidities that are associated with old age and how these interact with mental health problems. This interaction is complex because psychological distress can cause or exacerbate physical problems, and physical problems can exacerbate psychological distress. As a consequence, the mental health worker requires several things: a sound knowledge of pathophysiology; an understanding of how this pathology may influence mental health problems; and the skills to monitor such situations.

From an emotional perspective, older people usually have more mature cognitive processes that have developed from many years of interacting with other individuals from a variety of backgrounds. They will often have more understanding and hence more control over their affective states. Their life focus also changes from the time they have lived to the time they have left to live.

Help-seeking behaviours for the present cohort of older people are also changing and are likely to continue to change for the foreseeable future. Previously, older people might have sought help from their general medical practitioner, a friend or from the clergy. However, increasingly, they are becoming comfortable with acknowledging their mental health concerns and are more willing to seek help from mental health specialists. Although many different mental health problems affect older people, they often present in a superficially similar manner. This can make it difficult to arrive at an accurate diagnosis and prescribe the correct treatment.

SPECIAL POPULATIONS

There are certain vulnerable groups of older people who have a great need for mental healthcare. These include people who have chronic, lifelong mental illness, the homeless, people with an intellectual disability and prisoners.

Chronic mental illnesses such as schizophrenia or bipolar disorder do not usually abate in later life. Episodes of severe and disabling symptoms often intermingle with the general effects of ageing.

People with intellectual or developmental disabilities present with unique problems as they age as well. They have an elevated risk for mental health and behavioural problems (Cooper et al 2007). Most of these people have always lived at home and their primary carers—their parents—are either very old themselves or have died. Very few mental health workers have experience or specialist skills for this group of people. This type of dual diagnosis presents many complex care challenges (Taua & Farrow 2009).

Although older people are underrepresented among the homeless, the homeless population includes some older people with serious mental health or substance abuse problems (Australian Institute of Health and Welfare 2009). Men tend to be homeless more often than women, and as with all homeless people their physical health is generally poor. Sometimes, it is difficult to determine if homelessness caused the mental health problem or the mental health problem caused the homelessness. Either way, delivering good-quality mental healthcare is a very difficult proposition with this population.

It has been known for a long time that the mental health of the prison population is poor and ageing prisoners are presenting many problems to the prison system. The trend over the last few decades for harsher sentences has meant that the number and proportion of older prisoners serving long sentences have increased significantly (Allen 2003). The most common mental health problem in relation to imprisonment is depression. Prison staff are not equipped to deal with the serious mental health problems combined with the effects of ageing on a population that across the board began with a poorer health status than the non-prison population. Many older prisoners have been abandoned by their families and, not surprisingly, they have very few links with the wider community, making life once released from prison a particularly difficult prospect. Prison mental health services will need to adapt over time to better meet the needs of older prisoners with serious mental health problems.

SPECIAL CHARACTERISTICS OF CARERS FOR OLDER PEOPLE

Another feature that distinguishes OPMHS from general adult mental health services is the nature of the family context in which the older person lives. Older people with mental health problems often have spouses, adult children and grandchildren who may want to play a significant role in their care. Complex situations can arise where an older person with declining health wants to maintain control over their own life in the situation in which it is desirable for someone else, such as an adult child, to be actively involved.

When identifying the older person's supporters, the definition of carer needs to extend beyond individuals who are biologically related. It can include other people who either live with the older person or who have developed a relationship with them (e.g. a friend from a social network or a neighbour). The importance of such relationships should not be underestimated, although some may appear insignificant if taken at face value. For example, an elderly woman with mild cognitive impairment routinely lifted the blinds on her kitchen window every morning after closing them the previous night. This action indicated to her neighbour that everything was fine.

The profile of carers for older people is different from that for other age cohorts. Most carers are female, either older women caring for their husbands or daughters caring for one or both of their parents. When men are in the caring role, it tends to be a husband caring for his wife, rather than a son caring for one or both his parents. Women often have a more emotional involvement in a caring relationship and experience more strain and depression, whereas men tend to have a more task-orientated approach to care and more readily seek assistance with caregiving (Ekwall et al 2007, Yee & Schulz 2000). Depression and burden are higher in people who care for an older person with a mental health problem (e.g. dementia). How much time is spent caring for an older person varies and it has not been clearly established with research evidence. A recent study conducted in Germany of 357 carers established that a primary carer spent up to 2.1 hours per day with activities of living, instrumental activities of living and supervision, and well over half of the older people (57%) had more than one carer. Care time was significantly higher if the carer was the older person's partner (Neubauer et al 2008).

When assessing an older person, the carer is not only a source of information but is also integral to the whole process. They are often required to provide insights into the impact of functional loss on the older person and to assist with identifying what is placing stress on them. The primary carer should have their own mental health assessed and monitored because they are at risk of sleep disorders, depression, suicidal ideation, substance abuse and anxiety disorders, self-neglect and anger, which may lead to abuse and neglect of the older person. A person's capacity to care should be assessed, including taking into account what their vulnerabilities may be and whether there are any unresolved family conflicts that may impact on the carer role. Caring out of a sense of guilt or duty can increase the amount of emotional stress for the carer. There are a number of tools available to help with this (e.g. the Caregiver Well-Being Scale (CW–BS) (Tebb 1995), which is discussed in Ch 35).

CARER BURDEN

Burden is underreported and carer support services are underutilised. Poorer physical health and psychological problems, usually consisting of general psychological distress, depressive symptomatology, anxiety and inadequate coping skills are consistently linked to carer burden. There is frequently an adverse outcome after taking on a caregiving role, but there are many carers who find satisfaction in caring and value their commitment to the affected person. Caring can be associated with a sense of fulfilment and reward, feeling closer and more companionable to the care recipient, as well as with personal growth. Different carers are able to manage different stages of care. For example, caring for a person in the severe stages of dementia when they are bedridden may be easier than when they exhibited behavioural symptoms such as sleep disturbance and wandering that are present in moderate dementia. The Caregiving Hassles Scale (CHS) (Kinney & Stephens 1989) and the Burden Interview (BI) (Zarit et al 1980) are two examples of many scales that have been developed to measure carer burden. These are discussed further in Chapter 35.

INTERVENTION STRATEGIES TO SUPPORT CARERS

There are a variety of intervention strategies that can be implemented to assist the carer with their caring role. As caring is multidimensional, a multicomponent intervention program is usually necessary to effectively meet all the needs of carers. A recent study with carers of older people with dementia has demonstrated that a relatively simple intervention of five weekly counselling sessions and a 3-month support group reduced carer burden and significantly delayed a residential aged care facility (RACF) placement for 6 months. This time was delayed even further when the carers were adult children, particularly daughters (Andren & Elmstahl 2008). Some other strategies are:

- individual and family counselling
- family education
- support group participation, which can be an invaluable resource and can be found through local carer associations
- sustained availability of a case manager
- encouraging physical and social activities and harnessing secondary family support, which are positive measures to help reduce the impact of carer burden
- depending on the person's religious orientation, a clergy person may be of assistance to the carer
- internet services provided by carer organisations, which often have lots of information on their websites and links to other services for carers and healthcare workers, and
- chat rooms, which are useful for the sharing of information.

Telephone services, as well as the internet, are effective and suitable for people who have transportation difficulties.

Respite care allows the carer time to rest or pursue their own activities, such as shopping, paying bills or socialising. Respite services can be provided at a day centre, RACF, hostel, hospital or in the home. They can be provided in any combination of these on a planned or emergency basis. The duration of respite care can vary from hours to days to months. The spectrum of respite care ranges from impersonal 'sitting' services to structured, small group activities geared to individual needs and abilities. Respite services are often under-utilised for reasons as diverse as lack of knowledge about their existence and concern about the standard of care provided (Neville & Byrne 2007). The mental health worker can assist with the uptake of respite services by informing the carer about the services available, and by discussing the support the carer may need, how this need may be met by a respite service, and the quality of the services available (Neville & Byrne 2006, 2008).

Zarit and Zarit (2007) have developed an assessment and intervention model with the purpose of reducing carer burden and improving caregiving skills. The process begins with assessment of the older person and their carer. The primary carer is identified and the problems both parties are experiencing are noted. A medical history is taken, as well as details about the carer's and older person's knowledge about the presenting condition. The wider family context, support services and use of formal services are determined. Problems such as carer burden, carer distress and carer depression are also identified for future reference.

Once this information is gathered, goals for treatment can be set with the carer, and the process can move onto the treatment strategies and treatment modalities. The first of three treatment techniques is providing information about the illness and what treatment and care options are available. This step is carried out so that people can make informed decisions. The second treatment technique is problem solving for the management of problem behaviours that an older person may exhibit, as well as dealing with any stressors affecting the caring experience. The last treatment technique is providing support. This can be given by the mental health worker, other professional carers and service providers, plus family, friends and neighbours through assistance with tasks or giving emotional support. Some carers are hesitant of accepting support, usually based around a variety of reasons ranging from a sense of failure to not trusting others to be carers. Exploring reasons for the reluctance will help in designing solutions for this situation.

The treatment modalities in Zarit and Zarit's model (2007) start with counselling for the carer. This therapeutic relationship will provide a safe environment for the carer to express negative thoughts and feelings about their caring role and even delve into relationship conflicts that may exist. Family meetings are the second treatment modality because of the family being a fundamental source of support and assistance to the carer. Any disagreements over caring arrangements can be ventilated and how best to supply realistic, ongoing support worked through, such as arranging and paying for support if it cannot be physically provided. The final treatment modality is the support group, which can be an important adjunct to individual counselling and family meetings for the provision of long-term support. Support groups have a number of positive functions and therapeutic value. They allow carers to swap practical information concerning a range of matters, including treatments tried previously and professionals consulted. They lessen feelings of isolation and inadequacy, as the carer gets to hear first hand the experiences of other carers in similar circumstances and can learn that the range of feelings they experience are normal for people in their situation. Advice from peers is usually well accepted and support groups have a key function of encouraging people to take care of themselves.

There is often a broad spectrum of services available. Some carers will require minimal support and information, whereas others will need referral for specialist interventions and ongoing peer support groups. However, many older people and their carers are not aware of these services and therefore can remain housebound, depressed and bored. There is never any guarantee once people are aware of available services that they will take up on any of the suggested options.

When the question arises about institutional placement, it has usually come about from a combination of carer and older person factors. Personality and behaviour changes, including apathy, are particularly stressful and predictive of permanent placement (Yaffe et al 2002). Even if the option of permanent placement is taken up, it may not necessarily improve a carer's physical or mental health and reduce their 'burden of care'. They may have problems with 'letting go' their caring role, particularly if it has been part or all of their identity for a considerable period of time. They may continue to visit the older person for extended periods, sometimes every day.

Carers may develop excessive concern about the care their loved one is receiving or they may develop feelings of guilt regarding their decision to institutionalise their relative, and may see themselves as failing in their duty to care. Carers may also experience a sense of loss or grief. The sense of loss can arise from psychological and social causes. Loss can be of physical contact and intimacy, companionship, time for other people such as family and friends, personal freedom, sleep, leisure activities, work, career and financial security. Grief is the response to such losses and feelings may include anger, fear, despair, resentment and shame, and eventually acceptance.

SUMMARY

This chapter began by highlighting the important contribution that consumer and carer participation has in the delivery of mental healthcare. It then moved on to the special characteristics of consumers and carers of OPMHS. Within this population there are special groups of people such as those with chronic and severe mental health problems, the intellectually and developmentally disabled, homeless people and prisoners who bring unique challenges for the mental health worker. Older people often have carers, whether it be family members or friends. Caring for an older person with a mental health problem in the community is a complex undertaking that often requires the interaction of many services for it to be a success. At the personal level, caring can be a very satisfying role, but the burden created by such a role needs to be identified and acknowledged so that an appropriate level of support can be put in place.

FURTHER READING

Davidson PW, Prasher VP, Janicki MP (eds) 2003 Mental health, intellectual disabilities and the ageing process. Blackwell Publishing, Oxford
Qualls SH, Zarit SH (eds) 2009 Aging families and caregiving. John Wiley & Sons, Hoboken, NJ

USEFUL WEBSITES

Alzheimer's Australia: www.alzheimers.org.au
Carers Australia: www.carersaustralia.com.au
Carers New Zealand: www.carers.net.nz
Carers UK: www.carersuk.org/Home

Mental Health Carers Arafmi Australia: www.arafmiaustralia.asn.au
Mental Health Council of Australia: www.mhca.org.au
Mental Illness Fellowship of Australia: http://esvc000144.wic027u.server-web.com
Victorian Government Health Information: www.health.vic.gov.au/older

REFERENCES

Allen D 2003 Prisoner's health: key concerns. Nursing Older People 15(7):6

Andren S, Elmstahl S 2008 Effective psychosocial intervention for family caregivers lengthens time elapsed before nursing home placement of individuals with dementia: a five-year follow-up study. International Psychogeriatrics 20(6):1177–1192

Australian Health Ministers 2003 National mental health plan 2003–2008. Australian Government, Canberra

Australian Health Ministers Advisory Council 1996 National standards for mental health services. Australian Government Publishing Service, Canberra

Australian Institute of Health and Welfare (AIHW) 2009 Homeless people in SAAP: SAAP national data collection annual report. SAAP NDC Report Series 13. AIHW Cat. No. HOU 191. AIHW, Canberra

Cooper SA, Smiley E, Morrison J et al 2007 Mental ill health in adults with intellectual disabilities: prevalence and associated factors. British Journal of Psychiatry 190:27–35

Ekwall AK, Sivberg B, Hallberg IR 2007 Older caregivers' coping strategies and sense of coherence in relation to quality of life. Journal of Advanced Nursing 57(6):584–596

Human Rights and Equal Opportunity Commission 1993 Human rights and mental illness: report of the national inquiry into human rights of people with mental illness. Australian Government Publishing Service, Canberra

Kinney JM, Stephens MAP 1989 Caregiving Hassles Scale: assessing the daily hassles of caring for a family member with dementia. Gerontologist 29(3):328–332

Lelliott P, Beevor A, Hogman G et al 2001 Carers' and Users' Expectations of Services—User Version (CUES—U): a new instrument to measure the experience of users of mental health services. British Journal of Psychiatry 179(1):67–72

Lloyd C, King R 2003 Consumer and carer participation in mental health services. Australasian Psychiatry 11(2):180–184

Mental Health Council of Australia and Carers Association of Australia 2000 Carers of people with mental illness: final report. Commonwealth Department of Health and Aged Care, Canberra

Neville CC, Byrne GJA 2006 The impact of residential respite care on the behaviour of older people. International Psychogeriatrics 18(1):163–170

Neville CC, Byrne GJA 2007 Staff and home caregiver expectations of residential respite care for older people. Collegian 14(2):27–31

Neville CC, Byrne GJA 2008 Effect of a residential respite admission for older people on regional Queensland family carers. Collegian 15:159–164

Neubauer S, Hoole R, Menn P et al 2008 Measurement of informal care time in a study of patients with dementia. International Psychogeriatrics 20:1160–1176

Taua C, Farrow T 2009 Negotiating complexities: an ethnographic study of intellectual disability and mental health nursing in New Zealand. International Journal of Mental Health Nursing 18(4):274–284

Tebb S 1995 An aid to empowerment: a Caregiver Well-Being Scale. Health and Social Work 20(2):87–92

Yaffe K, Fox P, Newcomer R et al 2002 Patient and caregiver characteristics and nursing home placement in patients with dementia. Journal of the American Medical Association 287:2090–2097

Yee J, Schulz R 2000 Gender differences in psychiatric morbidity among family caregivers: a review and analysis. Gerontologist 40(2):147–164

Zarit SH, Reever KE, Bach-Peterson J 1980 Relatives of the impaired elderly: correlates of feelings of burden. Gerontologist 20:649–655

Zarit SH, Zarit JM 2007 Mental disorders in older adults: fundamentals of assessment and treatment. Guilford Press, New York

Chapter 10

CONSULTATION–LIAISON SERVICES TO RESIDENTIAL AGED CARE FACILITIES

INTRODUCTION

Community mental health teams for older people often provide consultation–liaison services to residential aged care facilities (RACFs). A consultation–liaison service has two components:

1. provision of consultations on individual residents, and
2. liaison with the RACF staff over problems being experienced by one or more residents.

These consultation–liaison services have been available in Australia and elsewhere in various forms for many years. Mental health problems occur commonly among RACF residents and there is a clear need for specialist services. This chapter summarises the types and prevalence of mental health problems likely to be encountered in an RACF. An important aspect of this role involves providing support to the staff who have direct contact and responsibility for the care of the residents to ensure that the best possible mental health outcomes for the older person are assured. This is a complex role with consideration having to be given to:

- the combination of mental and physical disabilities that exist for the older person
- continuity of treatment and effort put in by staff with a variety of qualifications and experience, and
- collaboration between multiple disciplines (e.g. the general practitioner and allied health professionals).

All of these facets have to be taken into account to ensure clear communication channels so that a comprehensive assessment can be completed and an appropriate treatment plan put in place. It is an important role, as it can improve the functioning of the older person and reduce the burden of caring experienced by the RACF staff.

RESIDENTIAL AGED CARE

In 2008, Australia had 175,472 places in 2830 RACFs, with an average of 57 places per facility (Australian Institute of Health and Welfare 2009). These places cater for people who are deemed to have low-care and high-care needs. Traditionally, RACFs were staffed and designed to deal with residents with chronic physical disabilities, rather than mental health problems. However, two factors have combined to generate a need for mental health consultation–liaison services. Firstly, the proportion of residents with dementia and associated psychological and behavioural problems has risen dramatically in the past two decades. Secondly, many older people with mental health problems were transferred to RACFs during the deinstitutionalisation of large mental institutions.

Estimates of the prevalence of mental health problems in RACFs have been subject to several studies. Brodaty et al (2001), in a study of 11 Sydney (Australia) nursing homes involving 647 residents using the BEHAVE–AD scale, established prevalence rates for the behavioural and psychological symptoms of dementia (BPSD), psychosis, depressed mood, activity disturbance and aggression (see Table 10.1). Neville and Byrne (2007), using the Dementia Behavior Disturbance Scale (DBDS), found that 89% of older people in residential respite care displayed one or more BPSD, although not necessarily all the time. The prevalence of all types of dementia was rated at 48% by the Australian Institute of Health and Welfare (2006); however, other studies have estimated that dementia can affect up to 90% of older people in residential care (Rosewarne et al 1997). A North American study found a 40% prevalence rate for anxiety in older people in RACFs (Larson & Lyons 1994). Despite these high rates, mental health problems are poorly recognised and treated in RACFs. When treatment is provided, it often consists solely of psychotropic medication prescribed by a general medical practitioner (Shea et al 1994).

Providing consultation–liaison in an RACF environment can be challenging for the mental health worker, as there are a number of potential barriers to be overcome (Craig & Pham 2006). These barriers include high staff turnover and clinical staff who are unlicensed or have limited education or training in mental health problems leading to poor understanding of symptoms and poor attitudes to mental health problems (Hsu et al 2005). This lack of understanding of mental health problems can also extend to visiting medical practitioners. In addition, financial constraints and staff recruitment issues may result in minimal staffing levels where only the basic physical needs of the residents are able to be met. Staff can also be concerned about accepting new services for fear of exposure of other problems that cannot easily be solved (Tourigny-Rivard & Drury 1987).

The consultation–liaison role involves working at the relationship with the older person, their family and the personnel involved in their care. The benefits of this approach have been found to include better diagnosis and management of a range of mental

Table 10.1 Prevalence rates of mental health problems in RACFs	
Mental Health Problem	**Prevalence Rate**
BPSD (at least one symptom)	89%
Psychosis	60%
Depressed mood	42%
Activity disturbances/aggression	82%
Dementia (all types)	48–90%
Anxiety	40%

Source: Brodaty et al (2001), Larson and Lyons (1994), Neville and Byrne (2007) and Rosewarne et al (1997).

health problems, identification of medication problems, improved tolerance of behavioural symptoms, increased use of new interventions and a reduction in hospital admissions (Fuller & Lillquist 1995, Goldman & Klugman 1990).

THE CONSULTATION–LIAISON PROCESS

The majority of consultation–liaison services are for assessment and treatment of behavioural symptoms (e.g. pacing and wandering, verbal abusiveness and disruptive vocalisations, physical aggression and resisting care). Kat et al (2008) examined reasons for consultation referrals in Dutch nursing home residents with dementia. Common reasons for referral included agitation, disinhibition and aberrant motor behaviour. These researchers noted their surprise that delusions, irritability and eating behaviour changes were not more common, considering the reasonably high prevalence rates of these symptoms that usually occur in this population. Conspicuous by their absence were common abnormal behaviours such as apathy, which are often considered less troubling to RACF staff.

The consultation–liaison process is complex and involves getting to know the working culture of the RACF, as many personnel as possible (clinical, administrative and domestic) and the major sources of referral. Initially, certain elements of this process have to be clarified (e.g. who the target for intervention is). It could be the system, the resident, the staff members or perhaps even family members if they are heavily involved in the care of the older person. Some family members experience persisting grief and remain devoted to the care of the older person even after permanent admission. They sometimes spend many hours every day of the week in attendance. The intervention may be delivered directly to the older person or indirectly through working with staff and relatives. Sometimes, if the problem is a systemic one (i.e. it is occurring frequently in a number of people), the level that may need to be addressed could be the facility management so that policies and procedures are modified to resolve the problem. A good guide on how to undertake the consultation process has been provided by Caplan (1970), and it can be easily applied to the consultation–liaison role. The steps are:

1. preparation
2. relationship development
3. problem assessment
4. formulation and delivery of interventions, and
5. follow-up.

Step 1: Preparation

Preparation is done on a number of levels. Firstly, undertaking this role requires up-to-date knowledge about mental health problems and their assessment and treatment. A sound clinical base will also incorporate knowledge about some more frequently encountered physical disease processes and problems affecting residents, such as diabetes, constipation, delirium, urinary tract infection, pain, Parkinson's disease and stroke, the medications usually prescribed and how these age-related pathologies may interact with mental health problems. Pharmacological knowledge includes side-effect profiles, how medications interact with each other and also that medication can create a delirium effect.

Secondly, knowledge of the working structure of an RACF is required. Normally, an RACF is run with a manager who is responsible for the operational matters and would be assisted by some administrative assistants. At that same level would be the Director of Nursing who would oversee clinical matters. The Director of Nursing may be assisted by a small number of other senior registered nurses who would be responsible for delegating care delivered by enrolled nurses and assistants-in-nursing or personal care attendants. It is the latter who undertake the manual tasks of caring and have most of the daily contact with the residents. These workers, although at times very experienced, have the least amount of training and often low education levels. The type of care environment needs to be understood as well (e.g. it may not be a secure or locked environment). Such knowledge is important in case the solution to a problem is relocating a person to a different care environment so their needs are met more appropriately.

Step 2: Relationship development

Relationship development or collaborations are essential for success. The best way to develop relationships is to explain the role of the consultation–liaison service, and be visible, accessible and responsive to people. This includes all of the people mentioned under step 1 and other healthcare professionals who may provide services to the RACF or to the resident specifically. Sometimes, an RACF has particular general medical practitioner/s and allied health professionals who service their RACF. Alternatively, the residents may have access to health professionals of their own choosing. All communication with these busy professionals needs to be clear and succinct, avoiding jargon. Verbal communication is ideal, but this must be supported with a written report that is placed in the clinical file. Access to the computer system may have to be sought, as there is an increasing use of electronic charting in RACFs.

Step 3: Problem assessment

Problem assessment usually begins with the person/staff member who made the initial referral for the consultation–liaison service. This person can elaborate on the reasons for the referral, give guidance on the best way forward and perhaps even indications for a solution. It is important to know who to involve so that any changes to be made can be supported and carried out effectively.

A thorough reading of the clinical file is essential to gain a medical history, pathology reports (blood, X-rays), biography, knowledge of past and current treatments including medications, timeframes in relation to behavioural changes and nursing care. The final and integral source of assessment information is the staff who are involved in direct care, family members who are in regular contact and the older person themselves, depending on their competency. If information is missing or conflicting, it may have to be verified from a number of different sources.

Step 4: Formulation and delivery of interventions

Formulation and delivery of interventions will vary according to the particular mental health problem, but there are several important issues to note. Presentation of information must take into consideration to whom the intervention is directed. Often the older person cannot be changed, but the attitudes and practices of the carers and/or service provider can be. The intelligence and education level of people concerned must be taken into account, with any information to be delivered pitched at that level. It may have to be given in a variety of forms, such as verbal, written, role modelled and practice sessions.

Step 5: Follow-up

Follow-up is vitally important. This is where all the stakeholders are consulted as to the success of the intervention. Changes to the interventions may have to be made in light of this feedback or extra support given.

INTERVENTIONS

The mental health worker providing a consultation–liaison service can intervene in the care of older people with mental health problems in a variety of ways and at different levels depending on the needs of the resident and the RACF. The main interventions centre on consulting, provision of direct care, staff training and education, and research.

Non-pharmacological interventions (except restraints) are the preferred first-line treatment before pharmacological interventions for mental health problems such as BPSD. Non-pharmacological treatments include such therapies as behavioural approaches and psychotherapy (see Ch 29). This tenet has come about because of a long and poor history for RACFs of overmedication, particularly antipsychotic drugs, overuse of physical restraints and very little use of other forms of treatment. In the past, physical restraints such as geriatric chairs and cuff belts were primarily used to control behavioural symptoms, falls and agitation. Restraints are still used in some circumstances, but this practice must be fully justified and special measures put in place to monitor its use (Department of Health and Ageing 2008).

Development and implementation of staff education programs on medications and regular medication audits that include prescribed and over-the-counter medications are two effective interventions to prevent polypharmacy. Medication audits can be carried out for the purpose of looking for medications that are an inappropriate choice, have an inappropriate dose or frequency of administration, that have been administered for an excessive duration and have not had adequate monitoring, particularly in relation to contraindications. Problems with overuse of antipsychotics and underuse of antidepressants have been identified. In an Australian study, Nishtala et al (2008) reviewed the evidence pertaining to the impact of medication reviews and medication education programs in RACFs and found that they are effective in reducing psychotropic drug prescribing.

Training an in-house OPMHS resource person was found to be a successful intervention in enhancing the care of older people with mental health problems in Canadian RACFs (McAiney et al 2007). Education sessions aimed at building the staff's capabilities through knowledge and skills relating to mental healthcare for older people were found to increase the staff's ability to detect and understand behavioural and psychological symptoms, mental health problems, and the ability to use a variety of assessment tools.

SUMMARY

RACFs have a high prevalence of mental health problems, which often go undetected or receive very little specialist attention. The provision of consultation–liaison services to an RACF is a very complex and challenging role that not only involves the older person but also knowledge of the structure and working culture of the RACF, as well as involvement of other healthcare professionals and family members. Sometimes, the intervention is not provided to the older person themselves, but rather to the people involved in their care. Such interventions can range from personalised treatment plans through to changing institution-wide policy and practice. Essentially, this role brings important knowledge and skills into an environment that does need a lot of support with the intended outcome of better quality and sensitive mental healthcare for the older person.

FURTHER READING

Department of Health and Ageing 2008 Report to the Minister for Ageing on residential care and people with older person's mental health service disorders. Department of Health and Ageing, Canberra

Melding P, Draper B 2001 Geriatric consultation–liaison psychiatry. Oxford University Press, Oxford

Smyer MA, Cohn MD, Brannon D 1988 Mental health consultation in nursing homes. New York University Press, New York

REFERENCES

Australian Institute of Health and Welfare (AIHW) 2006 Dementia in Australia: national data analysis and development. AIHW Cat. No. AGE 53. AIHW, Canberra

Australian Institute of Health and Welfare (AIHW) 2009 Residential aged care in Australia 2007–08: a statistical overview. Aged Care Statistics Series 28. AIHW Cat. No. AGE 58. AIHW, Canberra

Brodaty H, Draper B, Saab D et al 2001 Psychosis, depression and behavioural disturbances in Sydney nursing home residents: prevalence and predictors. International Journal of Geriatric Psychiatry 16:504–512

Caplan G 1970 The theory and practice of mental health consultation. Basic Books, New York

Craig E, Pham H 2006 Consultation–liaison psychiatry services to nursing homes. Australasian Psychiatry 14(1):46–48

Department of Health and Ageing 2008 Dementia resource guide. Department of Health and Ageing, Canberra

Fuller K, Lillquist D 1995 Geropsychiatric public sector nursing: placement challenges. Journal of Psychosocial Nursing and Mental Health Services 33:20–22

Goldman LS, Klugman A 1990 Psychiatric consultation in a teaching nursing home. Psychosomatics 31:277–281

Hsu M, Moyle W, Creedy D, Venturato L 2005 An investigation of aged care mental health knowledge of Queensland aged care nurses. International Journal of Mental Health Nursing 14:16–23

Kat MG, Zuidema SU, van der Ploeg T et al 2008 Reasons for psychiatric consultation referral in Dutch nursing home patients with dementia: a comparison with normative data on prevalence of neuropsychiatric symptoms. International Journal of Geriatric Psychiatry 23(10):1014–1019

Larson DB, Lyons JS 1994 The psychiatrist in the nursing home. In: Copeland JRM, Abou-Saleh MT, Blazer DG (eds) Principles and practice of geriatric psychiatry. John Wiley & Sons, New York

McAiney CA, Stolee P, Hillier LM et al 2007 Evaluation of the sustained implementation of a mental health learning initiative in long-term care. International Older Person's Mental Health Services 19(5):842–858

Neville CC, Byrne GJA 2007 Prevalence of disruptive behaviour displayed by older people in community and residential respite care settings. International Journal of Mental Health Nursing 16(2):81–85

Nishtala PS, McLachlan AJ, Bell JS, Chen TF 2008 Psychotropic prescribing in long-term care facilities: impact of medication reviews and educational interventions. American Journal of Geriatric Psychiatry 16(8):621–632

Rosewarne RC, Opie J, Bruce A et al 1997 Care needs of people with dementia and challenging behaviour living in residential facilities. Department of Health and Family Services, Canberra

Shea D, Streit A, Smyer M 1994 Use of specialist mental health services by nursing home residents. Health Services Research 29:169–185

Tourigny-Rivard M-F, Drury M 1987 The effects of monthly psychiatric consultation in a nursing home. Gerontologist 27:363–366

Chapter 11

THE THERAPEUTIC RELATIONSHIP

INTRODUCTION

The therapeutic relationship differs from ordinary human relationships in that its purpose is to allow the diagnosis and treatment of a health problem. It is usually assumed that both parties to the therapeutic relationship—the older person, and the health worker or health team—consent to the relationship and work constructively towards its development. However, there are particular challenges in mental healthcare generally and in caring for older people, particularly those with cognitive impairment, which can threaten the therapeutic relationship. This chapter deals with important concepts for the mental health worker attempting to optimise their therapeutic relationships with older people.

PERSON-CENTRED CARE

Person-centred care refers to the philosophy of caring for people as individuals, rather than as sets of problems or diagnoses. In order to deliver person-centred care, it is necessary to know quite a lot about the person for whom the care is being provided. Detailed information about the personal and developmental history of the older person is essential to this process. Once trust has developed between the mental health worker and the older person, this information should generally be straightforward to obtain. However, the mental health worker does need to maintain a sense of curiosity about the older person and be alert to opportunities to learn more about their broader life and experience. A person-centred approach is important also for people with dementia (Kitwood 1997). In this situation, considerably more effort may need to be made to track down collateral sources of information about the person's early life, their usual interests, and their likes and dislikes. However, this investment of time will often pay dividends in terms of the health worker's ability to understand the older person's behaviour in the context of their past life and usual habits.

Mental health workers often obtain a detailed account of the older person's current symptoms and past history of mental health problems when undertaking their initial assessment. However, when working under time pressure with very ill people, it is easy to neglect to seek a comprehensive personal and developmental history from each person. Nevertheless, it often turns out to be a false economy in the longer term not to have obtained this vital information early on in the therapeutic relationship. In older people, there is obviously quite a lot of personal history to obtain and it usually helps to use a template or structure to organise this information. Key headings will often include family relationships, history of childhood neglect or abuse, schooling, history of traumatic experiences, religious observance, military service, relationship history, occupational history, travel history, sport, hobbies, voluntary work and club memberships. Chapter 12 describes psychiatric history in more detail.

For some people and in some cultures, care is more appropriately delivered in partnership with the family or cultural group, rather than with the individual. Thus, in certain circumstances, it may not be appropriate to adopt a strict person-centred approach because group values and group processes are the cultural norm. Considerable judgment may be needed in order to decide whether to interview the person alone or with members of their family or cultural group. If in doubt, it is often worth doing both, thus allowing the person the opportunity to express their views without the influence of their supporters. Cultural issues are discussed in greater detail in Chapter 6.

THE SICK ROLE

The sick role is a sociological concept first described by Talcott Parsons in 1951 (Parsons 1951). It refers to sanctioned social deviance in which the sick person is exempt from normal social roles and is considered not responsible for their condition. In return, the sick person should try to get well by seeking technically competent help and by cooperating with health workers. As a concept, the sick role only works if the person has insight into their illness and the health worker accepts the person as being ill (Mechanic 1995). Problems arise with the sick role if the person denies that they have an illness or if the health worker does not accept that the person has an illness. Against this background have arisen the concepts of 'abnormal illness behaviour' (Pilowsky 1969, 1993, 1997) and 'abnormal treatment behaviour' (Singh et al 1981).

Abnormal illness behaviour refers to the situation in which the person either inappropriately affirms or inappropriately denies the presence of an illness. Abnormal treatment behaviour refers to the situation in which the doctor or other health worker either inappropriately affirms or inappropriately denies the presence of an illness. In community mental health practice, abnormal illness behaviour is commonly encountered. Many older people have little or no insight into their serious mental health problems and refuse to accept legitimate diagnosis and treatment. Similarly, many older people with dementia disagree with this diagnosis and do not see the need for the special arrangements, such as substitute decision making, that are put in place for them. As a consequence, involuntary treatment under mental health or guardianship legislation is often required.

Abnormal treatment behaviour is not uncommonly seen. For instance, abnormal treatment behaviour is seen when a mental health worker makes a diagnosis in the absence of the requisite diagnostic criteria or when they apply a treatment inappropriately.

THERAPEUTIC ALLIANCE

The therapeutic alliance refers to the cooperative relationship between a mental health worker and the older person that is intended to improve the outcome for the person. A strong therapeutic alliance is associated with improved adherence to prescribed treatments, including psychotherapy and medication. It is also associated with improved outcomes for older people. A satisfactory 'clinician–patient' relationship might itself have therapeutic effects (Priebe & McCabe 2008). The therapeutic alliance is a form of attachment behaviour and is more likely to develop if the mental health worker takes a warm and open approach towards the older person. Good eye contact, genuineness, active listening and summarising, and demonstrating respect for the person, are all likely to assist with the development of a therapeutic alliance.

However, some people have mental health problems that make it difficult for them to form productive attachments with mental health workers. This is particularly true for psychotic disorders associated with persecutory delusions, but also includes mood disorders with irritable or grandiose mood and severe neurotic disorders with obsessional rigidity. In addition, some people have had prejudicial early life experiences that make it difficult for them to trust others. In both these instances, the mental health worker needs to bring all their knowledge and skills to bear on the development of the therapeutic alliance. In such cases, a slow, steady approach with very careful attention to direct and honest communication style is likely to be important. People with intact cognitive function are likely to have long memories of their contact with mental health workers and if they have been treated poorly in the past may carry negative sentiment over into their current relationships with mental health workers.

In the mental health team for older people, the allocation of case managers to older people should take into account the likely fit between the two. In other words, some case managers are likely to have more success developing a therapeutic relationship with certain older people than with others.

TRANSFERENCE AND COUNTERTRANSFERENCE

The terms transference and countertransference are derived from Freudian psychoanalysis, but are now used in a much broader sense (Gabbard 2005). Transference reactions refer to the unconscious redirection of feelings from one person to another. Classically, transference was used to describe the transfer of feelings that the older person had towards their parents in childhood to the therapist during therapy. However, the term transference is now used more broadly to refer to any inappropriate redirection of emotion. Older people will sometimes develop tranference-based reactions to their mental health worker. For instance, the older person might start treating the worker as if they are their son or daughter. This might reduce the authority of the mental health worker.

Similarly, countertransference reactions refer to the redirection of the feelings of the therapist to the older person. Countertransference is now often used to refer to any inappropriate redirection of the therapist's emotions to the person. For example, therapists may develop feelings of anger or love towards a person, which must be understood as reflecting an issue or conflict within the person they are treating. Countertransference reactions can provide valuable information about the emotional state of the person and must be interpreted in that light. Therapists who fail to interpret their own countertransference reactions correctly are liable to commit boundary violations or otherwise manage older people inappropriately.

DEPENDENCY

People with a mental health problem are often dependent upon others for assistance. Like any other ill person, they are likely to be dependent upon their healthcare workers for specialised care and assistance. They may also be dependent upon family members or friends for assistance in their daily lives. These forms of dependency are normal and appropriate for an ill person. However, some people with mental illness come to rely too much on their mental health worker or on their family supporters. Mental health workers commonly develop negative countertransference feelings towards such pathologically dependent people and feel angry or put upon. Pathological dependency often reflects attachment problems earlier in life, as well as the impact of the current illness, and is likely to be reflected in multiple relationships with others in adult life. Thus, pathological dependency should communicate something important to the mental health worker about the older person.

On the other hand, some mental health workers encourage excess dependency upon them by older people. They may adopt an excessively paternalistic approach and not allow them room to make decisions for themselves or to exercise judgment within safe limits. In most mental health teams for older people, older people are discharged from the team back to their primary care providers, often a general practitioner and supporting community agencies, once an episode of care has been completed. This allows new people to be taken on and keeps the team's workload under some control. It also provides a limit to the duration of the therapeutic relationship, within which the clinician can work. Some clinicians are reluctant to give up their caring role because they have grown attached to older people. In such circumstances, a sensitive approach from the team leader may be required.

SABOTAGE AND SPLITTING

When dealing with mentally ill people, mental health workers commonly encounter interpersonally disruptive behaviour. This often takes the form of splitting or therapeutic sabotage. Splitting is a term derived from psychoanalysis which refers to a primitive defence mechanism. In splitting, people are 'split' into good or bad 'objects' and interpersonal interactions are affected by whichever of these is happening. People with severe personality disorders, particularly borderline personality disorder and narcissistic personality disorder, often exhibit splitting. However, when under stress, people with relatively normal personality function can also exhibit splitting.

Sabotage refers to deliberate or unconscious interference with therapeutic endeavours by the person or their family or other supporters. Sometimes, family members have a pathological investment in the person remaining ill or have a rigid view of the appropriate treatment. For instance, some family members might believe that the only interventions likely to work are biological treatments such as psychotropic medication or electroconvulsive therapy, whereas the treating team might believe that psychological or behavioural interventions are likely to have greater efficacy.

BOUNDARY ISSUES

Boundary violations and boundary crossings refer to deviations from professional behaviour in therapeutic relationships. Boundary violations occur when mental health workers abuse therapeutic privilege and exploit older people. The most obvious examples of this are when mental health workers develop sexual relationships with people in their care or when they exploit them for financial gain. Boundary violations are always unethical and, if revealed, often lead to criminal proceedings and professional deregistration. Boundary crossings are very different from boundary violations and refer to less severe deviations from normal professional behaviour. These include self-disclosure, accepting gifts and non-sexual touching.

It is important to note that although boundary crossing is not normally accepted in the setting of formal psychotherapy, it often has a strong therapeutic role in less formal settings, particularly when dealing with older people. Thus minor self-disclosure, accepting small gifts and non-sexual touching can be powerful techniques for increasing rapport with some older people. However, the therapeutic use of these techniques should be a topic of discussion when the mental health worker has their regular meeting with their professional supervisor.

COGNITIVE IMPAIRMENT

Cognitive impairment can have a profound impact on the development and maintenance of the therapeutic relationship, as most relationships are based on the memory of former interactions with a person. Fortunately, many people with dementia can recall enough of their past interactions with the clinician, including the emotional tone of past encounters, to allow a therapeutic relationship to develop or continue. By seeing the person with their spouse or other family supporter, the clinician can assist this process, as the significant other can provide the person with missing factual details and with essential emotional knowledge about the relationship.

However, in people with profound amnesia, even fragmentary continuity of memory is absent and the person lives in the moment. The clinician needs to adapt to this situation and work with the person and their family. In practice, this means introducing oneself and the clinical context to the person at every encounter and not assuming recollection of prior conversations. Greater formality and structure is often needed during clinical interviews.

INSIGHT

Insight refers to a person's knowledge of themselves—in other words, their self-awareness. In the therapeutic context it refers to the person's knowledge and understanding of their illness and its treatment. At one level, insight might refer to whether the person appreciates that their hallucinations are hallucinations or whether they experience them as real phenomena. At another level, insight might refer to the knowledge, gained over time, that their antipsychotic medication ameliorates their hallucinations, even if it does not banish them entirely. Sometimes, people have partial insight in that they deny their symptoms or that they are ill, but continue to attend appointments with their case manager or their doctor and continue to adhere to prescribed treatment. Insight is also used in the psychodynamic context, in which it is used to refer to the person's level of self-awareness of the factors that are influencing their mental state and behaviour.

CHALLENGING THERAPEUTIC RELATIONSHIPS

The development of a therapeutic relationship with an older person is often easier than with a younger person. Older people have had more life experiences than younger people and these can form the basis for a non-threatening conversation with a mental health worker. Many older people were brought up in an age of greater formality and this can work to the advantage of the mental health worker trying to gain some therapeutic traction. Most older people will not refuse to speak with a mental health worker who introduces themselves appropriately, treats them with respect, avoids the use of jargon and gives them sufficient time to respond. However, even when dealing with older people, there are some challenging situations that we should consider further.

One relatively common situation involves the development and maintenance of a therapeutic relationship with an older person who is under an involuntary treatment order. Such orders are necessary if an older person with a serious mental health problem does not have the capacity to consent to treatment because of their mental illness or if they unreasonably refuse treatment as a result of their mental illness. The imposition of an involuntary treatment order can sometimes lead to a severe distortion of the therapeutic alliance, particularly when the person views it as a breach of trust. It is thus critical that the mental health worker provides the person with a clear explanation of the reason for the involuntary order. In community teams, it is sometimes necessary for one member of the team to be the 'bad guy' to allow another member of the team to maintain their therapeutic relationship with the person.

MEASURING THE THERAPEUTIC RELATIONSHIP

Two 12-item scales have been developed to assess the therapeutic relationship (McGuire-Snieckus et al 2007). These are the STAR–P scale for use by patients and the STAR–C scale for use by clinicians. The STAR–P scale has three subscales: positive collaboration; positive clinician input; and non-supportive clinician input. Similarly, the STAR–C scale has three subscales: positive collaboration; positive clinician input; and emotional difficulties. The STAR scales have good psychometric properties.

SUMMARY

The therapeutic relationship is an essential ingredient in the provision of effective mental healthcare for older people. It needs to be developed in a considered and purposeful manner. The development of the therapeutic relationship within a person-centred framework requires detailed knowledge of the person's background. There are particular issues when dealing with older people with mental health problems, including dementia. These will often need to be discussed in supervision.

FURTHER READING

Booker D 2006 Person-centred dementia care. Making services better. Jessica Kingsley, London
Gabbard GO (ed) 1999 Countertransference issues in psychiatric treatment. In: Oldham JO, Riba MB (series eds) Review of Psychiatry Series. American Psychiatric Press, Washington, DC
Koubel G, Bungay H (eds) 2008 The challenge of person-centred care: an interprofessional perspective. Palgrave Macmillan, Basingstoke

REFERENCES

Gabbard GO 2005 Psychodynamic psychiatry in clinical practice, 5th edn. American Psychiatric Publishing, Washington, DC
Kitwood T 1997 Dementia reconsidered: the person comes first. Open University Press, Buckingham

McGuire-Snieckus R, McCabe R, Catty J et al 2007 A new scale to assess the therapeutic relationship in community mental health care: STAR. Psychological Medicine 37:85–95

Mechanic D 1995 Sociological dimensions of illness behavior. Social Science and Medicine 41:1207–1216

Parsons T 1951 The social system. The Free Press, Glencoe, IL

Pilowsky I 1969 Abnormal illness behaviour. British Journal of Medical Psychology 42:347–351

Pilowsky I 1993 Aspects of abnormal illness behaviour. Psychotherapy and Psychosomatics 60:62–74

Pilowsky I 1997 Abnormal illness behaviour. John Wiley & Sons, Hoboken, NJ

Priebe S, McCabe R 2008 Therapeutic relationships in psychiatry: the basis of therapy or therapy in itself? International Review of Psychiatry 20:521–526

Singh B, Nunn K, Martin J, Yates J 1981 Abnormal treatment behaviour. British Journal of Medical Psychology 34:67–73

Chapter 12

PSYCHIATRIC HISTORY TAKING

INTRODUCTION

Comprehensive psychiatric evaluation includes history taking, mental state examination, physical examination, laboratory investigations, neuroimaging, neuropsychological assessment, diagnostic formulation and treatment planning. This chapter is devoted to history taking from an older person in the community setting. In most clinical situations, the history provides more diagnostically useful information than the mental state examination and its value should not be underestimated. This chapter should be read in conjunction with the chapters on specific mental health problems.

SOURCES OF INFORMATION

History needs to be assembled from all available sources, taking into account the issues of consent and privacy. Likely sources of information include the older person, health workers such as doctors and community nurses, health records (hospitals, general practitioners, specialists, other health workers), family members, friends and neighbours, and police and other community agencies including pharmacies.

PREPARATION FOR THE INITIAL HOME VISIT

Prior to a domiciliary assessment visit, it is customary to telephone the person to discuss the referral and to ascertain their agreement to a home visit. If all goes well during this telephone call, a date and time can be made for the visit. If cognitive impairment is suspected, then a follow-up letter confirming the visit arrangements is likely to be well worth the extra effort. However, if the older person declines consent for a domiciliary visit, they should be offered a clinic visit. Some older people with persecutory ideation feel more comfortable seeing the mental health worker in a hospital or clinic setting. Some are embarrassed to receive visitors at home due to the presence of hoarded material or some other feature of their dwelling. If the older person declines contact with the older persons' mental health service (OPMHS), the referring person or agency should be recontacted to establish whether there are grounds to suggest that the older person is at immediate risk. If this is not the case, then the OPMHS might have to recontact the older person at a later date or decline the referral.

Prior to setting out for the home visit, the mental health worker needs to check that they have everything they will need. They should check that they have a fully charged mobile telephone and that their vehicle has sufficient fuel for the round trip, which in rural or remote settings could be several hundred kilometres. They need to let their administrative officer or supervisor know what their plans are so that an emergency plan can be instituted if they do not return to base within the expected timeframe. They need to check that they have the necessary assessment paperwork, including any forms that might be required for involuntary assessment or treatment under the local Mental Health Act. They need to check that they have a physical examination kit if that is to be part of their assessment.

ENGAGEMENT OF THE PERSON'S GENERAL PRACTITIONER

In many OPMHS, it is an operational requirement that the person's general practitioner (GP) agrees to the referral if the referral has not come from the GP in the first place. Although there may be occasional situations where this is not feasible or not appropriate, this is generally a sound principle. It encourages the OPMHS to liaise with the GP and is likely to assist the OPMHS to obtain a summary of the person's clinical history and other useful information about the person. It is likely also to make it much easier for the OPMHS to ask the GP to do the physical examination, arrange the blood tests, electrocardiogram (ECG) and neuroimaging (computed tomography (CT) or magnetic resonance imaging (MRI) brain scan). Sometimes, the GP will prefer to be present during the OPMHS domiciliary visit. Where this is possible, it is worthwhile scheduling the visit to fit in with the GP's availability. However, in recent years this has become less likely in many places and the person is more likely to be seen alone or seen with one or more family members, friends, neighbours or supporters. Nevertheless, engagement of the person's GP is an important aspect of the work of the OPMHS, and one that usually pays dividends for the person and the OPMHS in the long run.

THE HOME VISIT

Upon arriving at the person's home (or other residential accommodation), it is important to ensure that the person is aware of the names and roles of the personnel undertaking the home visit. There are several advantages to having two workers on initial assessment domiciliary visits. One important advantage is that there is safety in numbers. Another is that one worker can act as a chaperone for the other doing a physical examination. A third is that two workers can often interview the person and an informant simultaneously, thus reducing the total duration of the visit and preserving the confidentiality of both the person and the informant. Alternatively, the second worker can inspect the environment. When the person is highly distressed, one worker can comfort the person, while the other concentrates on obtaining what history can be reasonably attained under such circumstances.

Some OPMHS take the view that one of these two workers should be a medical practitioner, whereas other OPMHS take the view that two non-medical mental health workers can do a similar job. Of course, in some rural and remote regions, the OPMHS team will consist of a solo mental health worker and the luxury of having two workers present on initial assessment visits is simply not feasible.

Many older people living at home have a spouse, adult child, neighbour or other supporter present during the visit. Further information can often be obtained from that person, particularly where the person being assessed is cognitively impaired or lacking insight in the context of psychosis. Older people seen on domiciliary visits will sometimes want to give their history in the presence of a supporter, but sometimes will want to give it in private. The mental health worker should respect the person's wishes in this regard, if it is safe to do so. If there are two mental health workers on a home visit, one can take informants into another part of the house, enabling the older person to be seen alone.

The state of the home (or the environment if the person is homeless) will often tell much about the likely mental state of the person, even if they are unable or unwilling to divulge their history. It may also reveal risks or dangers to which the person is exposed.

VISITING A RESIDENTIAL AGED CARE FACILITY

When a domiciliary visit is being undertaken at a residential aged care facility (RACF), the dynamics are rather different from those that apply during a visit to the person's own home. Although residents in aged care facilities are entitled to visits from outside health workers, where possible such visits should be organised with both the older person and the facility's care manager. In many instances, it will be appropriate also to invite the older person's spouse or substitute decision maker to attend.

Assessment visits to RACFs will often be prompted by staff of the facility following an episode of abnormal behaviour by the resident. This commonly occurs in the context of dementia, but also in older people with mood disorders, psychotic disorders and personality disorders. In this situation, it is particularly important to establish who has the problem. Is the identified person psychologically distressed or mentally ill, or does the problem lie more with the staff's ability to manage or cope with the person's behaviour? This is an important distinction for it may be necessary to intervene with the staff rather than with the person.

Formal psychiatric history taking (as described below) with people with moderate or severe dementia will usually be limited to obtaining information from collateral sources such as staff, family members, GP records and hospital records. However, in such cases challenging behaviours often prompt the referral. There are various synonyms for these challenging behaviours, including disruptive behaviour, behaviours of concern, and behavioural and psychological symptoms of dementia (BPSD). Although an approach to the assessment of challenging behaviours is discussed separately (see Ch 28), it is important not to neglect those aspects of the standard psychiatric history that can still be obtained from informants other than the older person.

INTRODUCTION TO TAKING THE HISTORY

As history volunteered is often worth more than history extracted by interrogation, it is important to allow the older person sufficient time to tell their own story without too many interruptions from the interviewer. Exceptions to this principle include the highly circumstantial person who needs structure to provide a coherent story. Psychiatric history taking and many aspects of the mental state examination are usually undertaken simultaneously.

Early on in the domiciliary interview, the mental health workers need to make a tactical decision about how to approach the psychiatric interview. Some interviews will consist mainly of mental state examination activities because the person is unable

or unwilling to divulge their history. Other interviews will consist mainly of history taking because there is little cross-sectional evidence of any mental state abnormality. Some
interviews will be brief because the older person is unwilling to have the workers remain
in their home for a more extended period or because the older person becomes severely
fatigued or distressed. Some interviews will be extended in duration because the older
person is circumstantial in their speech or because they have some degree of cognitive
impairment.

On some domiciliary visits, the mental health workers will not be admitted to the
older person's home. The doors may be locked and the older person may be pretending
not to be home. Alternatively, the older person might be suspicious or delusional and
deny the workers access to their home. Sometimes, there will be a security grille or open
window through which a brief interview may be conducted.

If the workers gain admission to the home and are able to engage the older person
and/or their supporter, then it is often useful to see whether there is fresh food in the
refrigerator, whether there are signs of excessive alcohol consumption, and whether
the person has been taking their prescribed medication. It is often very useful to look
closely at the bottles and packets containing the prescribed medication—the amount
of medication remaining in the container can be reconciled with the dispensing date
on the container. Sometimes, people are on a large number of medications, including
more than one variety of the same drug (e.g. a brand-name version and a generic version), indicating that they might be taking twice the prescribed dose. Some people will
be on medications that interact or are mutually contraindicated (e.g. a cholinesterase
inhibitor such as donepezil and a drug with strong anticholinergic properties such as
amitriptyline).

Prior to the more formal part of the clinical interview, take the time to ensure that
the older person has their spectacles and/or hearing aid if they are required.

COMPREHENSIVE PSYCHIATRIC HISTORY

On an initial domiciliary visit, it might not be possible to gather all of the information
required for a comprehensive psychiatric history due to fatigue or reluctance on the
part of the older person. It often takes more than one consultation to obtain a comprehensive psychiatric history and this is facilitated by the development of a therapeutic
relationship with the older person, which might only be embryonic during an initial
consultation. In older people with more than mild cognitive impairment, much of the
psychiatric history will need to be obtained from other sources.

A comprehensive psychiatric history would include the following components:
- identification (name, age, marital status, occupation and/or income status, living
  arrangements, accommodation)
- referral information (name of referrer and mode of presentation)
- usual GP and other health practitioners (names and contact details)
- presenting complaints, which may come from the older person or other
  informants (list these briefly)
- history of the presenting complaints, which may come from the older person
  or other informants, depending upon the nature of the condition and the
  cooperativeness of the person (this should be one of the largest components
  of the history, and the information gathered under this heading will vary
  enormously: see chapters on individual mental health problems for details)

- psychiatric symptoms review (current symptoms), including:
  - mood symptoms
    — depressed or irritable mood; anhedonia (reduced interest or enjoyment)
    — hopelessness, helplessness, worthlessness
    — guilt, anger
    — manic/hypomanic or irritable mood; expansiveness
    — grandiosity
  - suicidal and quasi-suicidal thoughts, plans, intent, attempts
  - subintentional suicidality (placing oneself in harm's way—for example, not taking one's cardiac medication)
  - deliberate self-harm without suicidal intent (minor overdoses, cutting and burning)
  - homicidal thoughts, plans, intent, attempts
  - neurovegetative symptoms (sleep, appetite, weight, energy)
  - psychomotor symptoms (agitation or retardation)
  - speech abnormalities (pressured speech, poverty of speech)
  - anxiety symptoms and avoidance behaviour, including:
    — generalised anxiety
    — phobic anxiety
    — avoidance behaviour
  - obsessive-compulsive symptoms (obsessional thoughts or images, compulsive rituals)
  - perceptual abnormalities (e.g. illusions and hallucinations), with consideration given to all sensory modalities (e.g. auditory, visual, olfactory, gustatory, tactile and kinaesthetic)
  - thought content abnormalities (e.g. delusions, overvalued ideas and marked preoccupations), inquiring carefully for partition delusions (i.e. the delusion that people or things are behind or can pass through solid structures such as walls)
  - subjective problems with the form of thinking (e.g. thought blocking and problems with discourse)
  - cognitive symptoms (e.g. problems with concentration, memory and executive function), including:
    — an estimate of premorbid IQ (e.g. educational and occupational achievements)
    — an inquiry about subjective symptoms of cognitive impairment
  - subjective insight (What does the person think about their mental health?)
  - subjective judgment (What implications follow from their mental health problems?)
- adverse life events
- perceived and actual social support
- level of disability associated with symptoms
- past psychiatric history and response to treatment
- past medical, surgical and obstetric/gynaecological history
- medical systems review
- prescribed medication (including estimates of adherence) and medication-related adverse events (including allergies)
- over-the-counter and complementary medication

- substance use history, including:
  - caffeine
  - alcohol
  - nicotine
  - sedatives
  - amphetamines
  - cannabis
  - hallucinogens
  - opiates
- family genograms, including family of origin and family of reproduction
- family psychiatric and neurological history
- personal and developmental history, including family relationships, childhood neglect or abuse (physical, sexual, emotional), adult neglect or abuse (physical, sexual, emotional, financial), relationship history, occupational history, voluntary work, club memberships, travel history and military service, and
- premorbid personality, including attitudes to others, moral and religious attitudes, leisure activities and interests, fantasy life, usual mood and habitual pattern of reaction to stress.

SHORTCUTS TO HISTORY TAKING

The past medical, surgical and obstetric/gynaecological history can often be obtained from the person's GP. Most GPs now have computerised medical records and can readily print out a summary of their records, including a list of the person's medication and medication allergies. However, it is worth noting that some people will have consulted more than one GP or may have changed GPs recently without their records having followed them. Similarly, some people will have consulted medical and other specialists, some of whom might not yet have communicated with the GP. In integrated hospital and community OPMHS, clinical records held at the hospital might shed further light on the person's history.

Where the person being assessed has previously been a patient of the mental health service, much of the history will not have changed, and so in such cases it is worth requesting the clinical file as soon as a referral is received. Having this prior to the community consultation is likely to reduce the information-gathering burden on both the person and the mental health worker.

When the initial history is being obtained, it is sometimes helpful to use a history-taking template to avoid missing important components of the history. Such templates are particularly useful for beginning mental health workers. Commonly neglected aspects of history include a history of mania in people who are currently depressed and a history of substance abuse in older people. Most large mental health services now have these templates, although quite often they are not entirely suitable for OPMHS use without modification. In addition, templates often reduce psychiatric history taking to its 'bare bones' and do not encourage the mental health worker to allow the person to tell their own story in their own way. When people have been repeatedly asked standardised questions by different mental health workers, they tend to tell their story in a standardised way, rather than with all the nuances of personal experience that should accompany it. Person-centred care should be predicated on obtaining a personalised history.

BEHAVIOURAL AND PSYCHOLOGICAL SYMPTOMS OF DEMENTIA

Obtaining the history of behavioural abnormalities in people with dementia requires an approach that is different from that generally taken with older adults suspected of having other types of mental or behavioural disorders. This subject is dealt with in detail in Chapter 28. These behavioural and psychological symptoms of dementia (BPSD) are ubiquitous and generally increase in frequency and intensity as the dementia gets worse. They also occur in people with mild cognitive impairment. BPSD sometimes cause distress to the person with dementia, but more commonly cause consternation and distress to the caregiver. The presence of BPSD frequently contributes to the decision to place a person with dementia in an RACF environment. BPSD are of major concern to staff of RACFs. Fortunately, contemporary RACFs often keep excellent medical and nursing records on their residents, making assessment of BPSD relatively straightforward. However, it is worthwhile keeping the person's past psychiatric history and premorbid personality in mind when assessing their current behaviour.

SUMMARY

This chapter has provided a detailed overview of psychiatric history taking, with special emphasis on the domiciliary visit. It has emphasised the value of engaging the older person's GP prior to an initial home visit to reduce the burden of history taking. It has noted that history volunteered is more valuable than history extracted under interrogation. It has discussed the role of history-taking templates and their pitfalls.

FURTHER READING

Thomas A 2008 Psychiatric assessment of older people. In: Jacoby R, Oppenheimer C, Dening T, Thomas A (eds) Oxford textbook of old age psychiatry. Oxford University Press, Oxford

Chapter 13

THE MENTAL STATE EXAMINATION

INTRODUCTION

This chapter is devoted to the mental state examination of older people in the community setting. Mental state examination is often referred to as mental *status* examination in North America. Accurate mental state examination (MSE) with older people is quite an art and the mental health worker needs to obtain some experience before developing proficiency in this art. As noted in Chapter 12, near the beginning of a clinical interview with an older person, it is necessary to make a tactical decision about how much time and effort to devote to taking the history as opposed to undertaking the MSE. In people with moderate or severe cognitive impairment, most of the history will need to be obtained from other informants. In such instances, the mental health worker should concentrate on the MSE during the clinical encounter with the person. Similarly, in cases where the person is highly suspicious or uncooperative, the mental health worker should concentrate initially on the MSE.

In older people it is essential to conduct a detailed cognitive assessment as part of the MSE. This is covered in Chapter 14. Confusingly, one of the more commonly used cognitive assessment tools is called the Mini-Mental State Examination (MMSE) (Folstein et al 1975). The MMSE must not be confused with the MSE, despite the similarity in their acronyms. The MSE is much broader than the MMSE. Because of the importance of the cognitive component of the MSE in older people, this will be dealt with in detail in the following chapter, after discussing the essential features of the MSE in this chapter.

As was noted in Chapter 12, it is often preferable to see the person alone in case domestic violence or other types of elder abuse have been present. It also eliminates the risk that well-meaning supporters will assist the older person with their responses.

CULTURAL ISSUES

In transcultural situations (see Ch 6), it is preferable not to use family members as translators, as family members sometimes modify what the person says to save face or for other reasons. They also often try to make sense of what the person is saying, making it difficult for the mental health worker to identify formal thought disorder (see below). Thus, it is best to use accredited professional medical translators. However, it is important to ascertain the precise dialect that the person speaks before arranging for the translator to be present. Sometimes, there is no time to arrange this because an urgent situation has developed and the mental health worker will have to make do with family translators. However, in such situations, it is usually worthwhile doing a subsequent interview using a professional translator to check initial findings.

Sometimes, language is not an issue, but cultural issues are. In such circumstances, such as when assessing Australian Aborigines or New Zealand Maori, it is prudent to involve a transcultural mental health worker who is familiar with the cultural background of the person.

SENSORY IMPAIRMENT

The older person or their supporters should ensure that hearing aids are in working order and that spectacles and/or magnifying glasses are at hand if normally used. If the person is being seen at home, this should not usually be a problem. However, if the person is being seen in a community clinic or in a hospital outpatient department, the older person or their supporters should be advised to bring hearing aids and spectacles. Some community mental health teams for older people make it their practice to take a personal audio amplification system with them on home visits in case the person is deaf and without functioning hearing aids.

DETAILED MENTAL STATE EXAMINATION

The MSE starts as soon as you encounter the person, whether on the telephone, via a videolink or in person during a clinic attendance or a home visit. Much of the MSE can often be undertaken while obtaining the history from the person, and experienced mental health workers usually manage to conduct most of the MSE while engaging in friendly conversation with the person. It is often useful to commence proceedings with gentle inquiries about non-contentious issues. Many workers find it builds rapport to accept at least some offers of hospitality, such as a cup of tea or coffee, from the person.

General appearance and behaviour

Note the general appearance of the older person. Do they appear clean and well groomed? Have they dressed appropriately for the weather? Or have they neglected their appearance because of dementia or other serious mental illness? Perhaps they have a physical disability that limits their ability to care for themselves.

Is their attire so bright that elevated mood might be suggested or so dark and sombre that depressed mood might be indicated? Does their attire suggest that they belong to a particular subcultural group?

What is the person's gait and posture? Do they have the flexed posture and shuffling gait of Parkinson's disease or the small stepping gait of subcortical cerebrovascular disease? Is there evidence of disabling arthritis or stroke?

Note the state of the home. Is it appropriate to their needs? Is it clear of excessive junk and debris? Do they have ready access to the kitchen, bathroom and bedroom? Are there hazards such as loose rugs or open fires? Is there evidence of a reasonable diet? Are empty alcohol bottles lying around that might suggest excessive intake?

Abnormal motor behaviour

Look for evidence of the dyskinetic movements of tardive dyskinesia or of late-stage Parkinson's disease. In tardive dyskinesia there may be involuntary movements of the face, lips and tongue, or writhing or jerking movements of the trunk or limbs.

In Parkinson's disease there may be jerky or dance-like movements, usually after many years of treatment with L-dopa or other dopamine agonists. A dancing gait is also found in Huntington's disease.

Is the person pacing? This might reflect agitation in dementia or severe depression, or akathisia (motor restlessness) in someone on antipsychotic medication.

Is there evidence of mannerisms, stereotyped movements or posturing? These may occur in older people with early-onset schizophrenia or temporal lobe epilepsy.

Is there excessive checking or cleaning behaviour such as is often seen in obsessive-compulsive disorder?

Both psychomotor retardation and psychomotor agitation are often seen in severe depression in older people. Sometimes, gross motor retardation (e.g. lying in the fetal position) and fine motor agitation (e.g. wringing of the hands) occur together.

Level of conscious awareness

Conscious awareness can vary from full alertness to coma and death. The first stage on the downward path of consciousness from full alertness is known as clouding of consciousness. The person with clouding of consciousness often exhibits reduced alertness and may appear vague, lethargic or sleepy. However, they are easily rousable. In the next stage, the person is obtunded and only partially rousable. Next, the person is stuporous and is not rousable. In the final stage, coma, the person makes no purposeful response to stimuli.

The Glasgow Coma Scale (GCS) (Teasdale & Jennett 1974) is the standard measure of impaired consciousness that is used around the world. GCS scores range from 3 (deep coma or death) through to 15 (fully conscious and alert). It consists of three components: best eye response (scored 1–4); best verbal response (scored 1–5); and best motor response (scored 1–6). Scores of 8 or less indicate severe coma, whereas scores of 9–12 indicate moderate coma.

It is not uncommon for mental health workers to encounter older people at home or in residential aged care facilities (RACFs) who have a reduced level of consciousness.

Cooperativeness and rapport

One of the most important tasks of initial encounters with the older person is the development of rapport on which a therapeutic alliance can be built. Empathy with the person in their distress will assist the mental health worker to build rapport. Sometimes, however, empathy is difficult to achieve with a suspicious or angry person. Such individuals are often projecting on to the mental health worker negative feelings that have arisen because of their mental illness or the way they have been treated in the past by important figures in their own lives. In such circumstances, it is important for the worker to try to identify their own countertransference, or psychological reaction, towards the person. This may include unconscious hostile feelings towards the person that do not reflect the actual relationship between the person and the mental health worker. It is difficult to conduct a valid and reliable MSE with an uncooperative older person, so significant effort needs to be devoted to obtaining cooperation from the very beginning of the clinical encounter. Accurate reading of the worker's own countertransference towards the person will assist with the development of rapport.

Speech and language

Note whether the interview was conducted in English or in the person's own language by the mental health worker or via an interpreter. Note the presence of any dysarthria (slurred speech) or stuttering. Dysarthria is a feature of intoxication with drugs and alcohol, of cerebellar disease, and of tardive dyskinesia. Some older people with loose dentures or with a very dry mouth sound somewhat dysarthric. Look specifically for evidence of aphasia, which can sometimes be quite subtle. Look for word-finding difficulties, naming difficulties, difficulties understanding the interviewer (consider receptive aphasia) or difficulties in making themselves understood (consider expressive aphasia). Consider whether the person exhibits the normal musical quality of speech or whether this is absent (dysprosody). Aphasia and dysprosody occur in a variety of conditions, including stroke and dementia. Dysprosodic speech sometimes gives the impression that the person has a foreign accent.

Emotional state (affect and mood)

Affect refers to the superficial and immediate component of the person's emotional state. It may change from moment to moment and often in response to external events or the current social and emotional context. Affect is reflected in the person's facial expression, the musical quality of their speech (prosody), and their use of social gestures. Affect is not always in keeping with the person's thought content. In such cases, the affect is said to be incongruent. Incongruent affect is most commonly seen in early-onset schizophrenia and in mania, but may also be seen in some cases of frontotemporal dementia. Affect may be described as blunted in people with early-onset schizophrenia or flat in older people with depression. However, these affects overlap considerably with the facial appearance in Parkinson's disease, in drug-induced Parkinsonism, and in some cases of frontotemporal dementia. Some people with dementia due to Alzheimer's disease also have blunted affect, although this sign varies considerably from person to person.

Mood refers to the deeper and more enduring component of the person's emotional state. Although the person's mood is sometimes inferred from their affect, this is an unreliable practice. The best way to establish someone's mood is to ask them how they are feeling. Mood changes less in response to external events and is more likely to be modulated by the person's internal state.

A common aphorism says that 'affect is to mood as weather is to climate'. However, the terms affect and mood are sometimes used inconsistently and some writers do not distinguish between them in the way we have here. Confusingly, mood disorders are sometimes referred to as affective disorders.

Thought stream, possession, form and content
Thought stream

Abnormalities of thought stream include rapid speech with frequent discontinuities or inadequate connections. This is referred to as flight of ideas and commonly occurs in mania. Lesser versions of this are often referred to as pressure of speech or prolixity. Slowed speech occurs commonly in depression. In some cases, the person may be mute. People with psychotic disorders may exhibit a gross discontinuity of speech called thought blocking.

Thought possession

Thought possession refers to the perceived 'ownership' of thought. There are two main types of abnormal thought possession: obsessional thoughts and thought alienation. With obsessional thoughts, the person experiences thoughts and images as irrational, unwanted and intrusive. These obsessional thoughts and images are experienced as the product of their own mind. Although obsessional thoughts and images are most commonly found in obsessive-compulsive disorder, they may also occur in other conditions, including depression.

Thought alienation occurs in psychotic disorders such as schizophrenia and includes thought withdrawal, thought insertion and thought broadcasting. In thought withdrawal and thought insertion, the person experiences their thoughts as being under the control of an external force or agency, commonly another person. Thoughts are removed from or inserted into their mind by this external force. In thought broadcasting, the person experiences their thoughts as being involuntarily 'broadcast' to other people. People sometimes describe thought alienation as 'mental telepathy'. The internal experience of thought withdrawal may be associated with the observable phenomena of thought blocking.

Passivity phenomena

Passivity in this context refers to the experience that one is under the control of an outside force or agency. 'Made thoughts' are types of thought alienation. In 'made affect' the person experiences their emotional state as imposed on them from outside. In 'made acts' the person feels they are being made to do something by someone else, as if controlled like a marionette. In 'made volition' the person experiences their drive to act as imposed on them from an external agency.

Thought form

Abnormalities of the form of thought are referred to as formal thought disorder and sometimes abbreviated as FTD, although it is important to avoid confusing formal thought disorder with frontotemporal dementia, as both have the abbreviation FTD. In the present context, FTD refers to an abnormality of the structure of thought, rather than its content. The presence of FTD makes the person's thinking, as revealed in their speech and writing, less intelligible. The person makes grammatical, syntactical and semantic errors. When sequential thoughts have inadequate connections with one another, it is often referred to as 'loosening of associations'. In more severe cases this loosening of associations is referred to as derailment or asyndesis (complete separation of ideas). Sometimes, the entire structure of language is lost, leading to 'word salad' or incoherence. Or the person may make plays on the meaning or the sound of words, such as neologisms (made up words), punning or clang associations. When meaning is altered in an odd way, it is sometimes referred to as metonymic distortion. The person may weave into the conversation ideas that are not related to the topic of conversation, but have personal meaning for them. This is referred to as interpenetration of personal themes. Thus, there are many different manifestations of FTD, but all reduce the intelligibility of speech or writing. FTD is commonly found in early-onset schizophrenia, in mania and in organic mental disorders, including delirium. FTD is not commonly found in late-onset psychotic disorders.

When assessing a person in the community who may have FTD, it is useful to write down or otherwise record an example of their speech for later reference. If the person has been writing down their thoughts, ask to keep an example of their writing. One of the characteristics of FTD is that it is very difficult to recall later on if one has not kept a record of it.

It is important to appreciate that some older people with FTD actually have non-fluent aphasia, a neurological disorder seen mainly in people who have experienced a stroke or other types of coarse brain damage.

Thought content

Thought content refers to the dominant themes of the person's thinking. Abnormalities of thought content include delusions, overvalued ideas and marked preoccupations. Delusions are false, unshakeable beliefs that are out of keeping with the person's social, cultural and educational background. Overvalued ideas are abnormal beliefs that are neither delusions nor obsessions, but which dominate the person's life.

Delusional beliefs occur in a variety of different mental disorders, including delirium, dementia, schizophrenia, depression and mania. Overvalued ideas are associated with a more restricted range of non-psychotic disorders.

Delusional beliefs take many different forms. For example, persecutory delusions involve the belief that the person is being followed, harassed, spied on, poisoned, or otherwise abused. Delusions of guilt involve the belief that the person has done something wrong and deserves punishment. Other types of delusions include religious delusions, somatic delusions, erotomanical delusions, hypochondriacal delusions and delusions of jealousy. Delusions may be systematised in the sense that they are well organised and supported by related delusions. Some older people with persecutory delusions develop a delusional 'pseudo-community'; in effect, they believe there is a whole community of persecutors working against them wherever they go. In older people with dementia, so-called partition delusions may occur. Partition delusions and phantom boarders are described in Chapter 22.

Overvalued ideas are less prevalent than delusions and usually develop in the context of an abnormal personality. People with overvalued ideas become preoccupied with a single idea that gradually dominates their life. For example, in morbid jealousy the person becomes preoccupied with the idea that their spouse or partner is unfaithful and engages in a campaign to gather evidence to support this idea. Another example of an overvalued idea is dysmorphophobia. In this condition, the person believes that a part of their body is misshapen. For example, they may believe that their nose is too large and seek plastic surgery to make it smaller. Although overvalued ideas are sometimes seen as less severe than delusions, they nevertheless can lead to serious consequences for the person or their family.

It is preferable for the person to reveal delusions and overvalued ideas in general conversation with the mental health worker, as volunteered information is likely to be more reliable than information obtained through interrogation. However, often the worker must ask specific questions directed towards eliciting these abnormalities. Commonly used questions include: 'Are people out to harm you?', 'Do you have any special powers?' and 'Is anyone trying to influence you?' When directed questions like these are answered in the affirmative, it is essential that follow-up questions attempt to elicit examples of the person's beliefs. Once a likely delusional belief has been identified, the mental health worker should try to establish how strongly the person adheres to the belief.

Perception

Perceptual abnormalities include hallucinations, illusions and sensory distortions. These can be in any sensory modality, including auditory (hearing), visual (sight), olfactory (smell), gustatory (taste), tactile (touch) or kinaesthetic (movement). Illusions can be defined as sensory misperceptions. That is, the person with an illusion generates a false perceptual experience in the presence of an external stimulus. Someone who looks at variegated autumn leaves and sees a snake that is not actually there is having a visual illusion. Hallucinations can be defined as perceptions without objects. That is, the person with an hallucination generates a false perceptual experience without any external stimulus being necessary. The person who hears their name being called when they are waking up in the morning in an empty house is having an auditory hallucination.

Perceptual abnormalities occur commonly in normal older people, as well as in older people with physical and mental health problems. Thus, the presence of an illusion or hallucination does not necessarily indicate the presence of a mental health problem. However, people with mental health problems, such as delirium, dementia, depression, mania and schizophrenia, are much more likely to experience perceptual abnormalities than people without such a mental health problem. Visual hallucinations occur more commonly in organic mental disorders, such as delirium and dementia, than in so-called functional mental disorders such as schizophrenia. Visual hallucinations are part of the diagnostic criteria for dementia with Lewy bodies. Some older people with poor eyesight due, for example, to macular degeneration or glaucoma may develop a particular type of visual hallucination referred to as the Charles Bonnet syndrome.

One practical difficulty in eliciting perceptual abnormalities from people with mental health problems is that the person often lacks insight into their illusions or hallucinations. As a result, the person experiences the false perception as real. Some skill is required on the part of the mental health worker to elicit perceptual abnormalities. Detailed and persistent questioning is often needed. Commonly used questions include: 'Has anything strange or unusual happened to you recently?', 'Are people commenting on your behaviour?' and 'Are you able to see or hear things that no one else can see or hear?'

Sometimes, an older person may report an experience that resembles an hallucination, but it is actually something different. They may misidentify a real perception as something else. This misidentification is actually a cognitive error, rather than a perceptual abnormality. Another experience that might seem like an hallucination is visual agnosia, which is seen particularly in Alzheimer's disease. In visual agnosia the older person sees an object correctly, but fails to recognise it.

Cognition

Clinical cognitive testing is dealt with in Chapter 14. It consists of informal or formal tests of conscious awareness (see above), orientation to person, place and time, attention and working memory, recent and remote memory, several language functions, constructional praxis and frontal executive function.

Insight

There are various types of insight. However, the main types of insight that are assessed in the MSE are the person's insight into their current mental and physical health and insight into the need for treatment for their current mental and physical health problems.

Impaired insight makes the mental health worker's job much more challenging, and so it should be routinely assessed.

Judgment

Judgment refers to the capacity to choose between competing possibilities. Good judgment is rarely present in the absence of good insight, as judgment often depends upon insight. Judgment is sometimes tested by asking the person what they would do in certain situations (e.g. if they saw a fire in the cinema). However, this is less sensitive than asking the person and their family about their recent decision-making history. While poor judgment may be a sign of mental health problems, most people who exhibit poor judgment are not suffering from a mental health problem. As a consequence, a diagnosis of a mental health problem including dementia should not be made solely on the basis of poor judgment.

SUMMARY

This chapter has provided an introduction to MSE. It should be read in conjunction with Chapter 12 on psychiatric history taking. More details on MSE may be found in chapters on individual mental health problems.

FURTHER READING

Oyebode F 2008 Sims' symptoms in the mind: an introduction to descriptive psychopathology. Saunders, London

REFERENCES

Folstein MF, Folstein SE, McHugh PR 1975 Mini-Mental State: a practical method for grading the cognitive state of patients for the clinician. Journal of Psychiatric Research 12:189–198
Teasdale G, Jennett B 1974 Assessment of coma and impaired consciousness. A practical scale. Lancet 2:81–84

Chapter 14
CLINICAL COGNITIVE ASSESSMENT

INTRODUCTION

Clinical cognitive assessment involves the informal and formal testing of memory and other intellectual abilities in the context of the overall clinical assessment of the older person. It needs to be undertaken with most, if not all, people being assessed by an older persons' mental health service (OPMHS). Clinical cognitive assessment is not the same thing as formal neuropsychological testing, which should be undertaken by specialised personnel, preferably by clinical neuropsychologists. Most people being assessed by an OPMHS will not require formal neuropsychological testing. However, clinical cognitive assessment is a basic skill that all health workers within an OPMHS team should master.

CONTEXT OF COGNITIVE ASSESSMENT

The context of the interview and the response of the older person to initial history taking will determine the priority given to cognitive testing. However, most, if not all, older people will need to undergo some type of cognitive assessment.

Experienced mental health workers learn to integrate history taking, mental state examination (MSE) and some components of the cognitive assessment during their time with the older person. As a consequence, there will usually be no clear demarcation between history taking and MSE. In addition, the initial components of cognitive testing involve observing the older person responding to questions during history taking.

Cognitive testing during home visits sometimes poses challenges for the mental health worker. With any individual person seen in the community, the approach to clinical cognitive testing is likely to be influenced by the purpose of the interview and the history obtained from the person and at least one informant. It might also be informed by what the worker already knows about the person. For instance, the type of cognitive examination undertaken annually on a well-known, case-managed person might be different from the type of cognitive examination undertaken during the initial assessment of a newly referred person. Thus, it is appropriate to have a flexible approach to clinical cognitive assessment with a test selection strategy that is modified according to circumstances.

Although clinical cognitive assessment can be undertaken by experienced mental health workers without the assistance of standardised rating scales, in most cases the worker will use standardised measures. The advantage of using such scales is that it is easier to communicate the findings with other health workers and to make longitudinal comparisons by using the same scales each time. It is also easier to interpret scores in the light of normative data for potential confounders, like education and age, if one has used a standardised test.

Cognitive testing never takes place in a vacuum. Both the person and the clinician come to testing with preconceived notions of what will take place and both are often surprised. The person's level of cooperativeness and motivation is likely to be an important ingredient in the successful completion of valid and reliable cognitive testing. It is very difficult to test an uncooperative person, and in such circumstances the worker's time is often better spent working on the therapeutic alliance to prepare the way for cognitive testing at a later date. Meanwhile, the worker can make general observations of the person's mental state and behaviour that are likely to inform a broad judgment of the person's possible cognitive state.

When assessing an older person's performance on cognitive testing, it is important to consider the effort they put into it. Poorly motivated test taking generates falsely low scores and might lead to erroneous conclusions. Poor motivation might be due to the presence of a mental health problem such as depression or a contextual factor such as a compensation claim following a head injury. Sometimes, testing is conducted in less than optimal circumstances (e.g. in a very noisy environment), which does not allow the older person to do their best.

In Chapter 13, the distinction between the MSE and the Mini-Mental State Examination (MMSE) (Folstein et al 1975) was emphasised. This needs to be borne in mind by inexperienced mental health workers.

COMPONENTS OF CLINICAL COGNITIVE TESTING

When conducted under ideal circumstances with cooperative people, clinical cognitive testing should consist of the following components:
- level of conscious awareness
- level of cooperation with testing
- orientation to person, place and time
- attention and working memory
- recent and remote memory, including episodic (memory for personal events) and semantic (learned knowledge)
- language, including naming, comprehension, repetition, reading, writing and calculations
- visuospatial ability, including constructional apraxia and visual agnosia, and
- frontal executive function, including verbal fluency, trailmaking, similarities and differences, motor perseveration and cognitive estimates.

COMPONENTS OF MEMORY

The terminology for the various components of memory sometimes causes confusion. The ability to hold information in the mind for brief periods, either in the visuospatial sketchpad (imagine a jotting pad) or in the phonological loop (imagine a loop of audio tape), is now generally referred to as 'working memory'. Working memory has been likened to RAM in a computer. Material in working memory disappears when conscious effort is turned off, just like material stored in RAM, which disappears when the power is turned off. Neuropsychologists previously referred to working memory as 'short-term memory'. However, mental health workers often use the term 'short-term memory' to refer to 'recent memory' and the term 'long-term memory' to refer to 'remote memory'.

Neuropsychologists consider both recent and remote memory to be types of long-term memory. They further divide long-term memory into episodic memory (memory for events in the person's life) and semantic memory (memory for things that have been deliberately learned). Both of these are types of declarative memory (i.e. memory that the person knows about). There is another type of memory that is important in people with dementia: 'procedural memory'. This is a form of non-declarative memory that involves subcortical brain circuits. Procedural memory encompasses the acquisition of motor skills or routines, including automatic behaviours like riding a bicycle. It is also critical for learning in people with dementias that affect cortical circuits (e.g. Alzheimer's disease).

SCREENING INSTRUMENTS

It is important that screening is distinguished from diagnosis. Screening is designed to identify a subgroup of older people in which further diagnostic work-up is required. OPMHS often use a standardised approach to clinical cognitive assessment. Many services use long-established screening instruments such as the MMSE (Folstein et al 1975), although, in the United States, the Department of Veterans Affairs has supported the development of the Saint Louis University Mental Status (SLUMS) examination to replace the MMSE (Tariq et al 2006). In the United Kingdom, the cognitive section (CAMCOG–R) of the revised Cambridge Mental Disorders of the Elderly Examination (CAMDEX–R) (Roth et al 1999) has been used for many years. More recently, the revised version of the Addenbrooke's Cognitive Examination (ACE–R) (Mioshi et al 2006) has been adopted by some centres. The ACE–R includes the MMSE and executive function tests. In Canada, the Montreal Cognitive Assessment scale (MoCA) (Nasreddine et al 2005) has been developed to screen for mild cognitive impairment. In Australia, access to subsidised cholinesterase medication (donepezil, rivastigmine and galantamine) and to subsidised memantine under the Pharmaceutical Benefits Scheme (PBS) generally requires testing the person on the MMSE or on a more extended battery, the cognitive subscale of the Alzheimer's Disease Assessment Scale (ADAS–Cog) (Mohs et al 1983).

Regardless of which screening instrument is used, the work of diagnosis requires the knowledgeable integration of information from history taking, general MSE, cognitive examination, physical examination, laboratory tests and neuroimaging studies. In some older people, detailed neuropsychological assessment will also be required.

MINI-MENTAL STATE EXAMINATION

When the Mini-Mental State Examination (MMSE) was first introduced in 1975, it represented a significant advance because it allowed doctors and other clinicians without formal training in neuropsychology to administer a brief screening test to identify people who might be suffering from dementia. Although the MMSE is in widespread use around the world, and has been translated into many languages, it has some major deficiencies that mean that it should not be used as the sole clinical cognitive assessment tool in OPMHS. It suffers from so-called 'ceiling' and 'floor' effects, and is difficult to administer via an interpreter. Ceiling effects mean that some people score maximally despite having obvious cognitive impairment, whereas floor effects mean that some people, particularly those living in residential aged care facilities (RACFs), score zero, making it difficult to track their progress with this instrument.

MMSE items do not cover frontal executive function very well, whereas assessment of this is often essential in people presenting to an OPMHS, as frontal executive dysfunction often accompanies changes in mood, personality and behaviour. It is also commonly associated with impaired insight and poor judgment. Thus, if the MMSE is to be used as a routine cognitive screening test, it needs to be supplemented with tests of frontal executive function. In well-educated people, and those with a history of high occupational function, more difficult memory testing is prudent, as such individuals sometimes score maximally on the MMSE despite undoubted cognitive impairment.

Because the MMSE is so commonly used, it is worthwhile considering its items in more detail here. However, it is worth emphasising that the individual MMSE items do not measure single cognitive domains. The MMSE begins with five items that test orientation to time and five items that test orientation to place. Following the original publication of the MMSE in 1975, there has developed considerable variation in the precise wording of these items and in the scoring approach used. The nature of the items testing orientation to place is such that people examined at home are likely to score higher than those examined in less familiar environments, such as hospitals and clinics. This variability reduces the generalisability of scores obtained in different environments. The next item involves the registration of three words for later recall. The original three words, 'apple, table, penny', have now been over-learned by some people, including some with dementia, such that they may no longer be a valid test of new learning ability. The Standardised MMSE (SMMSE) (Molloy et al 1991) contains different words as well as alternative sets of equivalent words to allow valid retesting.

The MMSE then tests attention and calculation through the serial subtraction of 7 from 100 (usually referred to as 'serial sevens') or attention through spelling the word 'world' backwards. Confusingly, different versions of the MMSE impose different rules for interpreting the spelling of 'world' backwards. The MMSE then requires the person to recall the three words that they were asked to register before attempting the serial sevens and 'world' backwards items. The person is then asked to do a series of five language tasks. The first task is to name two objects, a watch and a pencil. The second task is to repeat a phrase: 'No ifs, ands or buts.' The third task is to follow a written instruction: 'Close your eyes.' The fourth task is to follow a three-part instruction: 'Take this piece of paper in your right hand, fold it in two with both hands and then place it on the floor.' In the fifth language task, the person is asked to write a sentence. Finally, to test constructional praxis, the person is asked to copy a diagram of intersecting pentagons.

When using the MMSE to monitor progress over time, it is important that a consistent method of administration is used and that consistent scoring rules are applied. For instance, one needs to decide whether the person will be scored as correct if they are only one or two days out in stating the date. The SMMSE and the ACE–R both have explicit scoring rules for the MMSE and for this reason might be preferred to the original MMSE by some teams. The other important issue is the use of alternative memory tasks. Although it is common practice for people to be given the same memory task (e.g. 'apple, table, penny') each time they are tested on the MMSE, this does not make good sense from a neuropsychological perspective unless the interval between testing occasions is at least 6 months, and preferably longer.

In older people, particularly those with some degree of cognitive impairment, performance on the MMSE often varies by time of day. Many older people do better on this test in the morning. As a consequence, it is important to standardise the time of day that testing takes place, if one is to make valid comparisons between testing occasions. Alternatively, it would be important not to over-interpret small changes in the MMSE score when testing has been undertaken at differing times of day.

When the MMSE was originally published in 1975, scores of 23 or less were found to be predictive of dementia in general medical inpatients in the United States. However, educational achievement has improved since then and scores higher than 23 are now commonly found in people with dementia. Under the Australian PBS, subsidised cholinesterase inhibitor therapy for mild to moderate Alzheimer's disease is available to people with MMSE scores of 10–24 inclusive. Normative data for the MMSE have been published for many countries, including Australia and New Zealand. Normal community-residing older people score 26 or over, even in advanced old age.

NEWER COGNITIVE SCREENING SCALES

A large number of new scales have been developed over recent years, including several by Australian researchers. Some of these will now be described.

The Informant Questionnaire for Cognitive Decline in the Elderly (IQCODE) (Jorm & Korten 1988) was developed as an informant-rated screening tool for dementia. The informant is asked to rate 26 items that compare the person currently with how they were 10 years earlier. The IQCODE is a very useful instrument for estimating the extent of cognitive decline without having to test the person directly. It is often used to supplement the use of screening tests such as the MMSE. It is invaluable when the person declines cognitive testing or when the informant has to be interviewed by telephone. There is also a short version of the IQCODE with 16 items. Both versions of the IQCODE generate scores between 1 and 5, with higher scores indicating greater likelihood of dementia.

The Rowland Universal Dementia Assessment Scale (RUDAS) (Storey et al 2004) has been developed for use via an interpreter in culturally and linguistically diverse populations. It includes six items that cover recall, body orientation, fist/palm alternation, copying a cube, crossing a road safely and verbal fluency for animals. Like the MMSE, the RUDAS requires no special equipment, and so is well suited to use within the OPMHS. The RUDAS underwent rigorous testing in community-residing older people, including many with limited education. Several items in the RUDAS test executive function, including 'crossing the road', 'animal generation' and 'cube copying'. Scores of less than 23 out of a possible score of 30 are highly predictive of dementia.

The Kimberley Indigenous Cognitive Assessment (KICA) test (LoGiudice et al 2006) has been developed for cognitive assessment in Indigenous people in the Kimberley Region. The KICA contains 16 items and generates scores between 0 and 39. Scores of 33 or less are highly predictive of dementia. The administration of the KICA requires several pieces of equipment, including a comb, a pannikin/cup, a box of matches, a plastic bottle with top, and a watch or timer. The KICA test and supporting documentation are freely available at www.wacha.org.au/kica.html.

Although, several other, even briefer, tests have been designed for use in the general practice setting (Brodaty et al 2006), these are unlikely to be useful in the OPMHS context, as a more thorough approach is needed.

MEMORY TESTING

One of the major deficiencies of the MMSE is its very easy memory test. The recall of three words is not sufficiently challenging for well-educated people suspected of having dementia. Even some poorly educated people with well-established dementia manage to learn the three words after several administrations of the MMSE. So clearly the MMSE needs to be augmented with a more difficult memory task.

Simple extensions to the MMSE include learning a name and address like the seven-part name and address in the CAMCOG–R or a complex sentence like the now some-what anachronistic Babcock sentence ('One thing a nation must have to become rich and great is a large secure supply of wood'). Alternatively there are the logical memory passages, verbal paired associates and word lists from the Wechsler Memory Scale, 3rd edn (WMS–III) or standalone word-list learning tasks including the Rey Auditory Verbal Learning Test (RAVLT), the California Verbal Learning Test (CVLT) and the revised Hopkins Verbal Learning Test (HVLT–R). The CVLT and HVLT–R employ words in semantic categories, adding another dimension to the testing. These word-list learning tests allow several different aspects of verbal memory to be tested, including free recall, delayed recall and recognition. In older people with Alzheimer's disease, impaired delayed recall is usually the earliest indicator of cognitive decline. In mild Alzheimer's disease, recognition memory is usually much better preserved than free or delayed recall, indicating that the problem is principally with retrieval rather than encoding.

In undertaking community-based assessments, a rapid, portable memory task is essential, limiting the usefulness of many of these word-list learning tasks that might be more efficiently used in clinic settings rather than community settings. For all but the simplest learning tasks, some degree of staff training is needed and some tests are best carried out by personnel with formal neuropsychological training.

One advantage of both the ADAS–Cog and the CAMCOG–R cognitive test batteries is that they have more difficult memory tasks than the MMSE and require very little staff training. The CAMCOG–R also has several straightforward executive function tests. However, both require specific equipment and scoring sheets, reducing their portability.

FRONTAL EXECUTIVE TESTING

Frontal executive function (or simply, executive function) is of critical importance in OPMHS. Frontal executive function covers planning, organising, making decisions and checking for errors. It is particularly important in novel or tricky situations where habitual responses may be inappropriate or even dangerous. Abnormalities of frontal executive function commonly accompany a range of mental health problems, including depression, dementia and psychosis. Executive dysfunction is one of the hallmarks of frontotemporal dementia and is frequently associated with impaired capacity to make decisions.

Before embarking upon executive function testing, it is important to reflect upon the clinical context in which the testing is being done. People with a change in personality or behaviour commonly have problems with executive function. Similarly, some specific symptoms are likely to suggest executive dysfunction. These include cognitive inflexibility, apathy, impaired volition and disinhibition. In addition, whenever other frontal lobe abnormalities such as aphasia are present, it is worthwhile undertaking executive function testing.

A wide range of test batteries and individual tests are available, but many require specific kits or forms that are unlikely to be readily at hand and may be expensive to purchase. Some tests are only meant to be used by clinicians with a particular type or level of training. Hence, we will concentrate here on tests that can be administered in the field without specialised equipment or much training. Here are some bedside tests of executive function:

- attention: digit span—forwards and backwards
- verbal fluency, including categories (e.g. animals and grocery items) and letters (e.g. FAS); these are timed tests
- motor perseveration: the Luria motor sequencing: fist/edge/palm or the go/no go test
- abstract thinking: similarities and differences (e.g. 'What is the similarity between an apple and a banana?' and 'What is the difference between a lie and a mistake?')
- planning (e.g. 'What would you do if …?'), and
- the Trailmaking test, particularly Trail B in which the person must alternate letters and numbers.

If time for testing of executive function was extremely limited, it would probably be best to use a test of verbal fluency, such as animals in 60 seconds and the Trailmaking test (Trails A and B), although the Trailmaking test does require standardised forms. Both of these tests are timed tests, and so a stopwatch or other timer is needed. Many mobile telephones have excellent countdown timers that can be used for this purpose. Alternatively, verbal fluency, and similarities and differences could be completed in 2 or 3 minutes. For all of these tests, there are age-based and education-based norms that need to be consulted when interpreting performance. There are several compendia of neuropsychological tests that include normative data that can be consulted (e.g. Strauss et al 2006).

More formal testing of frontal executive function is likely to entail neuropsychological tests such as the Wisconsin Card Sorting test, the Stroop or the California Older Adults Stroop Test (COAST), the Behavioral Assessment of the Dysexecutive Syndrome (BADS) (Krabbendam et al 1999) and the Dysexecutive Questionnaire (DEX) from the BADS. Specialist neuropsychologists should administer these tests.

FORMAL NEUROPSYCHOLOGICAL TESTING

Relatively few people seen by the OPMHS are likely to require formal neuropsychological testing because cognitive impairment is usually fairly obvious by the time a referral is made. However, neuropsychological testing is sometimes indicated to assist with a challenging differential diagnosis (e.g. possible frontotemporal dementia) to assess a younger person with possible dementia, or to provide a firmer basis for a medicolegal report. Specialist clinical neuropsychologists are often to be found in memory clinics, which are sometimes part of OPMHS in larger towns and cities.

The neuropsychologist will usually test the person in an office setting rather than in the person's own home. In this way, a quiet, distraction-free environment can be provided to maximise the person's performance. Testing might take up to several hours, and so adequate time must be set aside. The testing will often involve the WMS–III, and the Wechsler Adult Intelligence Scale, 3rd edn (WAIS–III), together with a variety of supplementary tests such as the Complex Figure of Rey, the Stroop and the Tower of London. Premorbid function is often estimated on the National Adult Reading Test (NART) (Nelson 1982) or on the Cambridge Contextual Reading Test (CCRT) (Beardsall 1998).

THE RESIDENTIAL AGED CARE FACILITY RESIDENT

Residential aged care facilities (RACFs) such as nursing homes and hostels pose potential difficulties for the mental health worker seeking to undertake valid and reliable cognitive testing. Environmental conditions in aged care facilities vary greatly, although many will have a quiet location with sufficient privacy to allow satisfactory cognitive testing to be completed. Others, however, will be noisy and will lack privacy. Another challenge in the RACF environment is people with very poor cognitive function. Such residents may score zero on the MMSE and similar scales. In our experience, between 10% and 20% of RACF people will score zero on the MMSE. Although cognitive scales are available for older people with severe cognitive impairment (e.g. the Severe Impairment Battery) (Panisset et al 1994), these do require specific equipment and are not always practicable in the RACF environment. Sometimes, quantitative cognitive testing is not possible and a rough estimate of cognitive function will need to be made at interview with the person and their carers. In such cases, there may be little doubt about the diagnosis and a functional assessment might be more useful than cognitive testing.

WRITING REPORTS

There are some important principles that should be borne in mind when writing reports that contain the findings from cognitive testing. The writer should clearly separate the test results from the interpretation of the results. The interpretation of results requires knowledge of the normative data for the test, including the impact of age and education on scores. The writer also needs to take into consideration the person's test-taking behaviour in interpreting the results. A certain degree of humility is often prudent, unless one is an expert neuropsychologist, as there is often more than one way to interpret the results of cognitive testing. In the context of an OPMHS, there are likely to be many people with reversible cognitive deficits due to delirium, depression, anxiety, mania or psychosis. The cautious mental health worker will postpone making a decision about whether cognitive impairment is likely to indicate dementia until any intercurrent episode of comorbid mental illness has resolved.

SUMMARY

In the community settings in which OPMHS workers often conduct cognitive testing, a screening test such as the MMSE augmented by a more difficult memory test and selected tests of frontal-executive function is prudent. However, some people will be so cognitively impaired that only the MMSE or a similar brief test can be carried out. All OPMHS clinical personnel should be familiar with the correct administration of cognitive screening tests.

FURTHER READING

Hodges JR 2007 Cognitive assessment for clinicians 2nd edn. Oxford University Press, Oxford
Kipps CM, Hodges JR 2008 Clinical cognitive assessment. In: Jacoby R, Oppenheimer C, Dening T, Thomas A (eds) Oxford textbook of old age psychiatry. Oxford University Press, Oxford

REFERENCES

Beardsall L 1998 Development of the Cambridge Contextual Reading Test for improving the estimation of premorbid verbal intelligence in older persons with dementia. British Journal of Clinical Psychology 37:229–240
Brodaty H, Low LF, Gibson L, Burns K 2006 What is the best dementia screening instrument for general practitioners to use? American Journal of Geriatric Psychiatry 14:391–400
Folstein MF, Folstein SE, McHugh PR 1975 Mini-Mental State: a practical method for grading the cognitive state of patients for the clinician. Journal of Psychiatric Research 12:189–198
Jorm AF, Korten AE 1988 Assessment of cognitive decline in the elderly by informant interview. British Journal of Psychiatry 152:209–213
Krabbendam L, de Vugt ME, Derix MMA 1999 The Behavioral Assessment of the Dysexecutive Syndrome as a tool to assess executive functions in schizophrenia. Clinical Neuropsychologist 13:370–375
LoGiudice D, Smith K, Thomas J et al 2006 Kimberley Indigenous Cognitive Assessment tool (KICA): development of a cognitive assessment tool for older Indigenous Australians. International Psychogeriatrics 18:269–280
Mioshi E, Dawson K, Mitchell J et al 2006 The Addenbrooke's Cognitive Examination Revised (ACE–R): a brief cognitive test battery for dementia screening. International Journal of Geriatric Psychiatry 21:1078–1085
Mohs RC, Rosen WG, Davis KL 1983 The Alzheimer's Disease Assessment Scale: an instrument for assessing treatment efficacy. Psychopharmacology Bulletin 19:448–450
Molloy DW, Alemayehu E, Roberts R 1991 Reliability of a Standardized Mini-Mental State Examination compared with the traditional Mini-Mental State Examination. American Journal of Psychiatry 148:102–105
Nasreddine ZS, Phillips NA, Bedirian V et al 2005 The Montreal Cognitive Assessment, MoCA: a brief screening tool for mild cognitive impairment. Journal of the American Geriatrics Society 53:695–699
Nelson HE 1982 NART: National Adult Reading Test: test manual. nferNelson, Windsor, UK
Panisset M, Roudier M, Saxton J, Boller F 1994 Severe impairment battery: a neuropsychological test for severely demented patients. Archives of Neurology 51:41–45
Roth M, Huppert FA, Mountjoy CQ, Tym E 1999 CAMDEX–R. The revised Cambridge Examination for Mental Disorders of the Elderly. Cambridge University Press, Cambridge
Storey JE, Rowland JTJ, Conforti DA, Dickson HG 2004 The Rowland Universal Dementia Assessment Scale (RUDAS): a multicultural cognitive assessment scale. International Psychogeriatrics 16:13–31
Strauss E, Sherman EMS, Spreen O 2006 A compendium of neuropsychological tests: administration, norms and commentary. Oxford University Press, New York
Tariq SH, Tumosa N, Chibnall JT et al 2006 Comparison of the Saint Louis University Mental Status Examination and the Mini-Mental State Examination for detecting dementia and mild neurocognitive disorder: a pilot study. American Journal of Geriatric Psychiatry 14:900–910

Chapter 15

PHYSICAL HEALTH ASSESSMENT

INTRODUCTION

As general medical conditions increase sharply in prevalence with advancing age, many people referred to older persons' mental health services (OPMHS), and many of their carers, will have one or more such conditions. Common conditions in later life include gastro-oesophageal reflux disorder, hypertension, ischaemic heart disease, type 2 diabetes mellitus, stroke, cancer, osteoarthritis, osteoporosis, chronic obstructive lung disease, impaired vision due to cataracts or macular degeneration, and impaired hearing (presbyacusis). Mental health problems can interact with physical health problems in various ways to increase the person's level of disability. For instance, some mental health problems, such as dementia or schizophrenia, can lead to reduced adherence with prescribed medications for general medical problems.

Because of its necessary use of technical medical language, this chapter is likely to be most relevant to clinical nurse specialists and junior medical personnel. It is beyond the scope of this book to go into great detail on physical examination. However, those interested in pursuing the matter further are advised to consult one of a number of excellent books on the subject (e.g. Talley & O'Connor 2005). For a shorter treatment of the subject, consult the brief article on physical examination in psychiatric practice by Garden (2005).

MEDICAL HISTORY

Much of the medical history, including past surgical and obstetric and gynaecological history, should be available from the person themselves and from records of the person's general practitioner (GP). However, it is worth running through a short list of general medical problems that are directly relevant to mental health. These include: hypertension, hypercholesterolaemia, atrial fibrillation, diabetes, myocardial infarction (heart attack), transient ischaemic attack (TIA), stroke, seizures, falls, head injury, syncope, other episodes of loss of consciousness, and surgical procedures involving cardiopulmonary bypass and general anaesthesia.

In older people certain 'geriatric syndromes' are common precipitants of medical presentations. These include confusion, falls and incontinence. These are not disease entities in themselves, but rather the final common pathways for a large number of disease states. Thus, the clinician must think broadly when confronted with one of these common syndromes.

There is a strong interaction between mental and physical health problems in that people with chronic physical health problems are more likely to develop mental health problems, and vice versa. For example, chronic physical ill health is a powerful predictor of both depression and anxiety symptoms in older people. In addition, certain acute medical conditions are commonly associated with depression. These include stroke and acute coronary syndrome. In addition, when older people with mental health problems are treated with psychotropic medication, this medication can lead to physical health problems. An example of this is drug-induced Parkinsonism, which can present as either falls or incontinence. Falls occur because of impaired gait and 'incontinence' because the older person cannot get to the toilet in time.

PERSONNEL INVOLVED IN THE PHYSICAL EXAMINATION

A general physical examination is an important component of the work-up of older people suspected of having a mental health problem. Ideally, the person's GP should carry this out prior to the person's referral to the OPMHS, or should accompany the mental health workers to the person's residence, but sometimes this is not feasible. As a consequence, staff of the OPMHS must either be able to undertake a general physical examination themselves or have access to an outside medical practitioner who is able to do one. Although GPs have a long history of performing brief physical examinations in people's homes, these seem to happen less commonly nowadays. If the OPMHS does not have its own medical personnel to undertake such examinations on home visits, consideration should be given to arranging for the older person to attend the GP's office or the local hospital outpatients department or emergency department for a physical examination. The person's case manager or the mental health workers doing the initial assessment may need to accompany the person to the doctor to request a physical examination. This is often also a suitable opportunity for blood to be drawn for screening laboratory tests and for an electrocardiogram to be performed (see below).

In better resourced OPMHS, the initial assessment can be done by two mental health workers, one of whom should be a medical officer who can undertake a screening physical examination. In some settings, experienced registered nurses carry out screening physical examinations. A screening physical examination should be informed by the history obtained from the older person and other informants, and what is already known about the person's general health. However, at a minimum, it is important to examine the person's level of consciousness, general appearance, vital signs (temperature, pulse rate, blood pressure, respiratory rate), eyesight, hearing, gait, speech, and cardiorespiratory and neurological status. All of these can be roughly assessed without having the person completely disrobe and most can be assessed with the person seated in a chair. Most mental health services now use a physical examination template to provide structure to screening examinations.

EQUIPMENT NEEDED FOR THE PHYSICAL EXAMINATION

Basic equipment needed for a physical examination includes:
- a thermometer
- a sphygmomanometer
- a stethoscope
- a watch with a sweep hand
- a tendon hammer
- a Snellen chart

- a tape measure
- a small torch
- urinalysis strips, and
- portable scales.

Additional equipment may include:

- an ophthalmoscope
- an auroscope
- a tuning fork (256 Hz)
- disposable tongue depressors
- disposable gloves
- a pulse oximeter
- a portable electrocardiogram (ECG) machine, and
- an alcometer.

FACTORS TO BE CONSIDERED IN THE PHYSICAL EXAMINATION

Consent

At common law, a physical examination without consent could constitute assault. Thus, the mental health worker should obtain the consent of the person, or their substitute decision maker, before undertaking a physical examination. This is particularly so when planning to do a physical examination during a domiciliary visit, as consent under these circumstances should not be assumed. When a substitute decision maker has given consent, the examiner should still attempt to obtain the person's assent.

Chaperone

It is generally prudent to have a chaperone present for all but the most superficial physical examinations. This advice holds true for female as well as male examiners and for male as well as female people who are being examined. The chaperone can assist with positioning the person and maintaining their dignity and privacy during the examination. The chaperone can also help minimise the risk of physical assault on the examiner in the case of an agitated, delusional or manic person, and can act as a witness to proceedings for the protection of both the person and the examiner.

Safety

The mental health worker should be alert to factors that might compromise their own safety and that of the older person, particularly when undertaking physical examinations on domiciliary visits with unfamiliar people. Sometimes, discretion is the better part of valour and the physical examination should be put off until another day. See also Chapter 18.

Evidence of elder abuse

The physical examination provides an opportunity to observe signs of physical abuse or neglect, which may be present if the older person has been the victim of domestic violence or some other type of physical abuse or neglect. Bruises of differing ages are a pointer to elder abuse just as they are to child abuse. Neglect may lead to chronic under-nutrition with weight loss and vitamin deficiencies.

Evidence of substance use

Some older people abuse alcohol over a long period and develop the normal sequelae of this. Some older people use illicit drugs, including amphetamines and cannabis. See also Chapter 24.

Level of consciousness

Assess whether the older person is fully conscious and alert or whether they exhibit a reduced level of consciousness. Reduced consciousness starts with clouding of consciousness (reduced awareness) and ends with coma and death. If the level of consciousness appears reduced, the Glasgow Coma Scale (GCS) (Teasdale & Jennett 1974) can be used to document the extent of conscious impairment. Reduced level of consciousness is often a medical emergency, requiring immediate action by the mental health worker.

General appearance

Assess the following:
- cachexia or obesity
- clothing (Is clothing appropriate for the climate? Are there any unusual features, such as clothes on back to front, too many layers, street clothes on over pyjamas in warm weather, or insufficient clothing in very cold weather?)
- personal hygiene (e.g. hair, nails and general dishevelment)
- dentition
- foot care, and
- height and weight.

Eyesight

Test each eye separately with the other eye covered using a Snellen chart (at 6 metres) or mini-Snellen chart (various distances, depending upon the font of the letters on the chart) for an estimate of visual acuity. The person should wear their usual spectacles during testing. If a Snellen chart is not available, ask the older person to read from a magazine or a newspaper, or ask the person to read the labels on their medicine bottles. Refer people with previously undiagnosed visual impairment for formal testing. Inquire about navigational difficulties that might be due to visual field defects.

Hearing

Whisper into each ear with the other ear covered by a hand for an estimate of hearing acuity. The person should wear their usual hearing aids during testing. Refer people with previously undiagnosed hearing impairment for formal testing.

Speech and language

Engage the older person in conversation and note any abnormalities of speech or language. Common abnormalities include dysarthria (slurred speech, which is often due to stroke or intoxication) and dysphasia (reduced ability to generate speech or understand speech, which may be expressive or receptive dysphasia, and is often due to stroke or dementia). A less common problem is dysprosody (loss of the musical quality or rhythm of speech, which is often due to stroke, head injury or Parkinson's disease). Dysprosody sometimes gives the clinician the impression that the person is speaking with a foreign accent. Other types of speech and language disorders are associated with longstanding mental illness, including the formal thought disorder associated with early-onset schizophrenia (see Ch 13).

Posture and gait

Note the seated posture of the older person. Ask the person to stand up, walk several metres, turn around, walk back and resume their seat. Look for abnormal seated posture, which might be due, for instance, to pain or discomfort, arthritis or other skeletal abnormality, stroke, Parkinson's disease or other neurological abnormality, or voluntary adoption of an abnormal posture. Look for abnormal gait, such as the shuffling gait, festination (shortening of stride and quickening of gait) and the absent arm swing of Parkinson's disease, the small stepping gait associated with deep white matter ischaemic changes in the brain, or the choreoathetoid movements and the so-called 'dancing gait' of Huntington's disease. The 'get up and go test' is also a straightforward test of locomotion.

Neurological examination

There may be clues to a neurological problem from the older person's speech and language function and their posture and gait. However, a more detailed neurological screening examination is warranted in all first presentations of mental health problems, including dementia, in later life.

The twelve cranial nerves can be screened quite simply and efficiently, as follows:

I	Ask the person about their sense of smell.
II	Test the person's eyesight with a Snellen chart.
III, IV and VI	Test the person's eye movements.
V	Test facial sensation by soft touch.
VII	Ask the person to smile and close their eyes tightly.
VIII	Test hearing and balance (ask them to heel–toe walk or stand on one leg).
IX and X	Ask the person to speak, to swallow, to say 'Ah' (look at their soft palate) and test their gag reflex with a tongue depressor.
XI	Ask the person to shrug their shoulders and turn their head.
XII	Ask the person to poke out their tongue.

The pyramidal tract can be screened by testing:

- the power in both arms and legs by asking the person to move them against resistance (this can be estimated even if the person is seated)
- the tone in both arms by moving them passively, and
- the deep tendon reflexes in both arms (triceps, biceps and supinator) and in both legs (patellar and, if possible, the Achilles tendon).

The extrapyramidal tract can be screened as follows:

- Use the finger–nose–finger test. Touch the person's index finger and ask them to touch the tip of their nose with their index finger, and then touch your index finger. Ask them to do this several times.

- Test for dysdiadochokinesia. Demonstrate this action for the person and ask them to copy it: tap the back of one hand with the palm of the other hand, and then with the back of the other hand; rapidly alternate between the front and back of the hand; repeat with the other hand.

Cardiorespiratory examination

This examination should include:
- vital signs (see above)
- colour (anaemia or cyanosis)
- finger clubbing and splinter haemorrhages
- peripheral oedema
- cough and audible wheeze
- nasal flaring and use of accessory muscles of respiration
- jugular venous pressure (JVP); the person needs to be lying at 45°
- apex beat, parasternal heave and thrills
- heart sounds and murmurs
- tracheal position
- chest movements with respiration
- percussion of lung fields and vocal fremitus, and
- breath sounds, crackles and wheezes, and vocal resonance.

Gastrointestinal examination

Look for:
- jaundice and anaemia
- spider naevi, and
- needle tracks.

The abdominal examination component of the gastrointestinal examination is difficult to complete during a domiciliary visit unless the situation allows the person to lie flat and remove at least some clothing. For the abdominal examination:
- observe the skin and sclerae for jaundice
- observe the abdomen for abnormal masses, particularly an enlarged liver
- observe for signs of portal venous congestion (caput medusae)
- percuss flanks for ascites (shifting dullness)
- palpate liver (with the person lying supine) and spleen (roll the person towards the examiner), and
- palpate for other masses.

A rectal examination is important in older people with a recent change in mental state, but it is sometimes difficult to achieve during a domiciliary visit.

Other components of the physical examination

Examination of other systems, including the musculoskeletal, endocrine and genitourinary systems may be challenging during a mental health domiciliary visit and is usually best left to those more expert, including the person's GP. However, urinalysis by dipstick is always worth doing in older people, as urinary tract infections are a common cause of mental state abnormalities.

REASONS WHY PHYSICAL EXAMINATIONS ARE SOMETIMES NOT DONE

Mental health workers sometimes feel incompetent to do physical examinations. If this is the case, the worker should obtain additional training and supervision or hand the task over to someone else. Other reasons why a physical examination may not be done include:

- insufficient time has been allocated (this is a logistical issue that needs to be resolved at team level)
- no suitable chaperone is available (this is a logistical issue that needs to be resolved at team level)
- the person does not provide consent (in this case, postpone the physical examination until consent is provided by the person or a substitute decision maker)
- the person is thought to be potentially assaultative (postpone the physical examination until the safety issue has resolved), and
- the worker did not bring the right equipment (this situation should be avoided by always carrying a physical examination kit on domiciliary visits).

MEDICATION REVIEW

The home visit provides an ideal opportunity to review the older person's use of medication, including prescribed drugs, over-the-counter (OTC) drugs and complementary substances. By taking into account the date of dispensing, it is often possible to estimate adherence to prescription medicine. It is preferable to ask the person and/or their carer to bring out their medication, whether it is in its original packaging or in a Dosette® box or Webster Pak®, to be examined. Not infrequently, the home visit will reveal inconsistencies between the list of medications in the GP's records or in hospital records and the medication actually being taken. As some OTC (e.g. pseudoephedrine) and complementary medications (e.g. St John's wort) have the potential to cause drug–drug interactions, it is important that these are audited as well.

LABORATORY INVESTIGATIONS

Laboratory investigations in older people presenting with mental health problems often reveal unsuspected abnormalities, including anaemia, hyponatraemia and vitamin deficiencies (especially vitamin B12, folate and vitamin D). Sometimes, these abnormalities reflect the cause of a change in mental state (e.g. severe hyponatraemia causing delirium), but more often they reflect the result of a change in mental state (e.g. low red cell folate due to dietary deficiency or low vitamin D due to lack of exposure to sunlight).

Routine blood tests (see Table 15.1) are often indicated in older people who have not recently had these done or in whom there has been a recent change in mental state or behaviour. After starting new treatment with psychotropic medication, targeted blood tests, and sometimes other investigations, are often indicated. Testing for syphilis and HIV is not usually undertaken unless risk factors are present. Specific consent and pre-testing counselling is required for these latter tests.

Table 15.1 Common laboratory tests used in screening older people		
Name of Test	Common Abbreviation	Condition Screened
Full blood examination	FBE or FBC	Anaemia
Electrolytes	E/LFT	Electrolyte abnormality
Urea and creatinine	U&E or E/LFT	Renal function
Liver function tests	LFT or E/LFT	Liver function
Glucose	BSL	Diabetes
Thyroid stimulating hormone	TSH	Hypothyroidism
Vitamin B12	Vit B12	Vitamin B12 deficiency
Red cell folate	RBC folate	Folate deficiency
Vitamin D	Vit D	Vitamin D deficiency
C-reactive protein	CRP	Inflammation

NEUROIMAGING

There is divided opinion about the role of neuroimaging in community OPMHS. Neuro-imaging in this context commonly means computed tomographic (CT) brain scans. CT brain scans use X-rays to provide structural information about the brain. They may be used with or without the administration of intravenous contrast material. CT brain scans are useful for providing an estimate of brain atrophy, for assessing the extent of cerebrovascular disease (including stroke and deep white matter ischaemic changes), and for excluding uncommon conditions such as brain haemorrhages, brain tumours and normal pressure hydrocephalus. CT brain scans are relatively inexpensive and widely available. However, like any X-ray procedure, they do expose the person to ionising radiation, which is a risk factor for cancer.

Less commonly used neuroimaging modalities include magnetic resonance imaging (MRI) brain scans and single photon emission computed tomographic (SPECT) brain scans. Because of their limited availability and expense, positron emission tomographic (PET) brain scans are rarely used in this context.

MRI brain scans do not involve ionising radiation and do provide better structural resolution than CT brain scans, but at present are more expensive and have several other significant limitations. MRI brain scans involve placing the person's head in the narrow tunnel of a powerful magnet and some people with claustrophobia are unable to tolerate this without sedation. In addition, the MRI brain scan commonly generates a rather loud tapping or knocking noise during some scanning sequences that can alarm or distress some people. Most importantly of all, many people with ferromagnetic metal in their bodies are unable to undergo an MRI scan for safety reasons. For instance, people with cardiac pacemakers, cochlear implants or vascular clips, and some people who have worked in occupations that involve metal grinding, are not able to have an MRI scan. Nevertheless, MRI scans produce better pictures than CT scans and are better than CT scans at picking up lesions involving the white matter (or 'wiring') of the brain, which are common in older people.

SPECT and PET brain scans provide information about the function of the brain. Their spatial resolution is considerably less than that provided by CT and MRI brain scans, and so SPECT and PET scans are usually only used in conjunction with a CT or MRI structural brain scan. Both SPECT and PET involve the injection of a radioactive tracer called a radioligand. This radioligand travels through the bloodstream to the brain and labels brain tissue. In the common situation the radioligand is fluorodeoxyglucose (FDG) and the brain images obtained reflect regional cerebral blood flow. Thus, through the use of SPECT or PET brain scans, the blood flow and function of various parts of the brain can be imaged. New PET imaging techniques allow certain components of the brain to be imaged. For example, a radioligand called Pittsburgh Compound B (PIB) causes the amyloid plaques in Alzheimer's disease to light up. PIB has the potential to enable presymptomatic identification of Alzheimer's disease. This might be important once effective preventive interventions for Alzheimer's disease have been identified, but for the time being it is mainly a research tool.

It is important to note that both structural and functional brain scans have significant limitations. In particular, an apparently normal CT or MRI brain scan does not exclude the dementia syndrome. Many younger people (aged 55–75 years) with dementia of mild to moderate severity have brain scans that are reported as normal.

ELECTROCARDIOGRAM

The electrocardiogram (ECG) measures the electrical activity of the heart via chest electrodes. It is useful to obtain an ECG in people being assessed for the first time, in people in whom an unexpected change in mental state has occurred, and in people about to be commenced on psychotropic medication. Sometimes, a change in mental state is the only symptom of an acute myocardial infarction or of an acute or recurrent cardiac arrhythmia. The person's GP or the GP's practice nurse should be able to do an ECG without delay. Alternatively, most general hospitals are able to undertake outpatient ECGs at short notice. Ultimately, it is hoped that more OPMHS personnel will obtain the training and equipment to enable them to do their own ECGs during domiciliary visits, as small, portable ECG machines become more widely available.

ELECTROENCEPHALOGRAM

The electroencephalogram (EEG) measures the electrical activity of the brain via scalp electrodes. It is a useful investigation if either delirium or epilepsy is suspected. However, there is no indication for the routine use of EEGs in the work-up of older people suspected of having a mental health problem.

NEUROPSYCHOLOGICAL TESTING

Most older people with mental health problems, including dementia, do not require formal testing by a neuropsychologist. However, neuropsychological testing can be very useful in certain specific situations. For instance, the pattern of deficits in people with less common types of dementia (e.g. frontotemporal dementia) can often be clarified by neuropsychological testing. When neuropsychological testing is undertaken, it is important that frontal executive function is tested as well as general verbal and non-verbal intellectual abilities, as frontal executive dysfunction is often relatively silent on standard brief cognitive assessments such as the Mini-Mental State Examination (MMSE) (Folstein et al 1975). Formal neuropsychological testing by an accredited neuropsychologist generally takes at least 4 hours (and often longer), is relatively expensive and is often not available outside of larger cities. Hence, it is generally reserved for cases of serious diagnostic uncertainty or cases in which forensic or other medicolegal issues have arisen.

COMMON GENERAL MEDICAL CONDITIONS

In this section we summarise some of the common general medical conditions found in older people. The material we present here is intended only as a guide to these mental health problems and not as treatment recommendations. The safe and effective management of general medical health problems seen in people being managed by an OPMHS requires detailed knowledge and clinical experience.

Hypertension

Hypertension, or high blood pressure, is a major risk factor for cerebrovascular disease (stroke, transient ischaemic attacks (TIA) and deep white matter ischaemia) and cardiovascular disease (angina pectoris, acute myocardial infarction and heart failure). Longstanding hypertension contributes to atherosclerosis, or 'hardening of the arteries', and kidney and eye disease. Fortunately, hypertension is easy to detect and relatively easy to treat in most people. While normal blood pressure can be up to 140/90 mmHg, epidemiological studies have demonstrated mortality and morbidity advantages down to a blood pressure of 115/75 mmHg.

Although there is some debate about how aggressively to manage hypertension in very old people (aged 80 years and older), it is generally considered appropriate to assiduously detect and treat hypertension in people under the age of 80 years. However, for otherwise well people aged 80 years and over, there is also likely to be benefit from good blood pressure control (Beckett et al 2008). A wide variety of medications are available to treat hypertension and people sometimes need to undergo several treatment trials before the ideal antihypertensive medication, or combination of medications, is found for them. Lifestyle interventions for hypertension include regular aerobic exercise (at least 30 minutes per day on most days), smoking cessation, weight reduction (each kilogram of weight reduction is associated with a 1 mmHg reduction in systolic blood pressure), and reduction in salt intake. Medications commonly used to treat hypertension include angiotensin converting enzyme (ACE) inhibitors, angiotensin II receptor antagonists, calcium channel blockers, diuretics and beta-blockers.

Hyperlipidaemia

Elevated lipids (cholesterol and triglycerides) are risk factors for cardiovascular disease, stroke and peripheral vascular disease. Levels of total blood cholesterol over 5.5 mmol/L are associated with increased risk. High cholesterol can be managed through diet, exercise and weight loss, and with drugs that are referred to as 'statins' (HMG–CoA reductase inhibitors). Although people taking statins have occasionally reported memory decline, current opinion is that there is no causal relationship between the two. It is important to note that many older people taking statins are people who already have vascular risk factors or a history of cerebrovascular disease and would be prone to memory impairment anyway. The statins are a highly effective class of medication for reducing elevated cholesterol.

Atrial fibrillation

Atrial fibrillation (AF) is the commonest cardiac arrhythmia in older people and is responsible for about one-third of all strokes. It also complicates ischaemic heart disease and contributes to heart failure. It can be treated in many cases by pharmacological or electrical cardioversion, and in some cases by radiofrequency ablation, usually by catheter. If this approach is ineffective, medication can be prescribed to slow the heart rate. In chronic AF, the risk of stroke can be reduced through the use of the anticoagulant warfarin or with aspirin, although aspirin is much less effective than warfarin for this purpose.

Acute myocardial infarction

Acute myocardial infarction (AMI) or 'heart attack' remains a common cause of death and disability among older people. It is frequently associated with depression and anxiety. AMI is caused by occlusion of one or more branches of the coronary arteries. This generally occurs against a background of narrowing of the coronary arteries, which has built up over many years. Sometimes, AMI is preceded by angina pectoris, which commonly manifests as chest pain on exertion, that resolves with rest or with sublingual nitrates. Although AMI classically presents with central crushing chest pain that radiates into the neck, jaw or left arm, in some older people AMI presents without chest pain but with an altered mental state. Prevention involves managing risk factors, including smoking, hypertension, hyperlipidaemia, diabetes, sedentary lifestyle and obesity.

Initial treatment of AMI is a specialised field and beyond the scope of this book. However, most older people who have suffered an AMI are managed initially in a coronary care unit (CCU) or a monitored ward bed. Following the acute phase of treatment, they are discharged home for an extended period of cardiac rehabilitation, which has physical and psychological components. People who have recently suffered an AMI are commonly commenced on maintenance treatment with aspirin and a beta-blocker. Other cardiovascular risk factors (especially hypertension and elevated cholesterol) are aggressively managed with medication. Smoking cessation is mandatory. AMI is commonly complicated by depression, and research has demonstrated that some of this comes on before the AMI and some comes on afterwards. AMI complicated by depression has a worse prognosis than AMI not complicated by depression. Treatment with selective serotonin reuptake inhibitor (SSRI) antidepressants is indicated in AMI complicated by major depression.

Stroke

Stroke (cerebrovascular accident or CVA) is a common cause of death and disability in older people and may be due to thromboembolism or to haemorrhage. More than 85% of all strokes are caused by thromboembolism. Several types of cerebrovascular disease, including stroke, are associated with dementia. Stroke is an important issue for mental health workers as there is an increased risk of stroke and death in older people taking antipsychotic medication. Many small strokes are asymptomatic, but over time the damage they cause contributes to cognitive impairment and then dementia. Subcortical cerebrovascular disease may lead to cognitive impairment and gait disorder, sometimes mimicking Parkinson's disease. It is important that mental health workers understand the usual risk factors for stroke, which include increasing age, cigarette smoking, hypertension, high cholesterol, diabetes, heavy alcohol intake, AF, and other heart or vascular disease. Medications taken to prevent stroke in people at high risk include aspirin, clopidogrel, dipyridamole and warfarin.

Diabetes mellitus (type 2)

Most older people with diabetes mellitus have type 2 diabetes. Type 2 diabetes is caused by insulin deficiency or insulin resistance and becomes more prevalent in later life. The main modifiable risk factors for this type of diabetes are overweight/obesity and sedentary lifestyle. Many older people with type 2 diabetes ultimately require treatment with insulin. The 1999–2000 Australian national diabetes survey, during which participants had their blood glucose level measured, found that approximately 850,000 Australians aged 25 years and over had type 2 diabetes (Australian Institute of Health and Welfare 2008). However, the prevalence of type 2 diabetes is estimated to be about three times higher in Indigenous than in non-Indigenous Australians. Similar patterns are found in Maori and Pacific Islander peoples. Type 2 diabetes is frequently complicated by cardiovascular disease, cerebrovascular disease, diabetic neuropathy, renal impairment and visual impairment. It sometimes leads to gangrene, necessitating lower limb amputations (Australian Institute of Health and Welfare 2008).

Osteoarthritis

Osteoarthritis (OA) is the commonest cause of disability after depression and dementia. It is quite uncommon before the age of 45 years and mainly affects people aged 65 years and over (Australian Institute of Health and Welfare 2007). It is estimated to affect around 7% of the Australian population and to affect more women than men. OA causes pain, stiffness and reduced movement of the affected joints. The hips, knees, hands, feet, spine and neck are the most commonly affected sites. Risk factors include injury to the joint, being overweight or obese, and certain types of repetitive use of the joints, such as squatting and heavy lifting (e.g. in the farming and construction industries). However, normal physical exercise is not a risk factor. Indigenous Australians have a lower prevalence of OA than non-Indigenous Australians. Management includes medication, exercise, physiotherapy, weight loss, mechanical aids and joint replacement surgery. Medication includes paracetamol and the non-steroidal anti-inflammatory drugs (NSAIDs). The dietary supplements glucosamine, chondroitin and omega-3 fatty acids are commonly used by people with OA. Joint replacement surgery for severe OA of the hip or knee is now considered a highly effective intervention.

Osteoporosis

Osteoporosis is a disease that most commonly affects people over the age of 55 years, more commonly women. Osteoporosis leads to reduced bone density, reduced bone strength and an increased risk of fractures with minimal trauma. Sites of osteoporotic fractures include the hip, wrist and spine. Known risk factors for osteoporosis include family history, low calcium intake, low vitamin D levels, smoking, excessive alcohol consumption, low body mass index (BMI), sedentary lifestyle, low oestrogen levels and long-term corticosteroid use. Osteoporosis is usually asymptomatic until a fracture occurs. The management of osteoporosis includes medication to promote bone formation and to reduce absorption of minerals from the bones. Commonly prescribed medications include calcium supplements, vitamin D and bisphosphonates. However, it is also important to promote regular weight-bearing exercise and to reduce the risk of falls by improving balance.

Parkinson's disease

Parkinson's disease (PD) is a progressive neurodegenerative disorder of unknown cause. PD leads to motor symptoms including flexed posture, reduced arm swing, shuffling gait and reduced facial expression. PD also leads to neuropsychiatric symptoms, including anxiety, depression and dementia. Both genetic and environmental factors are thought to be important in its aetiology. Treatment with dopamine agonists is generally quite effective early in the course of the disease, although it often ultimately leads to dyskinetic movements.

Gastro-oesophageal reflux disorder

Gastro-oesophageal reflux disorder (GORD) is highly prevalent among the citizens of developed nations and obesity is a risk factor. In Australia, the prevalence of frequent heartburn likely to reflect GORD has been estimated at 12% (Watson & Lally 2009). In the same study, an even greater proportion of the population (17%) reported taking medication for reflux symptoms, most commonly proton-pump inhibitors such as omeprazole. Frequent acid reflux can lead to oesophagitis and several more serious complications. Reflux is a common cause of dysphagia and can precipitate asthma.

Cancer

The term cancer is somewhat of a misnomer as it leads some to think that cancer is one condition that simply affects different organ systems in the body. In fact, the nature and prognosis of the many different neoplastic conditions that are collectively known as cancer vary enormously. Some, like basal cell carcinoma (BCC) of the skin, are relatively straightforward to treat, while others, like adenocarcinoma of the prostate in advanced old age, do not often cause death. Excluding BCC and squamous cell carcinoma (SCC) of the skin, the most common cancers in males are prostate cancer, bowel cancer, melanoma, lung cancer and lymphoma. In females, the most common cancers are breast cancer, bowel cancer, melanoma, lung cancer and lymphoma. Most types of cancer are more common in older people. The nature and treatment of cancer is a specialised subject that is beyond the scope of this book. However, it is worth noting that mental health workers sometimes need to work in collaboration with cancer care teams and with palliative care workers to provide optimal care.

SUMMARY

This chapter has summarised the physical assessment of the older person and outlined some of the common general medical health problems experienced in later life.

REFERENCES

Australian Institute of Health and Welfare (AIHW) 2007 A picture of osteoarthritis in Australia. Arthritis Series No. 5. AIHW Cat. No. PHE 93. AIHW, Canberra. Online. Available: www.aihw. gov.au/publications/phe/apooia/apooia.pdf 16 Jan 2009

Australian Institute of Health and Welfare (AIHW) 2008 Diabetes: Australian facts 2008. Diabetes Series No. 8. AIHW Cat. No. CVD 40. AIHW, Canberra. Online. Available: www.aihw.gov.au/ publications/cvd/daf08/daf08.pdf 16 Jan 2009

Beckett NS, Peters R, Fletcher AE et al 2008 Treatment of hypertension in patients 80 years of age or older. New England Journal of Medicine 358:1887–1898

Folstein MF, Folstein SE, McHugh PR 1975 Mini-Mental State: a practical method for grading the cognitive state of patients for the clinician. Journal of Psychiatric Research 12:189–198

Garden G 2005 Physical examination in psychiatric practice. Advances in Psychiatric Treatment 11:142–149

Talley NJ, O'Connor S 2005 Clinical examination, 5th edn. Churchill Livingstone, Sydney

Teasdale G, Jennett B 1974 Assessment of coma and impaired consciousness. A practical scale. Lancet 2(7872):82–84

Watson DI, Lally CJ 2009 Prevalence of symptoms and use of medication for gastroesophageal reflux in an Australian community. World Journal of Surgery 33:88–94

Chapter 16

FUNCTIONAL ASSESSMENT

INTRODUCTION

When an older person becomes mentally impaired, their ability to self-care is an area that usually becomes compromised. It is what a person cannot do that often concerns older people and their carers. Therefore, assessment of an older person should include their functional ability. The presence of functional impairment can have serious consequences. For example, if a person is unable to shop and cook, or even feed themselves, their nutritional health status can be severely compromised, which in turn affects the functioning of other body systems. The treatment plan and decisions are also heavily influenced by a person's functional ability.

FUNCTIONAL ASSESSMENT

Functional assessment is defined as:

> … a method for describing abilities and activities in order to measure an individual's use of the variety of skills included in performing the tasks necessary to daily living, vocational pursuits, social interactions, leisure activities, and other required behaviours (Granger 1984, cited in Dittmar 1997).

In order for an older person to undertake such tasks, they must be able to think in a logical manner, be oriented to time, place and person, be able to organise themselves physically and mentally, and have an understanding of the impact of the task on themselves and other people. For example, a person may be able to organise themselves to catch a bus, but it defeats the purpose if there is no bus to catch and they get angry at others because there is no bus.

Functional decline in older people may be due to single or multiple factors. It can involve cognitive, emotional, physiological or anatomical structure or function. The decline may be temporary, permanent or progressive (Dittmar 1997). In older people with dementia, for example, their functioning could be impaired because of cognitive impairment and the decline will be progressive and permanent. Conversely, an older person with severe depression may be functionally declined because of apathy or withdrawal. In this situation, their functional status might be temporary because once they receive treatment for the depression, their functioning could improve. Indeed, functional ability is an outcome measure for the effectiveness of treatment and also an important determinant for permanent placement in a residential aged care facility (Burns et al 2004).

ACTIVITIES OF DAILY LIVING AND INSTRUMENTAL ACTIVITIES OF DAILY LIVING

At a basic level, assessment of a person's functional ability involves activities of daily living (ADLs) and instrumental activities of daily living (IADLs). ADLs are basic self-care and self-maintenance skills. These include bathing, toileting, dressing, walking and the ability to transfer, for example, from a chair to a bed. IADLs are more complex, multi-faceted tasks that require a reasonable amount of planning and organising. These skills enable the older person to function independently in the community, and include using the telephone, handling finances, using public transport and shopping (see Table 16.1).

Additionally, this information is important as an indicator of whether or not an older person's health status is improving or declining and if treatment is effective. It also greatly assists in determining the management of the functional disability and the level of support the older person and/or carer may need. Fortunately, simple, reliable and useful tools for measuring functional ability are available. These tools assist with accurate assessment and the development of more precise interventions to organise and focus rehabilitative efforts. Examples of each of these scales are discussed below.

The Activities of Daily Living Scale

The Activities of Daily Living Scale (Katz et al 1963) is an extensively used scale for evaluating levels of severe physical disability, relevant mainly to people who are living in institutions and to older people. It is conceptually based on the biological model of human development, with the most complex functions being lost first. The six activities included in the index were found to lie in a hierarchical order. Katz further noted that, during rehabilitation, skills are regained in order of ascending complexity, in the same order that infants initially acquire them. These activities represent landmarks in the normal development of self-care.

Table 16.1 Important activities of daily living (ADL) and instrumental activities of daily living (IADL) skills	
ADLs (Harris et al 1996)	**IADLs (Lawton 1988)**
Walking inside	Using the telephone
Bed-to-chair transfers	Shopping
Getting on and off the toilet	Food preparation
Putting on and taking off shoes and socks	Housekeeping
Bathing	Laundry
Dressing	Mode of transportation
Continence (bladder and bowel)	Medication management
Eating	Handling finances
Mobility	

Through observation and interview, each activity is assessed on a 3-point rating scale of the person's ability to perform six activities (bathing, dressing, toileting, transferring, continence, feeding) unaided. The activities are rated as: (1) can be performed independently; (2) needs some assistance; or (3) needs total assistance or cannot do the activity. Reliability testing was good (Brorsson & Asberg 1984, cited in McDowell & Newell 1996).

The Barthel Index

The Barthel Index is probably the most commonly used ADL assessment scale (Mahoney & Barthel 1965). An informant such as a mental health worker assesses functional independence in personal care and mobility. The Barthel Index takes about 5 minutes to complete and is a valid and reliable scale. There are at least five versions of the Barthel Index available, so it is important to be aware of which one is in use. The original version consists of 10 items measuring:

1. feeding
2. moving from chair to bed (sitting up in bed) and return
3. personal grooming (face, teeth, hair, shaving)
4. getting on and off the toilet (attending to clothes, wiping and flushing)
5. bathing
6. walking on a level surface or propelling a wheelchair
7. going up and down stairs
8. dressing (shoe laces and zips)
9. bladder continence, and
10. bowel continence.

There is a scoring manual to accompany the scale. Scores range from 0 to 100, in steps of 5, with higher scores indicating greater independence. Even though an older person may score 100, this does not necessarily mean that they are independent because they may not be able to cook, clean or go out by themselves (McDowell & Newell 1996).

The Instrumental Activities of Daily Living Scale

The Instrumental Activities of Daily Living Scale is an extension of the ADL concept, allowing consideration to be given to problems more typically experienced by older people living in the community, such as mobility, difficulty in shopping, cooking or managing money. The movement towards community care for older people stimulated the development of functional assessment scales (McDowell & Newell 1996).

The Instrumental Activities of Daily Living Scale (Lawton 1988) assesses the functional ability of older people to perform activities that are of central importance in their everyday lives. These behaviours are among the most necessary for life preservation, but are the most likely to fail in the face of physical or mental health problems. Behaviours are categorised according to a hierarchy of complexity, in the sense of an increasing involvement of different systems of person and environment. The eight functions assessed include the ability to: use the telephone; shop; prepare food; do housekeeping; do laundry; travel; take medications; and handle finances at that point in time. The scale uses a 1–5-point rating scale measuring full ability to no ability. The score is summed with a higher score indicating a greater level of dependency. It has strong interrater and test–retest reliability (Lawton 1988).

AN OCCUPATIONAL THERAPY ASSESSMENT

A highly specialised, in-depth functional assessment can be undertaken by a qualified occupational therapist. In this context, the term 'occupation' encompasses more than vocation or employment, and refers to involvement in tasks that allow meaningful use of time and assumption of life roles (Fisher 1998, cited in Farhall et al 2007). To conduct an assessment, an occupational therapist will use one or a combination of the following strategies: interviewing; self-report questionnaires and rating scales; and performance-based assessments. Assessment information is obtained from the older person, family or significant others, and healthcare workers.

The purpose of the assessment (e.g. socialisation or falls) and where it is being undertaken (e.g. home or hospital) will influence the type of information gathered and what it will be used for. Generally, the type of information obtained can include occupational history, current occupational roles, activities that are associated with these roles and their meanings. How an older person uses their time is determined by detailing patterns and routines. Strengths and difficulties in regard to role performance are identified. An assessment is also made of the resources and supports that are available at home, within the local community or any other relevant places. Finally, desired roles, potential activities and skills necessary for participation in them are explored with the older person or the informant (Bland et al 2007).

SUMMARY

This chapter has discussed the important role functional assessment plays in the mental healthcare of older people. Loss of functional ability is a key indicator of some sort of pathology. The two main areas assessed are ADLs and IADLs. There are a number of tools available to assist in functional assessment and three commonly used tools were discussed in detail. The presence or absence of ADLs and IADLs helps to monitor health status and treatment effectiveness. Precise assessment pinpoints specific areas for attention and where additional support may be needed for the older person and most probably their family carer as well.

FURTHER READING

McDowell I 2006 Measuring health: a guide to rating scales and questionnaires. Oxford University Press, New York

USEFUL WEBSITE

Guidelines to minimise functional decline in older people: www.health.vic.gov.au/acute-agedcare/functional-decline-manual.pdf

REFERENCES

Bland R, Farhall J, Fossey E et al 2007 Specialised assessment skills. In: Meadows G, Singh B, Grigg M (eds) Mental health in Australia: collaborative community practice. Oxford University Press, Melbourne

Burns A, Lawlor B, Craig S 2004 Assessment scales in old age psychiatry. Martin Dunitz, London

Dittmar SS 1997 Overview: a functional approach to measurement of rehabilitation outcomes. In: Dittmar SS, Gresham GE (ed) Functional assessment and outcome measures for the rehabilitation health professional. Aspen Publishers, Maryland

Farhall J, Fossey E, Keeble-Devlin B et al 2007 Conceptual models used in mental health practice. In: Meadows G, Singh B, Grigg M (eds) Mental health in Australia: collaborative community practice. Oxford University Press, Melbourne

Harris BA, Jette AM, Campion EW, Cleary PD 1996 Validity of self-report measures of functional disability. Topics in Geriatric Rehabilitation 1(3):31–41

Katz S, Ford AB, Moskowitz RW et al 1963 Studies of illness in the aged: the index of ADL: a standardized measure of biological and psychosocial function. Journal of the American Medical Association 185(12):914–919

Lawton MP 1988 Instrumental activities of daily living (IADL) scale: original observer-rater version. Psychopharmacological Bulletin 24(4):785–787

Mahoney FI, Barthel DW 1965 Functional evaluation: the BARTHEL Index. Maryland State Medical Journal 14:61–65

McDowell I, Newell C 1996 Measuring health: a guide to rating scales and questionnaires. Oxford University Press, Oxford

Chapter 17

PSYCHOSOCIAL AND SPIRITUAL ASSESSMENT

INTRODUCTION

Psychosocial and spiritual assessments are addressed separately, but they can be interrelated in situations where active engagement and participation in spiritual experiences with other people enhances the psychosocial wellbeing of an older person. The underlying social integration that occurs when spiritual experiences are shared with others can be a protective factor against mental health problems. In this chapter, the term spirituality is used in a very broad sense to recognise that some people have spiritual experiences and practices, but do not subscribe to a recognised religion or system of faith and worship (e.g. Christian or Muslim).

PSYCHOSOCIAL FACTORS

Almost every aspect of an older person's mental health status is shaped by psychosocial factors. These factors influence the occurrence and course of a mental health problem, how a person behaves and adapts to being unwell, and how well they recover and remain healthy. Psychosocial factors are broad and include self-identity, self-esteem, sexuality, family life, household structure, education, working life, social and recreational activities, hobbies and interests, retirement, losses, socioeconomic status, transportation and access to services.

A framework that has stood the test of time for conceptualising people's needs, including psychosocial needs, is the work by Maslow (1970). According to Maslow, for normal human development to occur, the physical needs of nutrition and hydration have to be satisfied first and then the emotional needs of love, belonging and self-esteem can be met. After these basic needs are satisfied, then the person can continue to grow psychosocially by seeking meaning and fulfilment in their lives so they eventually reach the stages of self-actualisation and self-transcendence.

As people get older, how they perceive and address their psychosocial needs may influence their ability to remain independent, and how they deal with loneliness, social isolation and the development of mental health problems. Psychosocial support can vary enormously from a brief, weekly visit by one person for a housebound older person through to a person who has three or more social engagements outside the home almost every day. It is not the quantity of interactions but the quality that is the most important aspect. When an older person is struggling with mental health problems, it is high-quality psychosocial support that will act as a buffer in moderating the impact of the stress and will also have a strong influence on recovery. However, addressing an older person's psychosocial needs is not just a simple matter of introducing and encouraging the support of other people or networks. Unwanted and stressful social engagements can also be detrimental to an older person's mental health.

The reason assessment of this area is so important is that psychosocial support can mean a lot of different things to each and every person. Individual contacts and networks are used in different ways to satisfy the older person's needs. These needs can be human contact, emotional connectedness, personal growth, information, advice, the sharing of confidences and ideas through to general conversation. Satisfying one's needs leads to achieving purpose in life and, no matter what age, most people still want to have a purpose, to learn, contribute and be creative.

In undertaking a psychosocial assessment, the foremost question usually is what the older person perceives as their health concerns. Conversely, the mental health worker may want to focus on optimising physical functioning first because they can see the long-term benefits in such an approach, but this may not be what the older person wants. There may be a cognitive or emotional aspect to their health that the older person considers to be more important to them and their quality of life.

Identification and expression of such matters may not come easily to some older people. Through sensitive questioning, the mental health worker can create the opportunity to explore the older person's thoughts and feelings in relation to the psychosocial aspects of their life to determine which areas need strengthening and how this may be done. Many older people are very resourceful and recognition needs to be given for this. Some questions to explore psychosocial issues could be:

- What strategies have you used in the past to help overcome adverse events?
- Who do you turn to in crisis?
- Who do you call for everyday help, practically and emotionally?
- What do you see your strengths as?
- What do you see your weaknesses as?
- What are your goals and desires?
- How do you go about achieving your goals and desires?
- What do you fear?
- What do you not want to do?
- Do you feel as though you have reached your potential in family, work and public life?

Ecomaps

To determine the size, structure and strength of psychosocial networks, a good starting point is the use of an ecomap (Wright & Leahey 2000). The ecomap is an extension of the genogram, which outlines family relationships. The ecomap is a graphic depiction of contact, with not only family members, but also friends, social contacts, health services and any other significant contact. A lot of information can be contained in these diagrams. Information is recorded in squares or circles, which can be strategically placed or organised to show how all the relationships fit together. The strength of the relationships is signified by lines. Straight lines indicate strong relationships (the wider the line the stronger the relationship), while dotted lines indicate weak relationships and slashed

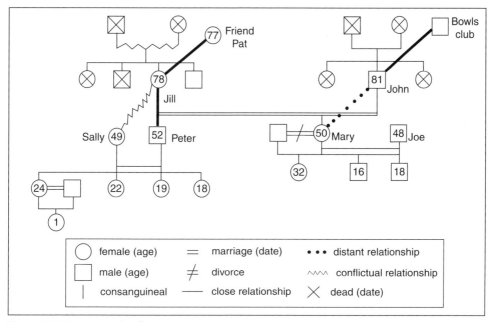

Figure 17.1 An example of an ecomap

lines indicate conflictual relationships. The frequency of contacts can also be noted on the diagram. See Figure 17.1 for an example of an ecomap.

Psychosocial assessment

There are a number of assessment tools that have been developed to assist in the collection of data in relation to psychosocial issues. A commonly used one is the Older American Resources and Services (OARS) scale (Duke University Center for the Study of Aging and Human Development 1978). This scale is discussed in more detail in Chapter 35.

SPIRITUALITY

In the 2006 census, nearly 70% of the Australian population reported they had a religion, 11% did not state their religious affiliation and 19% reported they had no religion (Australian Bureau of Statistics 2006). These data were limited to asking about 'religion' per se, rather than recognising that some people have spiritual practices and do not subscribe to a particular religion. However, it does highlight the fact that spirituality or religiosity is an aspect of life that many people consider important enough to note their affiliation with such practices. There are many definitions available on what spirituality means. MacKinlay (2001) has offered this definition:

> *That which lies at the core of each person's being, an essential dimension which brings meaning to life. It is acknowledged that spirituality is not constituted only by religious practices, but must be understood more broadly, as relationship with God, however God or ultimate meaning is perceived by the person, and in relationship with other people.*

Recently, more attention is being paid to the role of spirituality as a resilience and recovery factor in relation to mental health problems, particularly depression, anxiety and substance abuse. Some people choose to use their spiritual practice as a coping strategy when they are experiencing emotional difficulties. There is a significant amount of research evidence that indicates spiritual practice is associated with many positive mental health outcomes. Yohannes et al (2008) examined health behaviour, severity of depression and religiosity in older people admitted for rehabilitation (N = 173). It was found that religious attendance was associated with positive perceptions of health and less severe illness. Additionally, intrinsic religious activities were associated with less severe depression and lower likelihood of living alone.

Similarly, Blay et al (2008) examined religious characteristic associations with the use of tobacco, alcohol and depression. These researchers established that several aspects of religiosity reduced the odds of being a tobacco user by 51%, not having a religion increased the use of alcohol by 88% and participating in social religious activities reduced the risk of depression by 16%. Engaging in organised religious activities can act as a negator or provide a buffer against negative life experiences that occur in old age. The salutary aspects of religious participation have been identified as opportunities for friendship, a sense of connectedness and community, and as a means of contributing to the welfare of others (Neill & Kahn 1999).

Spiritual assessment

There are numerous scales that have been developed to assist in assessing an older person's spiritual needs. As it is a very complex topic, many of these scales have a specific focus. For example, some are rating scales, while others are inventories; some scales promote reflection and reminiscence, while others provide themes to aid in care planning or guide interventions. If a mental health worker intends on using an assessment scale, it would pay to be very judicious in the choice of scale and give due consideration as to whether or not it is culturally appropriate as well.

Spiritual needs

The reason it is important to consider an older person's spiritual needs is that if they are not being met they can experience the very negative and damaging feelings of anger, despair, hopelessness, grief, anxiety, fear, guilt and loss. Van Loon (2001) identified the following spiritual needs that may be encountered when caring for an older person:
- need for meaning and purpose in life
- love and belonging
- hope
- forgiveness
- a relationship with God, and
- transcendence of the human spirit.

Having to attend to an older person's spiritual needs can be a confronting idea, especially if the older person is from a different culture, religion or spiritual orientation to the mental health worker. It is certainly not expected that a mental health worker knows the liturgies and rituals of all the spiritual practices; however, it could be prudent to have some basic knowledge and understanding of key issues, rituals, behaviours, significant objects and dress codes of some of the main religions that may be encountered in the work day. Simple actions include: demonstrating respect, acceptance and tolerance of the older person's spiritual practice; organising a place where the older person feels comfortable to undertake their spiritual practice; allowing and assisting them to attend spiritual meetings and special events; and enlisting the support of their family, friends and spiritual guides or personnel.

On a personal level, sometimes spiritual needs can be met by just being present, offering physical comfort through touch in a professional sense (holding hands, hand on shoulder, arm around someone) and listening attentively and engaging in dialogue that will facilitate expression of spiritual needs.

Members of the clergy and pastoral carers have a specific focus of attending to a person's spiritual needs and can be important collaborators in the care of an older person. Furthermore, an older person seeking help from clergy rather than a mental health worker for an emotional or serious mental health problem is not uncommon (Pickard & Guo 2008). With the older person's consent, a mutual relationship based on knowledge and understanding of the important role and skills that clergy and mental health workers each have may improve the mental healthcare an older person receives.

SUMMARY

This chapter has considered the important topics of psychosocial and spiritual assessment. As these are very broad areas, the essential components have been identified and the mental health worker is encouraged to explore the different assessment formats that are available so that the one that is chosen is the one that is most suitable for the older person for whom they are caring.

FURTHER READING

MacKinlay E 2001 The spiritual dimension of ageing. Jessica Kingsley Publishers, Sydney
MacKinlay E 2006 Spiritual growth and care in the fourth age of life. Jessica Kingsley Publishers, Sydney

USEFUL WEBSITE

Centre for Ageing and Pastoral Studies: www.centreforageing.org.au

REFERENCES

Australian Bureau of Statistics (ABS) 2006 Census. ABS, Canberra
Blay SL, Batista AD, Andreoli SB, Gastal FL 2008 The relationship between religiosity and tobacco, alcohol use, and depression in an elderly community population. American Journal of Geriatric Psychiatry 16(11):934–943
Duke University Center for the Study of Aging and Human Development 1988 OARS multi-dimensional functional assessment questionnaire. Duke University, Durham, NC
MacKinlay E 2001 The spiritual dimension of ageing. Jessica Kingsley Publishers, Sydney
Maslow AH 1970 Motivation and personality. Harper & Row, New York
Neill CM, Kahn AS 1999 The role of personal spirituality and religious social activity on the life satisfaction of older widowed women. Sex Roles 40:319–329
Pickard JG, Guo B 2008 Clergy as mental health service providers to older adults. Aging and Mental Health 12(5):615–624

Wright LM, Leahey M 2000 Nurses and families: a guide to family assessment and intervention. FA Davis, Philadelphia

Van Loon A 2001 Assessing spiritual needs. In: Koch A, Garratt S (eds) Assessing older people: a practical guide for health professionals. MacLennan & Petty, Sydney

Yohannes AM, Koenig HG, Baldwin RC, Connolly MJ 2008 Health behaviour, depression and religiosity in older patients admitted to intermediate care. International Journal of Geriatric Psychiatry 23(7):735–740

Chapter 18
RISK ASSESSMENT

INTRODUCTION

This chapter gives an overview of risk assessment, with particular emphasis on falls, abuse and neglect of older people, and aggression. Risk assessment involves the consideration of risk factors, harm and likelihood (McSherry 2004). These factors are covered in this chapter, with the addition of intervention strategies and, in relation to abuse and neglect specifically, the different types are identified. In the final section, after aggression, there is a short discussion on the perplexing issue of self-neglect. Suicide is another important topic in regard to risk assessment and this is dealt with in Chapter 21.

FALLS

One of the most significant risks for older people relates to the incidence of falls. In Australia, for the year 2005–06, the estimated number of hospitalised injury cases due to falls in people aged 65 years and over was 66,800—a rise of 10% since 2003–04. Half of all fall injury cases for people aged 65 years and older occurred in the home (Bradley & Pointer 2008). Mild to serious physical injury can occur from falls, but with any fall the older person usually suffers some longer term psychological distress and fear of falling again. The result of this is that they reduce their activities, which can increase dependency, limit activities of daily living (ADL) and instrumental activities of daily living (IADL) function, increase morbidity and reduce their ability to socialise and overall quality of life (Kressig et al 2001).

Causative factors related to falls are multifactorial (i.e. intrinsic factors or extrinsic factors, or a combination of both, contribute to the problem). Listed below are some of these factors (American Geriatrics Society 2001, Lord et al 2007):

- *Age-related changes.* These include poor vision and hearing, less toe and foot lift while stepping, impaired balance, slower reaction time and continence issues (frequency, dribbling), loss of muscle strength and flexibility, and cognitive impairment.
- *Assistive devices.* Canes, walkers and wheelchairs can be cumbersome.
- *Medications.* These can cause orthostatic hypotension, visual and balance disturbances, dizziness, drowsiness and continence issues (frequency, dribbling). The effects of beta-blockers, antipsychotics, sedatives, diuretics and antihypertensives are known to increase the risk of falls.
- *Care-recipient-related factors.* These include substance abuse, dehydration and poor nutrition.

- *Footwear and clothing.* These include ill-fitting footwear, slippery or sticky shoe soles and loose, bulky clothing.
- *Disease-related symptoms.* These include orthostatic hypotension, continence issues (frequency, dribbling), reduced cerebral blood flow, oedema, confusion, ataxia, brittle bones, fatigue, weakness, paralysis and Parkinsonism.
- *Environmental hazards.* These include wet floors, waxed floors, clutter, poor lighting, mats, loose coverings and uneven flooring.
- *Carer-related factors.* These include improper use of restraints, poor supervision, and delays responding to the needs of the older person.

Falls assessment

There are numerous general and specific falls assessment instruments that have been developed over the years. A number of reviews assessing the value of these instruments have been undertaken. If the mental health worker intends to use one or more of the available instruments, it would be prudent to examine the reviews which summarise many of the characteristics and will make an informed choice somewhat easier. Reviews in this area have been conducted by Haines et al (2007), Lundin-Olsson et al (2003) and Perell et al (2001).

Prevention of falls

An enormous amount of effort has gone into prevention interventions and programs for falls (Lord et al 2007). A Cochrane Database Systematic Review to assess the effects of interventions to reduce the incidence of falls in older people living in the community found a number of interventions to be effective (Gillespie et al 2009). Over 100 trials involving 55,303 people were included in the review. The interventions likely to be beneficial in reducing the risk and rate of falls were tai chi and multiple component exercise (individual and group). Other prevention strategies such as multifactorial assessment and intervention, home safety interventions and vitamin D supplements still require further research to confirm their effectiveness. There was some evidence that falls prevention strategies can be cost effective.

ABUSE AND NEGLECT

Older people who have a mental health problem are a very vulnerable group of people and could be at risk of abuse and neglect. This is not a new problem, but awareness and unacceptability of it has grown in recent decades. It is a pertinent issue for mental health workers who have direct contact with older people and their carers in their homes and in residential aged care facilities (RACFs). It is imperative that if an abusive situation is suspected or recognised, it is acted upon promptly, but handled in a sensitive and professional manner.

Abuse and neglect often go undetected and there are many reasons as to why this happens. An older person, for example, may not be able to report the abuse due to cognitive impairment or communication difficulties caused by a stroke. They could be afraid of the perpetrator and fear retaliation, or if they lose the support of this person they may have to go into an RACF or some other form of supportive accommodation. Feelings of shame and embarrassment may prevail if it is a family member who is the perpetrator.

Also, it can be very difficult to differentiate normal ageing changes from signs of neglect and mistreatment. For example, weight loss and bruising and other such signs can be easily explained away as poor appetite or a fall (Anetzberger 2005, Carney et al 2003).

Elder abuse is defined as any pattern of behaviour that causes physical, psychological, financial and social harm to an older person (World Health Organization 2002). Abuse and neglect is a complex and multifactorial issue and can occur in a variety of ways. Determining the type of abuse will be helpful in planning how to intervene. It is generally categorised in the following ways:

- *Physical acts.* This category includes such physical acts as hitting, pinching, pushing and burning that cause pain and injury, as well as the use of restraints, force feeding, the presence of pressure sores and inappropriate use of medications.
- *Psychological acts.* These are acts that cause emotional pain and injury, and can be carried out by making threats, locking people up, keeping them isolated, the overuse of silence, making people feel rejected, ashamed and humiliated, verbal intimidation and harassment. The older person may respond by becoming withdrawn or agitated.
- *Sexual assault.* This includes such acts as sexual exhibition, rape, inappropriate touching, taking sexually explicit photographs, coerced nudity, and showing pornography.
- *Material exploitation.* This involves misuse or theft of money and possessions or not allowing a person to have control over their finances, making changes to legal documents, forging signatures, and improper use of power of attorney and guardianship.
- *Neglect.* This means failure to meet the needs of a dependent person. It can be active or passive. It can relate to nutrition, hydration, cleanliness, clothing, shelter, medical care, dental care and access to other health services (e.g. home help and domiciliary nursing care). Neglect is the most common form of elder abuse.
- *Abandonment.* This occurs when a person who has taken on the responsibility of caring for an older person leaves them to fend for themselves for an unreasonable extended period of time.

The extent of this problem is very difficult to determine, as it is often not reported. However, a recent national prevalence study of elder abuse was conducted in private households in England, Scotland, Wales and Northern Ireland (Biggs et al 2009). Of the 2111 respondents, 2.6% reported abuse by family members, close friends or healthcare workers. The predominant type of reported abuse was neglect (1.1%), followed by financial abuse (0.6%), with 0.4% of respondents reporting psychological abuse, 0.4% physical abuse and 0.2% sexual abuse. Women were significantly more likely to have experienced abuse than men.

Risk factors

The older the person is, the greater the risk of neglect. Other risk factors are cognitive impairment, including dementia, functional impairment and shared living situations, particularly in isolated areas.

The perpetrators often have a mental illness, abuse substances or are somehow dependent on the older person. They are usually family members, such as a spouse or adult children and grandchildren.

There may be a history of abusive behaviour and violence within the family. For example, the care recipient may have abused their spouse or children for many years and now it is time for revenge.

Carer burden is also a significant risk factor. If a carer is not getting enough support financially, emotionally and physically, or even simple recognition for their caring role, they can become very resentful (Choi & Mayer 2000).

The abuser

The characteristics of the abuser are no different from other abuse cases involving children and domestic violence situations. Abusers are usually reluctant for the victim to be interviewed on their own. Patterns of abuse are made difficult to determine by seeking medical help from many different sources, or the abuser refuses to seek help so the situation is not noticed. The abuser can appear overly concerned or indifferent to the condition of the victim, and they can be threatening to healthcare professionals who are involved in the case (e.g. threaten legal action).

Carer abuse

Another issue that is worth mentioning is carer abuse. One such case comes to mind where an elderly gentleman was refusing to leave hospital after minor surgery as he was scared of going home to his wife who had dementia and regularly assaulted him and he did not know what to do. The older persons' mental health service (OPMHS) assessed the man and his wife and instituted some aggression management strategies.

The assessment process

Kurrle (2001) has provided a comprehensive framework for the assessment, management and intervention of elder abuse cases, as follows:

- The older person has the right to refuse to answer questions or be examined, and to remain in the situation if that is their choice.
- Interviewing the older person by themselves and in private is essential, as it may be very difficult to admit to abuse in front of other people, particularly the perpetrator.
- The interview should be undertaken by an experienced person with highly developed interpersonal skills, as it requires the development of a trusting relationship and the use of tact and sensitivity.
- Detailed, accurate and timely documentation is essential.
- In cases of physical and sexual assault, a physical examination will need to be undertaken and the results detailed (see Ch 15).
- Cognitive assessment should also be undertaken using the tools outlined in Chapter 14. This assessment is very important as a baseline for evaluating the information received and involvement in decision making.
- Functional and psychosocial assessments (see Chs 16 and 17) are also important to provide the baseline for interventions and future planning.
- If possible, information can also be gained from the referral source and other people who may be involved in some way (e.g. other family members and carers).

It is not the role of the mental health worker to pass judgment or apportion blame in these situations. If the abuser has identified needs in relation to counselling, more practical support and the handing over of affairs to another person or the Adult Guardian, then these interventions need to be actioned. In Australia, elder abuse is a recognised issue and there are specialised services available to assist in dealing with these matters. Examples of such services are listed below under 'Useful websites'.

Interventions

Kurrle (2001) also advises on useful interventions. These include crisis care if the victim needs immediate removal from an abusive situation. This could be in hospital or an RACF. If practical support is required to assist with carer burden, this could be in the form of community support provided under the home and community care program. Depending on the identified needs, it could be home nursing, help with incontinence, home-delivered meals, housekeeping, home maintenance, assistance with shopping, transportation and/ or respite care. Respite care could be in-home, day centre or residential. Counselling for the victim and abuser would also be appropriate. This could be on a one-to-one basis, family or group therapy and, if warranted, attendance at support groups. If the situation is not redeemable, the only option could be permanent placement in some form of alternative accommodation, which for an older person is most likely to be an RACF.

Legal intervention and perhaps criminal charges may be necessary depending on the actual abusive situation. In some jurisdictions, reporting of abuse cases is mandatory. Physical, sexual and financial abuse can be very obvious and readily proved, whereas psychological abuse and cases of mild to moderate neglect may be less easily determined. For example, the only way a wife may be able to manage her husband who has dementia and is aggressive is to oversedate him. In making decisions with such matters, it is ideal if a mental health worker can rely on the support of a multidisciplinary team or at least another health professional. Legal intervention could involve revoking power of attorney arrangements, taking out a domestic violence order or having the perpetrator evicted from the older person's premises. If the older person's cognitive assessment has revealed significant deficits, then they may have to be made incapable of decision making and their affairs handled by a guardianship office.

As is often the case, there are no clearcut answers in many of these situations and decisions are often made based on ethical principles of autonomy and beneficence. Within the principle of autonomy are the notions of respect, informed consent and self-determination. If a competent older person decides not to do anything about an abusive situation in which they are the victim, this decision must be respected. On the other hand, health professionals are also guided by the principle of beneficence, which is to promote good and prevent evil and harm. This is the balancing act of weighing up the harms and benefits when making a decision. It is also helpful for the mental health service to have a protocol in place on how to deal with elder abuse and neglect. Such a protocol should also include support for the healthcare workers through debriefing and supervision sessions.

Routinely inquiring about the topic and screening for it would aid in detection as well. Fulmer et al (2004) provided a review of existing elder abuse screening tools, assessment instruments, protocols and guidelines that can be administered to the care recipients or the carers. A comparative analysis, attributes and limitations of the various instruments is given to assist in the choice of the most suitable instrument for the healthcare worker's needs. The authors encourage the use of the instruments to ensure a thoughtful, thorough, consistent and balanced judgment is made in relation to this issue, which could easily become subjectively clouded. The instruments would be an asset, particularly for mental health workers who have limited experience in elder abuse.

AGGRESSION

Aggression is an overt behaviour with clear aggressive intent that is directed at either people or objects. It is made clear that the behaviour is not accidental. Behaviours such as hitting, kicking, biting, spitting, throwing things and verbal abuse are included within the category of physical aggression. Such behaviour may have several adverse consequences, including injury to self and others, and the use of physical and chemical restraints (Patel & Hope 1992).

Aggression is one of the most frequently used reasons for referral to an OPMHS and earlier admission to an RACF (Lyketsos et al 1999). The presence of physical aggression has been reported in 15–45% of community-dwelling older people with dementia (Lyketsos et al 1999). A higher incidence has been found in RACFs, with reports of 76.5% (Brodaty et al 2001).

Risk factors

McSherry (2004) identified risk factors from a review of aggression and violence studies. The factors have been categorised according to whether they are static (historical and fixed) or dynamic (changeable). Static risk factors give an indication of the long-term likelihood of aggressive behaviour (i.e. *risk status*), whereas dynamic risk factors provide an estimate of short-term likelihood of aggression or *risk state* (Carroll 2007). Dynamic factors can be the focus of interventions. Static risk factors include:
- history of aggression
- male gender
- mental health problems (diagnosis): dementia, depression, schizophrenia, personality disorder and substance abuse, and
- loss (e.g. spouse, retirement).

Dynamic risk factors include:
- mental health problems (symptoms of): delusions and hallucinations, substance abuse, and behavioural and psychological symptoms of dementia
- non-compliance with treatment
- demands and expectations, confrontations and ready availability of weapons
- troubled interpersonal relationships
- hearing and vision problems, physical illness, impairment in activities of daily living, speech difficulties and memory problems
- poor social networks, lack of education and work skills, itinerant lifestyle, poverty and homelessness, and
- anger and fear.

Assessment

In a crisis situation the best approach is expert clinical judgment. In a non-crisis situation, assessment is usually carried out over a period gaining information from as many sources as possible, including the older person. An analysis of the behaviour is needed, including type, intensity, frequency, pattern, who is involved, where and when it occurs, the history of the presenting problem, a medical and psychiatric history, and an assessment of the environment (Wells & Wells 1997). There are rating scales for aggression that will support and augment assessment and treatment. For example, the Ryden Aggression Scale (RAS) (Ryden 1988) and the RAGE (Patel & Hope 1992) are specific tools for older people, particularly if dementia is present. Depending on the purpose of assessment, there are other tools that have been developed for risk assessment in the general population that may suit. The Historical Clinical Risk–20, which examines static and dynamic factors, is one such example (Webster et al 1997).

Intervention

Aggressive behaviours are overt and therefore can be closely observed and monitored. This makes behavioural strategies likely for intervention. The care plan will aim at reducing the behaviour and also giving the carer, be it a family member or mental health worker, skills to manage the behaviour. Behaviour therapy is covered in detail in Chapter 29. The treatment of specific mental health problems and psychotherapeutic treatment for psychosocial problems are also covered in later chapters.

SELF-NEGLECT

Self-neglect is a perplexing issue where an older person neglects their self-care and often at the same time is neglectful of their home environment by hoarding and living in squalor (McDermott 2008). Sometimes, these older people can have a mental health problem and other times it is not able to be determined. They are usually quite happy, going about their business, but it is their neighbours and the local council workers who voice grave concerns about the older person's safety and the safety of the neighbourhood. This is when the older person comes to the attention of the OPMHS and other healthcare agencies. Coming to a satisfactory solution requires a collaborative intra-agency approach, while remaining respectful of the older person's right for autonomy and privacy. Neville (1995) and Snowdon et al (2007) provide comprehensive accounts and advice on dealing with this issue.

SUMMARY

The chapter has covered risk assessment of falls, elder abuse and aggression. Many strategies have been put forward so the management of these dilemmas is easier to navigate. As a mental health worker, one has to be able to recognise risk factors and signs if a problem is occurring and know how to intervene effectively. All the matters addressed in this chapter are very complex; therefore, the mental health worker has to proceed sensitively and cautiously so that interventions are appropriately based on professional and ethical principles.

FURTHER READING

Journal of Elder Abuse and Neglect
Kosberg JI 2007 Abuse of older men. Howarth Press, New York
Lord S, Sherrington C, Menz H, Close J 2007 Falls in older people: risk factors and strategies for prevention. Cambridge University Press, Cambridge

Maden A 2007 Treating violence. Oxford University Press, Oxford

Pritchard J 2007 Working with adult abuse: a training manual for people working with vulnerable adults. JKP Resource Materials, London

USEFUL WEBSITES

Aged Care Australia: www.agedcareaustralia.gov.au. This organisation provides information on falls prevention.

Australian Network for the Prevention of Elder Abuse: www.sa.agedrights.asn.au

Department of Health (UK), Best practice in managing risk: principles and guidance for best practice in the assessment and management of risk to self and others in mental health services: www.dh.gov.uk/en/Publicationsandstatistics/Publications/PublicationsPolicyAndGuidance/DH_076511

Elder Abuse Prevention Association: www.eapa.asn.au. This organisation also provides a toll free number (1800 550 552) to the Complaints Investigation Scheme, so an abuse situation can be reported and options discussed. This call can be made anonymously, or can be kept confidential.

REFERENCES

American Geriatrics Society 2001 Guideline for the prevention of falls in older persons: American Geriatrics Society, British Geriatrics Society, and American Academy of Orthopaedic Surgeons Panel on Falls Prevention. Journal of the American Geriatrics Society 49:664–672

Anetzberger G 2005 The reality of elder abuse. Clinical Gerontologist 28(1/2):1–25

Biggs S, Manthorpe J, Tinker A et al 2009 Mistreatment of older people in the United Kingdom: findings from the first National Prevalence Study. Journal of Elder Abuse and Neglect 21(1):1–14

Bradley C, Pointer S 2008 Hospitalisations due to falls by older people, Australia 2005–06. Injury Research and Statistics Series No. 50. Cat. No. INJCAT 122. AIHW, Adelaide

Brodaty H, Draper B, Saab D et al 2001 Psychosis, depression, and behavioural disturbances in Sydney nursing home residents: prevalence and predictors. International Journal of Geriatric Psychiatry 16:504–512

Carney M, Kahan F, Paris B 2003 Elder abuse: is every bruise a sign of abuse? Mount Sinai Journal of Medicine 70(2):69–74

Carroll A 2007 Are violence risk assessment tools clinically useful? Australian and New Zealand Journal of Psychiatry 41(4):301–307

Choi N, Mayer J 2000 Elder abuse, neglect, and exploitation: risk factors and prevention strategies. Journal of Gerontological Social Work 33(2):5–25

Fulmer T, Guadano L, Dyer CB et al 2004 Progress in elder abuse assessment instruments. Journal of the American Geriatrics Society 52(2):297–304

Gillespie LD, Robertson MC, Gillespie WJ et al 2009 Interventions for preventing falls in older people living in the community (review). Cochrane Collaboration

Haines TP, Hill K, Walsh W et al 2007 Design-related bias in hospital fall risk screening tool predictive accuracy evaluations: systematic review and meta-analysis. Journals of Gerontology A: Biological Sciences and Medical Sciences 62(6):664–672

Kressig RW, Wolf SL, Sattin RW et al 2001 Associations of demographic, functional, and behavioral characteristics with activity-related fear of falling among older adults transitioning to frailty. Journal of the American Geriatrics Society 49(11):1456–1462

Kurrle S 2001 Assessment of elder abuse. In: Koch S, Garratt S (eds) Assessing older people: a practical guide for health professionals. MacLennan & Petty, Sydney

Lord S, Sherrington C, Menz H, Close J 2007 Falls in older people: risk factors and strategies for prevention. Cambridge University Press, Cambridge

Lundin-Olsson L, Jensen J, Nyberg L, Gustafson Y 2003 Predicting falls in residential care by a risk assessment tool, staff judgment, and history of falls. Aging Clinical and Experimental Research 15(1):266–274

Lyketsos CG, Steele C, Galik E et al 1999 Physical aggression in dementia patients and its relationship to depression. American Journal of Psychiatry 156(1):66–71

McDermott S 2008 The devil is in the details: self-neglect in Australia. Journal of Elder Abuse and Neglect 20(3):231–250

McSherry B 2004 Risk assessment by mental health professionals and the prevention of future violent behaviour. Australian Institute of Criminology, Canberra

Neville C 1995 Community mental health nursing and the elderly client: a case presentation. Australian and New Zealand Journal of Mental Health Nursing 4:190–195

Patel V, Hope RA 1992 A rating scale for aggressive behaviour in the elderly: the RAGE. Psychological Medicine 22:211–221

Perell KL, Nelson A, Goldman RL et al 2001 Fall risk assessment measures: an analytic review. Journal of Gerontology: Biological Sciences and Medical Sciences 56(12):M761–M766

Ryden MB 1988 Aggressive behavior in persons with dementia who live in the community. Alzheimer Disease and Associated Disorders 2(4):342–355

Snowdon J, Shah A, Halliday G 2007 Severe domestic squalor: a review. International Psychogeriatrics 19(1):1–15

Webster CD, Douglas KS, Eaves D, Hart SD 1997 The HCR–20: assessing risk for violence, version two. Simon Fraser University, British Columbia

Wells C, Wells J 1997 Reducing challenging behaviour of elderly confused people: a behavioural perspective. In: Norman IJ, Redfern SJ (eds.) Mental health care for elderly people. Churchill Livingstone, New York

World Health Organization (WHO) 2002 Toronto declaration on ageing. WHO, Toronto

Chapter 19

THE OLDER PERSON WITH CONFUSION

INTRODUCTION

The main causes of confusion among older people are dementia, delirium and amnestic disorder. These conditions are not mutually exclusive and it is not uncommon for one person to have both dementia and delirium. This chapter contains key information relevant to the assessment and management of the older person with these organic mental health problems. It should be read in conjunction with Chapter 28, which deals in more detail with the behavioural and psychological symptoms of dementia.

CLINICAL CONTEXT

Older people with confusion are seen in many different settings. Acute delirium often presents in the hospital emergency department or in general medical or surgical wards. However, it may also present in the residential aged care facility (RACF) setting. Dementia is commonly seen during domiciliary visits, in the general hospital setting, in the memory clinic or in the RACF setting. Amnestic disorder is generally seen in the emergency department or in general medical and surgical wards. In some places, older people with uncomplicated dementia are seen primarily in memory clinics, whereas in other places they are seen by older persons' mental health services (OPMHS). Regardless, all mental health workers need to be familiar with these three conditions.

CASE VIGNETTE

Mrs X, an 82-year-old widow, has been referred to the OPMHS by her daughter, who is concerned about her memory and thinking ability. The daughter says her mother has a 4-year history of insidious decline in her memory in association with word-finding difficulties and topographical disorientation. In addition, she has begun to have difficulty with instrumental activities of daily living (IADL), such as using the telephone and calculating change at the corner store. Mrs X denies any major difficulties, just saying: 'What do you expect at my age?' Recently, Mrs X scraped the side of another car while parking at the local shopping centre. She has also been accusing her daughter of stealing things from her house. Mrs X is reluctant to attend the outpatient clinic and her daughter has requested a domiciliary assessment.

EPIDEMIOLOGY

Dementia

The prevalence of dementia in Australia and most developed nations is approximately 6.5% among people aged 65 years and over. The prevalence rises exponentially with age, doubling every 5 years after the age of 65 years. The incidence of dementia (the number of new cases per year) also rises exponentially with age, with a similar doubling every 5 years.

Amnestic disorder

Although the true prevalence of amnestic disorder is not reliably known, an Australian autopsy series found signs of the Wernicke-Korsakoff syndrome in 2.8% of brains, the highest prevalence ever reported (for a review see Harper et al 1995). However, more recent research has suggested that the fortification of flour with thiamine might have reduced the prevalence of this condition (Harper et al 1998). The syndrome of amnestic disorder is sometimes considered to be a subtype of dementia, although by definition it is not associated with the global cognitive impairment associated with dementing illnesses.

Delirium

Delirium is also known as acute confusion or acute brain syndrome, and these terms highlight the acute nature of the condition. The community prevalence of delirium is not reliably known, but it is present in 15–35% of older hospital inpatients, either on admission or within 3 days of admission.

CLINICAL FEATURES

Dementia

The cardinal feature of dementia is decline from a previous level of cognitive performance involving memory and at least one of the following: aphasia, apraxia, agnosia and executive dysfunction. Aphasia is a language and communication disorder; apraxia is an abnormality of complex movement despite normal peripheral motor function; and agnosia is an inability to recognise objects despite normal sensory function. Executive dysfunction involves abnormalities in planning, organisation, initiation and checking of behaviour. In most cases of dementia, there is progressive and irreversible deterioration in cognitive function. However, some cases of dementia are caused by acute insults to the brain, such as head injury or encephalitis. In such cases, there may be the prospect of some improvement in cognitive function over several months following the acute event.

Amnestic disorder

In amnestic disorder, clinical impairment is restricted to memory function, rather than the global cognitive impairment found in dementia. People with amnestic disorder have particular difficulty with new learning, while other cognitive functions remain relatively intact. In severe cases of amnestic disorder, the person is completely unable to make new memories and remains like this permanently.

Delirium

Delirium is characterised by the acute onset of global cognitive impairment, fluctuating clouding of consciousness, altered day/night cycle, psychomotor agitation (one-third of people) or psychomotor retardation (two-thirds of people). Delirium is considered a neuropsychiatric emergency because quick action may prevent a poor outcome for the person and may even prevent death. Delirium is a clinical chameleon and can mimic other conditions, such as dementia, psychosis, anxiety, depression and mania.

AETIOLOGY

Dementia

Most cases of dementia are caused by Alzheimer's disease or cerebrovascular disease, or a combination of the two (so-called mixed dementia). However, there are more than 70 other diseases that cause dementia, including frontotemporal lobar degeneration (FTLD), dementia with Lewy bodies (DLB), alcohol-related dementia, Parkinson's disease, traumatic brain injury (TBI), normal pressure hydrocephalus (NPH), hypoxic encephalopathy, Huntington's disease, herpes simplex encephalitis and Creutzfeldt-Jakob disease (CJD).

Alzheimer's disease is associated with progressive brain atrophy. Microscopic examination of the brain in this condition reveals neuronal loss, accumulation of extracellular neuritic plaques and intracellular neurofibrillary tangles, and a variety of other neuropathological features. In addition, there is massive loss of synapses, particularly acetylcholine synapses. Although the underlying aetiology of Alzheimer's disease is still being studied, the common late-onset sporadic form of the disease appears to be caused by a combination of advancing age, susceptibility genes such as the gene for apolipoprotein E, and environmental factors. Putative environmental factors include reduced brain reserve due to poor education and lack of cognitively stimulating activities.

Various types of cerebrovascular disease are associated with dementia, including multiple infarcts (strokes), subcortical damage to cerebral white matter (deep white matter ischaemic changes), hypoxic encephalopathy, small strokes in strategic locations (e.g. the thalamus), and several rare inherited vascular syndromes, including CADASIL (cerebral autosomal dominant arteriopathy with subcortical infarcts and leukoencephalopathy).

Amnestic disorder

There are many different causes of amnestic disorder, although only one common cause in the developed world—thiamine (vitamin B1) deficiency, which is often associated with alcohol dependency. Recent research indicates that the characteristic brain changes of this focal syndrome may also be present in alcohol-dependent people who present clinically with more generalised dementia. The Wernicke-Korsakoff syndrome is at least partially reversible in many people once thiamine replacement has been implemented and alcohol intake has ceased. Uncommon causes of thiamine deficiency include bulimia nervosa, hyperemesis gravidarum (excessive vomiting during pregnancy) and chronic gastrointestinal disease. Rare causes of amnestic disorder include carbon monoxide poisoning and herpes simplex encephalitis.

Delirium

Delirium may be caused by any acute medical problem that either primarily or secondarily affects the brain. Common causes in older people include intercurrent infections, organ failure, metabolic disease, prescribed medication and alcohol withdrawal. Other common causes include stroke, acute myocardial infarction and cancer. Common intercurrent infections include those of the urinary tract, lungs and skin. Organ failure includes cardiac failure, respiratory failure, renal failure and hepatic failure. Metabolic disease includes diabetes mellitus. Drugs with powerful anticholinergic effects, such as older-style antidepressants (tricyclics), antipsychotics, antiparkinsonian agents and drugs to treat urinary incontinence, are particularly likely to precipitate delirium in older people otherwise predisposed to this condition

COMORBIDITY

The principal comorbid mental health problem with delirium is dementia, whereas the principal comorbid mental health problem with amnestic disorder is alcohol dependence. The situation with dementia is more complex, as the condition has multiple comorbidities. Dementia is frequently associated with both mood disorder due to a general medical condition and subsyndromal depressions that we might label minor depression. It is also associated with anxiety, delusions and hallucinations.

DIFFERENTIAL DIAGNOSIS
Dementia

Differential diagnoses include:
- delirium
- amnestic disorder
- aphasic stroke
- depressive pseudodementia
- intellectual impairment, and
- oversedation with prescribed medication.

Amnestic disorder

Differential diagnoses include:
- dementia, and
- dissociative amnesia.

Delirium

Differential diagnoses include:
- dementia
- psychosis

- anxiety
- depression, and
- mania.

ASSESSMENT
History overview

It is important to obtain a reliable history if one of these three cognitive disorders is suspected. This history should be obtained from an informant who has regular contact with the older person. It would be unsafe to conclude that an older person was not suffering from one of these three conditions without speaking with an informant.

The critical distinction between dementia and delirium is in the history of onset. Most cases of dementia have a slow and insidious onset, whereas most cases of delirium have a rapid onset (over hours or days). Textbooks often describe a 'stepwise' deterioration in cases of multi-infarct dementia, but most cases of vascular dementia do not have this history. The course of onset of amnestic disorder is more varied.

Dementia of recent onset or rapidly progressive dementia raise additional issues. Such dementias may be due to remediable causes, such as severe depression or subdural haematoma, or due to unusual causes, such as cerebral vasculitis or CJD. As a general principle, people with dementia of recent onset (weeks to a few months) should be referred urgently for neurological review.

The person with delirium exhibits fluctuations in their level of consciousness and in the expression of their other symptoms. They may have lucid intervals in which they seem normal. In contrast, the person with dementia usually exhibits a much more stable state of mind. However, there are some exceptions to these general rules. The first is that dementia and delirium can coexist; the second is that many people with dementia exhibit so-called 'sundowning' (late afternoon deterioration) and alterations in their sleep continuity; and the third is that many people with DLB show brief alterations in their level of consciousness.

Amnestic disorder is suspected when the person presents with acquired memory impairment in the absence of global cognitive decline. There is usually dense anterograde amnesia as well as retrograde amnesia. Confabulation often occurs in amnestic disorders.

History: specific types of dementia
Dementia of the Alzheimer's type

The initial symptoms in dementia due to Alzheimer's disease are quite variable. Often the earliest manifestations are subtle changes in personality, mood, motivation or volition, rather than obvious cognitive impairment. These symptoms may be wrongly thought by others to be deliberately put on and may sometimes lead to marital disharmony or separation. In addition, the person with early dementia due to Alzheimer's disease may develop clinically significant anxiety or depression. They may also experience panic attacks or panicky feelings.

However, sooner or later the person develops clear evidence of insidiously worsening cognitive impairment. In most cases, this involves impaired recent memory, topographical disorientation and executive dysfunction (problems with planning and organisation particularly). This is often followed by word-finding difficulties (aphasia) and difficulties with object recognition (agnosia). As all of these symptoms get worse, the person develops more problems with instrumental activities of daily living (IADLs) and with the behavioural and psychological symptoms of dementia (BPSD). Ultimately, the person develops difficulties with even basic activities of daily living (ADLs) and requires assistance with personal care. If the person lives long enough with dementia, they become mute, doubly incontinent and unable to walk.

Vascular dementia

The clinical history in vascular dementia is often surprisingly similar to that in Alzheimer's disease. Although the classically described 'stepwise' deterioration does occur, most cases of vascular dementia seem to exhibit a rather slow, steady trajectory of decline. However, there is more often a history of stroke, transient ischaemic attack (TIA), syncope or pre-syncope. In addition, there is often a history of hypertension, atrial fibrillation, acute myocardial infarction, angina pectoris, peripheral vascular disease or aneurysm. Often there is also a history of diabetes mellitus and cigarette smoking. Mood changes are more common in vascular dementia than in Alzheimer's disease. The rate of progression in vascular dementia is usually much slower than in Alzheimer's disease.

Dementia with Lewy bodies

In dementia with Lewy bodies (DLB), there is often a history of gait disorder, including bradykinesia, rigidity and tremor associated with a history of falls. Hallucinations, particularly visual hallucinations, occur commonly. There may also be a history of very short-lived fluctuations in the level of consciousness, which often manifest as attentional difficulties. Otherwise, the symptoms are similar to those found in Alzheimer's disease. The rate of clinical progression in DLB is often noticeably faster than in Alzheimer's disease or in vascular dementia.

Frontotemporal dementia

Frontotemporal dementia often presents in quite a different way from the other dementias. The history is usually one of marked personality change, including loss of tact and social graces. There is often a history of disinhibited behaviour, including inappropriate aggression or sexual behaviour. The person may exhibit apathy and impaired volition. In some cases, there will be a history of prominent aphasia (language difficulties) in the absence of much memory impairment. In those cases associated with motor neurone disease, there may be swallowing difficulties.

Mental state examination

Look for the following:
- *Attention.* It is poor in delirium, but often normal or near normal in dementia and amnestic disorder.
- *Orientation.* It is usually impaired in all three conditions.
- *Language.* It is often disorganised in delirium, aphasic in dementia and normal in amnestic disorder.
- *Memory function, especially new learning ability.* It is impaired in all three conditions.
- *General intellectual functions.* For example, calculations, similarities and differences, and verbal fluency are usually impaired in dementia and delirium, but intact in amnestic disorder.

- *Perceptual abnormalities.* Illusions and hallucinations occur commonly in dementia and delirium, but are uncommon in amnestic disorder.
- *Abnormalities of thought content.* Delusional beliefs, overvalued ideas and marked preoccupations are common in dementia and delirium, but uncommon in amnestic disorder, although confabulations may sometimes be difficult to distinguish from delusions.
- *Insight.* It is often impaired in all three.
- *Judgment.* It is often impaired in all three.

Clinical cognitive testing

An important issue in relation to clinical cognitive testing is that the tests used should be tailored to the person being tested. A highly intelligent and well-educated person with an excellent occupational record may require testing with more challenging tests than someone without these attributes. In contrast, someone suspected of low cognitive function (whether innate or acquired) will need to be tested on less challenging tests. It follows that test performance should be compared with normative data for the person's age and educational background.

Screening with the Abbreviated Mental Test Score (AMTS), the General Practitioner Assessment of Cognition (GPCOG), the Psychogeriatric Assessment Scales (PAS) or the Mini-Mental State Examination (MMSE) is generally warranted for almost all people seen by an OPMHS. However, these screening tests do not provide a broad coverage of cognitive functions and need to be supplemented with other tests in many people, including a more difficult word-list learning test such as the revised Hopkins Verbal Learning Test (HVLT–R). In addition, further tests of frontal executive function such as the Trailmaking test (Trails A and B) and the category fluency test (animals in 60 seconds) are usually warranted.

Another approach would be to use the cognitive section of the Cambridge Mental Disorders of the Elderly Examination (CAMDEX), which is referred to as the CAMCOG–R, or the more recently developed Addenbrooke's Cognitive Examination–Revised (ACE–R). Both the CAMCOG–R and the ACE–R are relatively brief test batteries that augment the MMSE. However, neither the CAMCOG–R nor the ACE–R has a difficult auditory verbal learning test suitable for people with high premorbid function. All of these tests must be administered in a standardised way and their results should be interpreted in light of published normative data. Most people seen by an OPMHS do not need full neuropsychological testing and all clinical personnel need to be familiar with the administration of cognitive screening measures.

Another measure with considerable utility in the assessment of older people who might have dementia is the Informant Questionnaire for Cognitive Decline in the Elderly (IQCODE). This comes in a 26-item original version and a shorter 16-item version that is suitable for all screening purposes. The IQCODE is completed by an informant (usually a family member) who has known the person for at least 10 years. The informant is asked to compare the person's cognitive ability now with what it had been like 10 years earlier. The IQCODE works as well as the MMSE in predicting who will meet diagnostic criteria for dementia.

The Confusion Assessment Method (CAM) is a straightforward measure of the diagnostic criteria for delirium. For optimum results, however, it needs to be completed by an experienced clinician.

The formal assessment of people suspected of suffering from amnestic disorder involves detailed assessment of memory, using either a standardised battery such as the Wechsler Memory Scale, 3rd edn (WMS–III), or a combination of tests such as a word-list learning test (e.g. the HVLT–R, the California Verbal Learning Test (CVLT) or the Rey Auditory Verbal Learning Test (RAVLT)) and a non-verbal test such as the incidental recall test using the Complex Figure of Rey. The administration and interpretation of these tests is best left to clinical neuropsychologists or to experienced clinical psychologists with training in neuropsychology.

Physical examination

A physical examination is an important component of the assessment of any older person who might be suffering from dementia, amnestic disorder or delirium. In the person with probable dementia, it is important to rule out intercurrent general medical problems that might be adding to the person's level of disability. In addition, the physical examination sometimes provides clues as to the underlying disease diagnosis, particularly in cases of vascular dementia, DLB, dementia due to normal pressure hydrocephalus, and dementia in the context of Parkinson's disease or Huntington's disease. In the person with probable dementia, the physical examination should concentrate particularly on the neurological and cardiovascular systems.

A physical examination in the case of likely delirium is often essential in discovering the underlying medical problem causing the delirium.

A physical examination in the case of likely amnestic disorder is important to rule out the Wernicke-Korsakoff syndrome, as this has a specific treatment—high-dose thiamine (vitamin B1). This syndrome is characterised acutely by Wernicke's encephalopathy, which is a quiet delirium accompanied by ataxia and ophthalmoplegia. The chronic Korsakoff's syndrome is characterised by impaired new learning ability together with confabulation.

In cases of suspected dementia, a screening physical examination can be undertaken by team members during a domiciliary visit. Alternatively, the person's general practitioner can be asked to undertake one. The physical examination for suspected dementia should also concentrate on the cardiovascular and neurological systems. However, it is prudent for the psychogeriatric team to at a minimum check the person's vital signs, including lying and standing blood pressure.

Acute Wernicke's encephalopathy is more likely to be seen in the emergency department or in temporary accommodation for people with alcohol dependency than on domiciliary visits by the OPMHS team. However, it is important for medical staff to be aware of the physical findings in this condition. The person is often ataxic, with contributions to this coming from damage to both the cerebellum and the vestibular apparatus. There is often horizontal or vertical nystagmus and weakness of the lateral rectus muscle causing internal strabismus (squint). The person will complain of diplopia (double vision). Conjugate gaze may be affected and in severe cases the pupils may be miotic (constricted) and non-reactive, and all eye movements absent.

Laboratory investigations

Routine screening blood tests should include full blood examination (FBE or FBC), serum biochemistry (E/LFTs), including electrolytes, glucose, urea, creatinine and liver function tests, thyroid stimulating hormone (TSH), serum vitamin B12 and red cell folate. Syphilis, hepatitis and HIV serology should be reserved for people with risk factors for these conditions. If amnestic disorder is suspected, serum thiamine should be tested.

All older people presenting with confusion should undergo urinalysis with a dipstick system. If abnormalities are evident, then further investigations including blood tests and a mid-stream urine for microscopy and culture are likely to be warranted.

In older people presenting with confusion of unknown cause, particularly when the duration of the confusion is uncertain, it is prudent to obtain an electrocardiogram (ECG) and a troponin or CK–MB level to exclude a recent myocardial infarction. Acute myocardial infarction in older people may present in the absence of chest pain.

The electroencephalogram (EEG) is often useful in the work-up of people with suspected delirium because in this condition it may show a significant excess of slow-wave activity. In contrast, in dementia and amnestic disorder, the EEG is either unremarkable or shows minor non-specific abnormalities.

Neuroimaging

The main types of neuroimaging are computed tomography (CT), magnetic resonance imaging (MRI), single photon emission computed tomography (SPECT) and positron emission tomography (PET). In practice, CT, MRI and SPECT are in common use, whereas PET is restricted to research uses and special clinical situations. CT scans use X-rays to produce structural images of the brain, whereas MRI scans use the interaction between a powerful magnetic field and radio frequency waves to produce structural images of the brain. By contrast, SPECT and PET scans both use radioisotopes to produce functional images of the brain.

CT brain scans are the most commonly utilised neuroimaging modality in older people with dementia, delirium or amnestic disorder because they are relatively inexpensive and widely available. MRI scans produce better quality images, particularly of cerebrovascular disease, and are the preferred neuroimaging modality in older people. However, they are more expensive and less widely available than CT scans. In addition, some older people are not able to undergo an MRI scan because of the presence of ferromagnetic metal implants or fragments. Furthermore, some people are reluctant to enter the MRI scanner because of its narrow aperture.

In dementia due to Alzheimer's disease in older people, structural brain scans (CT and MRI) often show symmetrical shrinkage of the brain together with widening of the cerebral sulci (the gaps between the cerebral gyri) and dilation of the cerebral ventricles (the cerebrospinal fluid-containing spaces within the brain). The hippocampi are usually disproportionately atrophic. However, such changes also occur to a lesser extent with normal ageing and it is not yet possible to reliably diagnose Alzheimer's disease on a single structural brain scan.

CT and MRI brain scans are undertaken during the work-up of people suspected of having dementia to assess the extent of cerebrovascular disease and to exclude rare causes of dementia including brain tumour and multiple sclerosis. In some cases of frontotemporal dementia, structural brain scans may reveal lobar atrophy.

Structural brain scans are often normal in older people with delirium or amnestic disorder.

In research settings, special radioligands (a biologically active molecule with a radioactive tracer attached) are being used to image beta amyloid in people suspected of having Alzheimer's disease. However, this technique does not yet have the specificity to be useful clinically.

Rating scales

A very large number of rating scales have been developed to rate older people with dementia or delirium. Scales to measure BPSD suitable for use by nurses have been reviewed (Neville & Byrne 2001). The short list below includes some of the commonly used scales. The authors have found these scales useful in various community settings when assessing older people who may have cognitive impairment. See also Chapter 35 for more on rating scales.

Cognitive screening

Commonly used scales for cognitive screening include:
- the Mini-Mental State Examination (MMSE)
- the Rowland Universal Dementia Assessment Scale (RUDAS)
- the Montreal Cognitive Assessment (MoCA)
- the Hopkins Verbal Learning Test–Revised (HVLT–R)
- the cognitive examination component of the Cambridge Mental Disorders of the Elderly Examination (CAMCOG)
- Addenbrooke's Cognitive Examination–Revised (ACE–R), and
- the Informant Questionnaire for Cognitive Decline in the Elderly (IQCODE).

Behavioural and psychological symptoms

Commonly used scales for behavioural and psychological symptoms include:
- the Dementia Behavior Disturbance Scale (DBDS)
- the Neuropsychiatric Inventory (NPI)
- the NPI–NH (Nursing Home version)
- the NPI–Q (Quick version)
- the Cornell Scale for Depression in Dementia (CSDD), and
- the Cohen-Mansfield Agitation Inventory (CMAI).

Other useful scales

Other useful scales are:
- the Modified Barthel Index (MBI)
- the Disability Assessment for Dementia (DAD)
- the Zarit Caregiver Burden Scale (ZCBS), and
- the Confusion Assessment Method (CAM).

TREATMENT OUTLINES

Dementia

The treatment outline for dementia is as follows:
- Most people with dementia can be managed in the community.
- Dementia complicated by severe depression or psychotic symptoms, or by marked behavioural abnormalities, may require hospitalisation.
- Where relevant, psychoeducation may be provided for the person, the family and health workers.

- If the dementia is mild, consider implementing memory optimisation strategies (for example, see Sargeant & Unkenstein 2001)
- The person will require a driving assessment. These are often provided by specialist occupational therapy clinics. The assessment should include:
  o a history of the person's driving performance (e.g. from family)
  o an off-road assessment, and
  o an on-road individualised driving test.
- Capacity and legal issues (will, enduring power of attorney, advance health directive) should be assessed.
- Consider respite care (day, in-home, twilight, overnight, holiday).
- Conduct a carer assessment (for burden, distress, depression).
- Make contact with Alzheimer's Australia (for information, support, counselling, respite, advocacy).
- Assess residential care options (low care, high care, secure).
- Assess non-pharmacological behavioural management, including:
  o consider any challenging behaviours in the light of the person's premorbid personality and usual habits
  o define and identify target behaviour
  o chart the frequency of behaviour
  o consider the care environment
  o consider carer behaviour (this is a frequent precipitant of the person's behaviour)
  o consider simple measures (e.g. distraction, massage with aromatherapy oil, individualised music), and
  o undertake formal behaviour modification using the A–B–C (antecedent–behaviour–consequence) approach: stimulus control and contingency management.
- Consider use of cholinesterase inhibitors (donepezil, rivastigmine, galantamine) to enhance cognitive function. Overall, these drugs are modestly effective for the symptomatic treatment of cognitive impairment in Alzheimer's disease. It is important to advise the person and the family about the modest efficacy and adverse effects (especially the initial gastrointestinal effects) of these drugs. These drugs are contraindicated in uncontrolled asthma, active peptic ulcer disease and heart block. Initiate treatment at the lowest available dose and wait at least 1 month before increasing the dose. Then review cognitive performance after 2–3 months of treatment.
- Consider use of an NMDA-receptor antagonist (memantine). Overall, this drug is modestly effective for symptomatic treatment of cognitive impairment in Alzheimer's disease. It is important to advise the person and the family about modest efficacy and adverse effects. Memantine must be titrated up from the starting dose of 5 mg daily to a final dose of 10 mg twice daily over 4 weeks.
- Consider use of antidepressant medication (e.g. sertraline, citalopram, moclobemide) for dementia complicated by clinically significant depression. Watch for hyponatraemia (low serum sodium concentration).
- Where necessary for physical aggression, marked agitation or distressing psychotic symptoms, consider use of atypical antipsychotic medication (low-dose risperidone, with a starting dose of 0.25–0.5 mg once or twice daily). Watch for Parkinsonism, which may develop after several months of treatment. Review with the mindset of stopping the drug after 3 months of treatment.

Amnestic disorder

The treatment outline for amnestic disorder is as follows:

- Admit urgently to hospital if delirium is present (this is often the quiet delirium of Wernicke's encephalopathy).
- If the Wernicke-Korsakoff syndrome is suspected, administer thiamine 100 mg by intramuscular injection and follow with thiamine at a dose of at least 300 mg per day orally.
- Assess the person for other nutritional deficiencies and replace as necessary (e.g. protein, vitamin B12, folate, magnesium, zinc).
- Provide general treatment measures for delirium (see below).
- If amnestic disorder is present in the absence of delirium and the Wernicke-Korsakoff syndrome is suspected, administer thiamine at a dose of at least 300 mg per day.
- Provide alcohol detoxification measures.
- Consider ongoing management and relapse prevention for alcohol dependence.
- Assess and treat other associated conditions (e.g. gastrointestinal disease).
- If amnestic disorder does not appear to be due to thiamine deficiency, work-up the person for other causes (usually undertaken on an inpatient basis).

Delirium

The treatment outline for delirium is as follows:

- Some older people with mild delirium with a clear cause (e.g. a person with an otherwise uncomplicated urinary tract infection or a person with terminal cancer receiving palliative care) can be managed in the home or RACF environment. However, in most other cases, it is prudent to admit the person with delirium to hospital without delay. The person with delirium of unknown aetiology is usually managed on the general medical ward.
- Nurse in an orientating environment with familiar objects.
- Encourage contact with family and friends.
- Provide excellent general medical and nursing care.
- Provide fluids, nutrition and vitamins as needed.
- Identify and treat underlying medical condition(s).
- Consider short-term symptomatic use of low-dose antipsychotic medication (e.g. haloperidol 0.5 mg or risperidone 0.5 mg) if psychotic symptoms are highly distressing or if behaviour is dangerous.
- Give regular oxazepam (e.g. 15–30 mg up to four times per day) if the suspected aetiology is withdrawal from benzodiazepines or alcohol.

PREVENTION

If the onset of dementia could be delayed by 5 years, this would lead over time to almost a halving of its prevalence. Unfortunately, this seems a rather distant prospect. The main hope at present is that current vaccine trials that target the putative disease mechanism underlying Alzheimer's disease will lead both to an effective treatment and a preventive measure. Otherwise, one must turn to epidemiological studies of risk factors for dementia for data on potential preventive measures. However, those that have undergone rigorous randomised controlled trials, such as oestrogen, non-steroidal anti-inflammatory drugs

(NSAIDs) and vitamin E, have all failed to demonstrate preventive effects. Oestrogen has been associated with an increased risk of dementia in older women. Clinical trials of physical activity and effortful mental activity are now underway.

SUMMARY

The older person with confusion is core business for the clinician working in an OPMHS. Although most such older people will have dementia, it is important to remain vigilant for those with delirium or amnestic disorder, as both the latter conditions require an urgent medical response.

FURTHER READING

Burns A, O'Brien J, Ames D (eds) 2005 Dementia, 3rd edn. Hodder Arnold, London

Inouye SK, van Dyck CH, Alessi CA et al 1990 Clarifying confusion: the confusion assessment method. A new method for detection of delirium. Annals of Internal Medicine 113(12): 941–948

Kitwood T 1997 Dementia reconsidered: the person comes first. Open University Press, Buckingham

Lindesay J, Rockwood K, Macdonald A 2002 Delirium in old age. Oxford Medical Publications, Oxford

Mace NL, Rabins PV 2006 The 36-hour day: a family guide to caring for people with Alzheimer's disease, other dementias, and memory loss in later life, 4th edn. Johns Hopkins University Press, Baltimore

Wei LA, Fearing MA, Sternberg EJ, Inouye SK 2008 The Confusion Assessment Method: a systematic review of current usage. Journal of the American Geriatrics Society 56(5):823–830

REFERENCES

Harper C, Fornes P, Duyckaerts C et al 1995 An international perspective on the prevalence of the Wernicke-Korsakoff syndrome. Metabolic Brain Disease 10(1):17–24

Harper CG, Sheedy DL, Lara AI et al 1998 Prevalence of Wernicke-Korsakoff syndrome in Australia: has thiamine fortification made a difference? Medical Journal of Australia 168(11):542–545

Neville CC, Byrne GJA 2001 Rating scales for disruptive behaviour in older people with dementia: which is best for nurses to use? Australasian Journal on Ageing 20(4):166–172

Sargeant D, Unkenstein A 2001 Remembering well: how memory works and what to do when it doesn't, 2nd edn. Allen & Unwin, Sydney

Chapter 20

THE OLDER PERSON WITH MOOD SYMPTOMS

INTRODUCTION

Depression is one of the most common mental health problems to affect older people and it usually responds well to treatment. Despite this fact, it remains underrecognised and undertreated. There appears to be a pervasive myth, at least in developed countries, that depression and old age go together because at this time of life there is a decline in physical health and older people experience significant losses, such as the loss of meaningful employment and death of a spouse. On the other hand, many older people are very satisfied with their life and look forward to what older age will bring (Nierenberg 2001). Mental health workers are in the ideal position to be aware of the key symptoms of depression, to know that older people respond to antidepressant medication and that psychological treatments may also be successful in both effecting a remission and in preventing a relapse in the longer term.

This chapter begins with a case vignette that illustrates a common presentation of an older person with depression who has been referred to an older persons' mental health service (OPMHS). It highlights how events that have occurred earlier in an older person's life can contribute to depression. It considers the family support that is often needed and an approach to treatment planning.

This chapter considers the prevalence of depression in older people and the clinical features of depression, and then provides a detailed outline of the clinical management of depression. Although depression is a risk factor for suicide, suicide is addressed in a separate chapter (see Ch 21), as is the closely associated topic of anxiety (see Ch 23). This chapter ends with a discussion about mania. Mania may present for the first time in an older person and it is often associated with serious comorbidity.

CASE VIGNETTE

Michael, aged 83, had been referred to the OPMHS by his general practitioner (GP) for treatment of depression. The GP had tried to treat Michael's severe depression with a combination of antidepressant and antipsychotic medication, but Michael had experienced serious complications, including frequent falls. In the initial interview, the following history emerged. Michael had been born in Australia and was of

Anglo-Saxon origin. Although retired for a considerable number of years, he had spent his working life as a motor mechanic. Nowadays, he occupied his time by meticulously maintaining his house and garden. He had been married to Doris for 55 years and they had three sons, all of whom were well established with their own families and businesses in the same town as their parents. The family relationships were assessed as being functional and close.

Over the past month, Michael had become increasingly irritable, anxious and worried that a petty theft he had committed as a young apprentice would be uncovered and that his life savings and family home would be taken away in order to pay compensation. He continually watched out the front window of his house at passing cars, expecting them to be the police. He thought the mental health worker undertaking the interview was an undercover police officer and that various objects around the room were secret radio devices. Michael's appetite and sleeping habits had deteriorated and he continually ruminated over his past misdeed. However, he was otherwise in good health.

After routine physical tests, Michael was admitted voluntarily as an inpatient for electroconvulsive therapy (ECT). He was assessed by the OPMHS as suffering from a severe major depressive disorder with psychotic features. This was the first time the family had been in contact with a mental health service and they needed extensive explanations and reassurance about the care and treatment that was planned for Michael. He responded well to ECT and on returning home his treatment included continuation treatment with an antidepressant medication, regular interpersonal therapy sessions at the OPMHS, and home visits by a mental health worker.

Key issues at assessment

Key issues included:
- first contact with a mental health service (no previous mental health problems)
- good social circumstances
- 4-week history of irritable mood and agitation
- poor response to antidepressants and antipsychotics
- recurrent falls
- guilty ruminations
- psychotic symptoms, and
- poor sleep and appetite.

EPIDEMIOLOGY

Depression is a global health problem and soon it will rate as the second largest cause of disease burden (World Health Organization 2001). The age-adjusted community prevalence of clinically significant depression in older Australians is 8.2% (95% CI = 7.8–8.6%), with the rate for men at 8.6% (95% CI = 7.9–9.2%) and women at 7.9% (95% CI = 7.4–8.4%). The male and female age-adjusted rate for 'major depressive episode' is 1.8% (95% CI = 1.6–2.0%) (Pirkis et al 2009). However, in environments where there is a concentration of older people, such as RACFs, the prevalence of depressive illness increases, with reported figures around 10% (O'Connor 2006). It is also well established that up to 30% of older people who are medical patients in general hospitals have major depression (Cole 2008). Recent spousal bereavement, functional impairment and physical illnesses, such as myocardial infarction, stroke and cancer, all increase the likelihood of an older person developing a depressive illness (Pfaff et al 2009).

Depression can present with varying severity. Criteria for major depression, dysthymia and adjustment disorders with depressed mood are outlined in *The Diagnostic and Statistical Manual of Mental Disorders* (American Psychiatric Association 2000) (see the box below). Differentiating between the different types of depression depends upon the duration and number of symptoms. Dysthymia is a chronic low-grade depression, while adjustment disorders with depressed mood are depressive reactions to adverse life events that do not meet diagnostic criteria for major depression. Major depression is the most clinically significant and will be the focus of this chapter.

DSM–IV DIAGNOSTIC CRITERIA FOR A MAJOR DEPRESSIVE EPISODE

The diagnostic criteria are a 2-week history of depressed or irritable mood and/or reduced interest or pleasure together with a total of at least five of the nine listed symptoms:

1. depressed or irritable mood
2. reduced interest in usual activities or reduced ability to experience pleasure (anhedonia)
3. poor sleep (insomnia or hypersomnia)
4. altered appetite or weight (reduced appetite and weight loss or increased appetite and weight gain)
5. impaired concentration
6. reduced energy or fatigue
7. psychomotor agitation or retardation
8. hopelessness and guilt, and
9. suicidal thoughts or behaviour.

RISK FACTORS

Risk factors for depression include:

- a previous history of depression
- mild symptoms of depression
- family history (particularly early-onset depression)
- a childhood history of emotional, physical or sexual abuse
- premorbid personality (particularly high levels of trait neuroticism)
- bereavement
- limited social support
- stroke and cerebrovascular disease
- acute myocardial infarction (if depression is untreated, there may be an increased mortality rate)
- chronic insomnia, and
- medication (e.g. benzodiazepines, corticosteroids, interferon, gonadotrophin-releasing hormone antagonists, propranolol and some chemotherapy).

CLINICAL FEATURES

The clinical features of depression vary quite widely in later life.

Thought content symptoms

Thought content symptoms include:
- *Anhedonia.* There is an inability to experience pleasure where pleasure was previously experienced. The person may withdraw from family, friends, hobbies and activities.
- *Demoralisation.* The person is not confident in their abilities.
- *Pessimism.* The person believes that something bad will happen and there is no hope for the future.
- *Worthlessness.* The person believes they are undeserving of attention and concern.
- *Hopelessness.* The person believes they have nothing to look forward to and there is nothing they can do to help themselves.
- *Helplessness.* The person believes no one else can help them.
- *Guilt.* The person has distorted beliefs about current or past failings or blames themselves for some untoward event.

Neurovegetative symptoms

Neurovegetative symptoms include:
- *Sleep disturbance.* In older people, sleep disturbance generally involves insomnia, although occasionally hypersomnia can also be a symptom of depression. Insomnia in depression can include difficulty getting off to sleep, frequent waking during the night, or waking early in the morning.
- *Appetite disturbance.* In older people with depression, appetite disturbance usually involves reduced appetite, although occasionally it can involve increased appetite. The older person does not enjoy food, eats less and loses weight.

Sleep and appetite disturbance and lethargy are common accompaniments, but these are also found in older people who are not depressed, so these are not strong discriminatory symptoms.

Behavioural symptoms

Behavioural symptoms include:
- *Psychomotor retardation.* The person has slowed monotonous speech, increased pauses before answering (speech latency), reduced facial mobility, slow body movements, decreased amount of speech (poverty of speech) or muteness.
- *Fine motor agitation.* The person is not able to sit still, paces, wrings hands, and pulls hair or clothes.

Other symptoms

Crying is an uncommon symptom in depression, but older people with depression may become overly distressed to seemingly minor life occurrences where previously they would have been quite stoical. The older person may also display excessively 'needy' or dependent behaviour. The mental health worker needs to distinguish between dependent behaviour as a manifestation of a lifelong personality style or dependent behaviour as a result of psychological regression in depression.

Depression may also present somatically. This is a common presentation for people from non-Anglo-Saxon backgrounds. The older person may present with symptoms indicative of cardiorespiratory, gastrointestinal or neurological illness. As a consequence, medical assessment, with a detailed physical examination, laboratory investigations and neuroimaging, is often needed to rule out these disorders. However, the mental health worker needs to be mindful that actually experiencing and reporting a greater number of physical symptoms is common for an older person with depression.

Another clinical feature to be aware of is 'smiling depression'. The socially ingrained habit of many older people of being polite, pleasant and smiling, particularly on initial interactions with people, can mislead the inexperienced mental health worker into thinking the older person could not possibly be depressed (Neville & Byrne 2009). Some older people deny feeling depressed, even though they have many other symptoms of major depression.

COMORBIDITY

Depression is often complicated by anxiety disorders, substance-use disorders, physical disorders, dementia and delirium. Approximately 35% of older people with a major depressive disorder also meet the criteria for generalised anxiety disorder. If the generalised anxiety disorder is not treated alongside the depressive disorder, there is an increased risk of delayed remission, early relapse or recurrence. Substance-use disorders are relatively common in older people and it usually involves abuse of alcohol and/or benzodiazepines, and this may complicate depression. Depression is common after a person suffers a stroke or myocardial infarction or is diagnosed and treated for cancer. The presence of depression complicates the outcomes for physical disorders.

Depressive symptoms often coexist with vascular dementia and vascular cognitive impairment and are common in the mild and moderate stages of dementia. It is frequently reported that depression is an early feature of dementia with the suggestion that the neurodegenerative changes in the ageing brain lead first to late-onset depression and then to dementia. Depression and cognitive impairment (usually dementia) are risk factors for the development of delirium and a significant number of older people with delirium (up to 25%) have undiagnosed dementia (Fick et al 2002).

DIFFERENTIAL DIAGNOSIS

A common feature of depression, dementia and delirium is that they are all underrecognised and undertreated, and differentiating between these three syndromes is sometimes difficult. Table 20.1 sums up some of the key differences.

Other common disorders that are easily mistaken for depression include anxiety, Parkinson's disease and the excessive sedation caused by certain medications or combinations of medication (polypharmacy). Cancer and chronic infections may present in a similar manner to depression. People who have suffered a stroke are often tearful and emotional, but this emotionality should not be confused with depression. Of course, stroke is commonly complicated by depressive disorder.

Table 20.1 Comparison of depression, delirium and dementia

Defining Dimension	Depression	Delirium	Dementia
Onset	Abrupt or gradual (develops over weeks to months)	Sudden (develops over hours or days)	Slow and insidious (develops over several years)
Aetiology	Multifactorial (genetic, physiological, psychosocial)	Related to general medical conditions or psychosocial changes	May be linked genetically and to specific medical conditions, such as HIV or Parkinson's disease
Duration	Acute: from 2 weeks to 6 months Chronic: many years	A couple of days to weeks	Until death (months to years)
Progression	Self-limited or chronic without treatment	Fast and fluctuating, but temporary if underlying condition is treated	Slow, stable with a continuous and permanent decline in abilities and cognition
Symptoms	Do not fluctuate	Fluctuate rapidly	Tend not to fluctuate
Cognitive changes			
Consciousness	Clear	Clouded	Clear
Orientation	Unaffected	Disorientated	Alters in accordance with severity of dementia
Speech	'I don't know' is a common response	Incoherent or unable to respond	May use confabulation, repetition, aphasia in later stages
Thought content	Negative	Confused	Disorganised and sometimes delusional

(Continued)

Table 20.1 Comparison of depression, delirium and dementia—cont'd			
Defining Dimension	Depression	Delirium	Dementia
Perception	May be distorted	Misinterpretations common	Occasionally distorted
Attention span	May experience some difficulty	Reduced	Fluctuates
Affect	Flat	Labile	Labile and apathetic
Memory	Generally unaffected	Impaired	Impaired
Insight	May be some impairment	May have some if lucid	Only in early stages
Judgment	Poor	Poor	Poor
Psychomotor activity	Agitation or retardation	Abnormally increased or reduced	Often normal
Behaviour	Fatigued, apathetic, occasionally agitated	Varies from agitation to unresponsiveness	May or may not have behavioural symptoms
Sleep	Early morning wakening	Often disturbed	Often disturbed
Activities of daily living	Not inclined	Unable	Struggles

It is important also to differentiate between depression and grief. Older people are exposed to many grief-provoking situations, such as losing a loved one, job retrenchment, reduced income, and the presence of physical illness and disability. Grief, with its various cultural expressions, is a normal process and it should only be medically treated if the usual symptoms become more severe and persist for more than a few months.

ASSESSMENT

The principles of assessing an older person with depression rely on taking a systematic approach, which begins with an extensive history, mental state examination (MSE) and physical examination, together with selected laboratory investigations. Rating scales for depression such as the Geriatric Depression Scale (GDS) (Sheikh & Yesavage 1986) and the Cornell Scale for Depression in Dementia (CSDD) (Alexopoulos et al 1988) are also useful adjuncts for the assessment process. It is worthwhile asking the older person whether they have ever been depressed before, as a history of depression greatly increases the probability that their current symptoms are part of a depressive syndrome (Cole 2008).

It is often appropriate for the mental health worker to conduct the initial assessment with the older person alone, particularly if there is suspicion of elder abuse or domestic violence. With the older person's permission, the involvement of others such as family members, neighbours, their GP and any other health professionals who have been in contact with the older person is extremely important for the provision of corroborating evidence. Due consideration must also be given to the older person's level of cognitive function, as well as their ability to see and hear.

History

Initially, it is important to establish if the depression has been a recent occurrence or whether it has been present at other times in the older person's life. Because the aetiology of depression involves a complex mix of biological, psychological and social factors, it is logical to take a life-span approach to history taking, starting from birth (they may have been adopted) and early development, to schooling, relationships with parents, siblings, friends, spouse and children, and experience of major generational-specific events (e.g. childhood poverty during the Great Depression of the 1930s and war experiences during World War II, the Korean War and the Vietnam War). Even in people of advanced years, it is important to inquire about a history of childhood abuse and neglect, as these may have an enduring impact on the risk of depression.

The severity, development and duration of the current episode need to be determined along with the response to any previous treatment the older person may have had. Other factors that need to be determined include premorbid personality, family history of depression, the current symptom profile and the effect on daily functioning. Factors that are maintaining the depression need to be determined. These could include such things as avoidance behaviour (e.g. avoiding social situations), alcohol and drug abuse, and dysfunctional interpersonal relationships. Resilience factors also need to be assessed. These might include high intelligence, good education, extensive social supports, low neuroticism, good general health, sound financial security, and religious beliefs or other types of spirituality.

Mental state examination

Many aspects of the MSE will help in determining whether an older person is depressed. To get maximum accuracy, it is important to give the older person plenty of time to respond to the questions. The mental health worker must take particular care to obtain information regarding severe depressive symptomatology, such as suicidal ideation and psychotic features. Any evidence of cognitive impairment needs careful documentation and investigation.

Physical examination

After detailing current and past physical problems and medications, the conduct of a physical examination, including a neurological examination, is very important to exclude other pathologies or to determine if present physical problems are triggering the depression. If the mental health worker has not been trained to do this themselves, they should arrange for it to be completed by another member of the team or by the older person's GP.

Laboratory investigations

Routine laboratory investigations include urea, serum electrolytes and folate (may be indicative of undernutrition), complete blood count with platelets (may indicate anaemia, vitamin B12 deficiency or alcohol excess), vitamin B12 estimation and thyroid function test (depression is strongly associated with hypothyroidism).

Rating scales

General adult depression scales are considered inappropriate for older people because symptoms indicative of depression in young people, such as sleep disturbance, weight loss and pessimism about the future, may occur in older people as normal effects of ageing or as the result of physical illness. Older people also have more agitation and psychotic and bodily complaints (with no determined physical cause) than younger people. A general description of two depression rating scales suitable for older people with and without dementia is as follows.

Geriatric Depression Scale

The Geriatric Depression Scale (GDS–15) (Sheikh & Yesavage 1986) is a 15-item, brief questionnaire devised from the original 30-item GDS. It is a useful screening tool in the clinical setting to facilitate detection of depression, to measure the severity of depression and to monitor changes in depression during treatment. The GDS does not rely on somatic symptoms. The GDS may be used with healthy, medically ill, and mildly to moderately cognitively impaired older adults. It has been used extensively in community, acute and long-term care settings. Participants are asked to respond to the questions by answering 'yes' or 'no' in reference to how they felt on the day of scale administration. Scores of 0 to 5 are considered as not indicating depression, while scores of 6 to 15 indicate depression. Scores on the GDS have been found to increase significantly with the level of depression. Completion time is 10 minutes.

Cornell Scale for Depression in Dementia

The CSDD (Alexopoulos et al 1988) is a 19-item clinician-rated scale for depressive symptoms in dementia. The items are rated on the basis of observation and on their presence in the last week. It is a 3-point scale—absent (0), mild (1), severe (2)—for a total of a possible 38 points. Suggested cutoff scores are given, with a score of 12 or greater indicating depression. It has high interrater reliability and consistency, as well as correlating significantly with severity of depression. It is sensitive to change, with major depression improving with treatment. Completion time is 15 minutes.

TREATMENT PRINCIPLES

The goal of treatment is for the older person to return to their baseline mental health status or to where residual physical symptoms are explicitly related to an underlying chronic physical illness rather than to depression. For mild depression, non-pharmacological interventions are often sufficient. However, for moderate or severe depression, a combination of pharmacological treatment and non-pharmacological treatment is usually required. Initial treatment is usually conducted in the community, unless it is not safe to treat the older person at home.

In more severe depressive illnesses, hospitalisation and the use of ECT may be required. In such circumstances, the older person and their family members will require extra support from the OPMHS. It has been shown that when the primary care practitioner collaborates with a mental health worker or team, there are more positive outcomes of care (Unutzer 2002). The mental health worker needs to appreciate that response to treatment of depression in older people often takes considerably longer than in young or middle-aged people.

Although non-pharmacological treatments are often better tolerated than pharmacological treatments, a multimodal approach has been found to be ideal in the treatment of depression and in the prevention of relapse. Some treatments are briefly mentioned in this chapter, with more detailed discussion provided in Chapters 29–31.

Pharmacotherapy

Pharmacotherapy has proven useful in moderate to severe depression, particularly when there are symptoms of sleep and appetite disturbance, suicidal thoughts and/or psychosis (delusions and hallucinations). Due to pharmacokinetic and pharmacodynamic changes in older people, they are often more susceptible to adverse effects during antidepressant therapy. Thus, smaller doses of antidepressant medication are often appropriate, particularly at initiation of treatment. Antidepressant medication can take up to 12 weeks to be effective in older people and the older person needs to be warned not to expect instant results. Several different medication trials or combinations of medications may be needed before the optimal treatment regime is established (see Ch 30).

The most common antidepressant medications used in older people are the selective serotonin reuptake inhibitors (SSRIs). Second-line agents are the serotonin and noradrenaline reuptake inhibitor (SNRI) medications, followed by the older tricyclic antidepressants (TCAs) and monoamine oxidase inhibitors (MAOIs). Because of a more severe side-effect profile and poorer tolerance in older people, the TCAs and MAOIs are now generally only used if the depression is unresponsive to newer antidepressants. Combining antidepressant medication with psychotherapy has been found to be very effective for older people. Lithium has also been used to augment antidepressant medication in the treatment of depression. In depression complicated by psychotic symptoms, treatment will usually require combination pharmacotherapy with antidepressants and antipsychotics, or treatment with ECT.

Psychotherapy

Psychotherapy has been found to be effective in group settings and also on an individual basis (see Ch 29). Group therapy is especially appealing for older people who lack sufficient support through their social network. Psychotherapy is particularly useful for the symptoms of anhedonia, demoralisation, pessimism, worthlessness, hopelessness, helplessness, guilt and other problems associated with depression, such as low energy levels, interpersonal problems and treatment compliance issues. These types of interventions increase the rate of recovery and are fundamental in maintaining improvement and preventing relapse.

Cognitive behaviour therapy (CBT) has the goal of altering negative thought patterns and behaviours. Behaviour therapy (BT) has been found to be as effective as CBT. BT commonly utilises the principles of operant conditioning to develop a structured plan for daily activities. Interpersonal psychotherapy (IPT) is particularly useful when helping older people with grief and family issues, as well as resolving conflict or assisting with problem solving and decision making.

Electroconvulsive therapy

Electroconvulsive therapy (ECT) is a well-established, safe, effective and accepted treatment for depression in older people. It is particularly effective when depression is complicated by psychotic symptoms, high suicide risk, inadequate intake of food and fluids, and when depression has failed to respond to trials of antidepressant and antipsychotic medication. ECT is administered under general anaesthesia. Electrodes are placed strategically on a person's scalp and an electrical stimulus that causes a seizure is administered through the electrodes. The person receiving ECT does not experience any pain. Approximately 5–10 minutes after the seizure, the older person wakes up and is monitored for confusion, agitation, headache and any changes in cognition or memory. If the older person has dementia and there is a coexistent depression being treated with ECT, the mental health worker must monitor the older person for delirium and amnesia post-ECT (see Ch 31).

Other treatment options

Other novel treatment options such as exercise, yoga, qigong, meditation, relaxation, music, tai chi, St John's wort, light therapy and acupressure have been used for the treatment of depression in older people. A review of randomised controlled trials for complementary and alternative treatments for depression in older people found that tai chi and acupressure were modestly effective for depression, anxiety and sleep disturbance (Meeks et al 2007). Given the small evidence base for these complementary therapies, there is plenty of scope for more research into these treatments.

Care for the caregiver

An important component of care that is provided by mental health workers is monitoring the mental health of the primary caregivers. These people are essential in the recovery of the older person with depression, yet they are also at risk of developing depression themselves through the strain of caring and poor morale. Therefore, part of every treatment plan should involve assessment of the primary caregivers for depression, as well as the provision of both practical and supportive interventions (Zarit & Zarit 2007).

TREATMENT SUMMARY

Multimodal approach: psychology and pharmacology

A treatment summary is as follows for a multimodal approach:

1. CBT, behaviour therapy and interpersonal therapy
2. exercise, tai chi and acupressure
3. antidepressants/antipsychotics and St John's wort, and
4. ECT.

PREVENTION OF DEPRESSION

Prevention of depression is of fundamental importance because the effectiveness of available treatments for depression in older people is relatively modest. Improvement and recovery are slow and the chance of relapse and recurrence are high (Cole 2008). The contributing environmental factors for depression have been identified as social and economic difficulties and poor health. Thus, preventive strategies lie with improving the general welfare and standard of living of older people. Early detection and treatment of physical illness and pathological grief by the older person's GP is likely to be one effective preventive strategy for depression. Maintaining or establishing strong social support networks is equally important. Public awareness campaigns and training for health professionals so that they are highly skilled at screening, detecting and treating depression are additional important preventive strategies (Cole 2008) (see Ch 26).

MANIA IN OLDER PEOPLE

Mania and hypomania episodes are the hallmarks of bipolar disorder and distinguish it from unipolar major depressive disorder. Bipolar disorder, in which there are usually alternating episodes of mania and depression, is primarily classified according to the severity of the manic symptoms. Episodes of major depression in bipolar disorder are often indistinguishable from episodes of major depression in major depressive disorder. Four distinct subtypes of the manic syndrome have been proposed by Shulman and Herrmann (2002):

1. *Primary bipolar disorder.* This type includes that which manifested early in life and persists into old age.
2. *Latent bipolar disorder.* This type includes people who have developed mania in late life after many earlier episodes of depression.
3. *Secondary mania (disinhibition syndromes).* This type is very late onset where there is no prior history and can be in association with a general medical disorder or an organic mental disorder.
4. *Unipolar mania.* This type involves manic-only episodes.

Epidemiology

The prevalence of mania in older people living in the community is reported at <0.1% (Weissman et al 1996). In a study conducted in Western Australia with patients diagnosed with bipolar disorder (N = 6182), it was found that 8% were aged 65 years or over at the time of first contact with mental health services (Almeida & Fenner 2002). A 35-year study conducted in the UK found 10% of people aged 60 years and over had an onset of mania (Kennedy et al 2005). Greenwald et al (1992) found that bipolar disorder was present in 9.7% of RACF residents, although this figure seems remarkably high and might reflect local factors. In later life, bipolar disorder is more likely to affect women (Almeida & Fenner 2002, Sajatovic et al 2005), but, overall, the prevalence of bipolar disorder declines in later life (Kennedy et al 2005). The ethnic distribution of this condition is uncertain (Depp & Jeste 2004). Bipolar disorder is often a serious, chronic and very debilitating disorder, and sometimes leads to permanent functional impairment and heavy use of medical services.

Clinical features

The clinical features of bipolar disorder in older people do not differ that much from younger people. However, with older people, there can be significant associated changes in cognitive function. The common clinical features include:

- elevated or irritable mood
- hostility
- overactivity
- pressure of speech
- reduced requirement for sleep
- grandiose or persecutory thought content
- poor insight and judgment, and
- inappropriate behaviour such as financial and sexual indiscretions.

Comorbidity

Older people with bipolar disorder commonly have a number of comorbid conditions and this makes making a clear diagnosis of mania difficult. These comorbid conditions include cerebrovascular disease, diabetes and other neurological disorders (Depp & Jeste 2004, Tohen et al 1994). Sajatovic et al (2005) found that late-life bipolar disorder is associated with a mean of 3.7 comorbid medical conditions, substantial health service usage (average length of stay 14.8 days per admission) and polypharmacy usage. Psychiatric comorbidity extends to substance abuse, post-traumatic stress disorder, personality disorders, anxiety and dementia (Depp & Jeste 2004, Sajatovic et al 2006).

Differential diagnosis

Mania in older people needs to be distinguished from disorders that can also present with irritable mood, emotional lability, sleep disturbance and impaired social judgment, such as dementia, delirium and agitated depression (Forester et al 2006).

Assessment

The mental health worker should take a detailed history from the person with probable bipolar disorder. This should include their lifelong history of symptoms of mental disorder, their use of substances, and their social and occupational history. The presence of impaired insight or cognitive impairment may make it necessary to obtain corroborating evidence from another person who knows the older person well. An MSE would also be undertaken and these assessment processes could be augmented with a rating scale. The Young Mania Rating Scale (Young et al 1978) and the Mania Rating Scale (Bech et al 1978) have been used in studies for older people with mania, but it is unclear whether these have been adequately validated with this group.

Treatment principles

The clinical features of mania, such as lack of insight and judgment, and irrational behaviour, make hospitalisation almost inevitable. This is primarily done to ensure the older person's safety, as they are often vulnerable to physical, financial and sexual abuse when in a manic state.

Non-pharmacological therapies

The efficacy of non-pharmacological therapies such as psychotherapy for the manic aspect of bipolar disorder in older people has not been well addressed in the treatment literature. Individualised psychological treatment plans may be developed from the approaches described in Chapter 29. However, in many instances, there will be practical difficulties in implementing such treatment plans while the older person's mood remains significantly elevated. Symptoms such as extreme overactivity and excessive excitement can compromise the physical health status of an older person and medical resuscitation may sometimes be needed.

Pharmacological therapies

Major depression in bipolar disorder is treated as described earlier in this chapter, although antidepressant medication is generally used in combination with a mood stabiliser to minimise the risk of precipitating a manic episode.

Mania can be treated with atypical antipsychotic medications to reduce symptoms and improve functional status (Sajatovic et al 2008a). The mood stabilisers lithium, valproate and carbamazpeine are also used to reduce the frequency, severity and duration of episodes (Sajatovic et al 2008b). Lithium therapy has to be monitored closely in older people through regular serum-level estimations, as elevated serum levels can be toxic. For the prevention of relapse, there is often a need for long-term pharmacological therapies. The older person and their family should be provided with information regarding the early signs of relapse. These may vary from person to person.

Older people with mania who do not respond to treatment with antipsychotics and mood stabilisers may require treatment with ECT (Shulman 1994).

SUMMARY

Depression in older people is one of the mental health problems that can be successfully treated with a combination of psychological therapies and antidepressant medication. Mania in older people is also responsive to treatment, although empirical research lags behind clinical practice.

FURTHER READING

Baldwin RC, Chui E, Katona C, Graham N 2002 Guidelines on depression in older people: practising the evidence. Martin Dunitz, London
Manthorpe J, Illife S 2005 Depression in later life. Jessica Kingsley, Philadelphia

USEFUL WEBSITES

Australian National Depression Initiative: www.beyondblue.org.au
Black Dog Institute: www.blackdoginstitute.org.au

REFERENCES

Alexopoulos GS, Abrams RC, Young RC et al 1988 Cornell Scale for Depression in Dementia. Biological Psychiatry 23(3):271–284
Almeida OP, Fenner S 2002 Bipolar disorder: similarities and differences between patients with illness onset before and after 65 years of age. International Psychogeriatrics 14(3):311–322

American Psychiatric Association 2000 The diagnostic and statistical manual of mental disorders, 4th edn. American Psychiatric Publishing, Washington DC

Bech P, Rafaelsen OJ, Kramp P, Bolwig TG 1978 The Mania Rating Scale: scale construction and inter-observer agreement. Neuropharmacology 17(6):430–431

Cole M 2008 Brief interventions to prevent depression in older subjects: a systematic review of feasibility and effectiveness. American Journal of Geriatric Psychiatry 16(6):435–443

Depp CA, Jeste DV 2004 Bipolar disorder in older adults: a critical review. Bipolar Disorders 6:343–367

Fick DM, Agostini JV, Inouye SK 2002 Delirium superimposed on dementia: a systematic review. Journal of the American Geriatrics Society 50(10):1723–1732

Forester B, Antognini FC, Stoll A 2006 Geriatric bipolar disorder. In: Agronin ME, Maletta GJ (eds) Principles and practice of geriatric psychiatry. Lippincott Williams & Wilkins, Philadelphia

Greenwald BS, Kreman N, Aupperle P 1992 Tailoring adult psychiatric practices to the field of geriatrics. Psychiatric Quarterly 63:343–362

Kennedy N, Everitt B, Boydell J et al 2005 Incidence and distribution of first-episode mania by age: results from a 35-year study. Psychological Medicine 35(6):855–863

Meeks TW, Wetherell JL, Irwin MR et al 2007 Complementary and alternative treatments for late-life depression, anxiety, and sleep disturbance: a review of randomized controlled trials. Journal of Clinical Psychiatry 68(10):1461–1471

Neville C, Byrne GJA 2009 Depression and suicide in older people. In: Nay R, Garratt S (eds) Older people: issues and innovations in care. Elsevier, Sydney

Nierenberg AA 2001 Current perspectives on the diagnosis and treatment of major depressive disorder. American Journal of Managed Care 7(11):S353–S366

O'Connor DW 2006 Do older Australians truly have low rates of anxiety and depression? A critique of the 1997 National Survey of Mental Health and Wellbeing. Australian and New Zealand Journal of Psychiatry 40(8):623–631

Pfaff JJ, Draper BM, Pikis JE et al 2009 Medical morbidity and severity of depression in a large primary care sample of older Australians: the DEPS–GP project. Medical Journal of Australia 190(7Suppl):S75–S80

Pirkis J, Pfaff J, Williamson M et al 2009 The community prevalence of depression in older Australians. Journal of Affective Disorders 115(1–2):54–61

Sajatovic M, Bingham R, Campbell EA, Fletcher DF 2005 Bipolar disorder in older adult inpatients. Journal of Nervous and Mental Disease 193(6):417–419

Sajatovic M, Blow FC, Ignacio RV 2006 Psychiatric comorbidity in older adults with bipolar disorder. International Journal of Geriatric Psychiatry 21:582–587

Sajatovic M, Calabrese JR, Mullen J 2008a Quetiapine for the treatment of bipolar mania in older adults. Bipolar Disorders 10:662–671

Sajatovic M, Coconcea N, Ignacio RV et al 2008b Aripiprazole therapy in 20 older adults with bipolar disorder: a 12-week, open-label trial. Journal of Clinical Psychiatry 69(1):41–46

Sheikh RL, Yesavage JA 1986 Geriatric Depression Scale (GDS): recent evidence and development of a shorter version. Clinical Gerontologist 5:165–173

Shulman K 1994 Mania in late life: conceptual and clinical issues. In: Chui E, Ames D (eds) Functional psychiatric disorders of the elderly. Cambridge University Press, Melbourne

Shulman KI, Herrmann N 2002 Manic syndromes in old age. In: Jacoby R, Oppenheimer C (eds) Psychiatry in the elderly. Oxford University Press, Oxford

Tohen M, Shulman KL, Satlin A 1994 First-episode mania in late-life. American Journal of Psychiatry 151:130–132

Unutzer J 2002 Diagnosis and treatment of older adults with depression in primary care. Biological Psychiatry 52(3):285–292

Weissman MM, Bland RC, Canino GJ et al 1996 Cross-national epidemiology of major depression and bipolar disorder. Journal of the American Medical Association 276:293–299

World Health Organization (WHO) 2001 The world health report 2001: mental health: new understanding, new hope. WHO, Geneva

Young RC, Biggs J, Ziegler V, Meyer D 1978 A rating scale for mania: reliability, validity, and sensitivity. British Journal of Psychiatry 133:429–435

Zarit SH, Zarit JM 2007 Mental disorders in older adults. Guilford Press, New York

Chapter 21

THE OLDER PERSON WITH SUICIDAL THOUGHTS

INTRODUCTION

Some of the highest rates for suicide are found among older people, particularly men. Yet despite this fact, older people are often left out of discussions on suicide for a number of reasons (Mitty & Flores 2008). These include more emphasis given to youth suicide because the young carry a higher economic burden and, where ageist attitudes prevail, feelings of wanting to die and hopelessness are sometimes considered normal for older people. Unfortunately, these attitudes also manifest in clinical practice where it may not be considered important to ask an older person about suicidal feelings and, consequently, they are less likely to be offered assertive treatment (O'Connell 2005).

There has been a significant decline in late-life suicides over the last decade or so (Australian Bureau of Statistics 2007). However, the increased prevalence of depression and suicide attempts among middle-aged people, particularly the large number of baby boomers who are now beginning to reach the status of being older people, may be suggestive of a generational effect that will carry over into the coming decades, boding late-life suicide as a looming major public health concern. Suicide is a tragic event for all the people involved, including mental health workers. The purpose of this chapter is to highlight the trends and themes concerning suicide and older people, and create an awareness of risk factors and the role they have in the prevention of suicide. Effective interventions are also detailed to reduce the morbidity and mortality associated with suicide in older people.

CASE VIGNETTE

Tom is a 67-year-old, unmarried, retired farmer. He had been discovered by his neighbour early one morning preparing to hang himself from a tree in the backyard. The neighbour had rung the police who took Tom to the local hospital's emergency department. Tom was admitted voluntarily to the psychiatric unit. He had been there for a week and was being discharged home. He had been referred to the older persons' mental health service (OPMHS) on admission for intensive follow-up on discharge. Staff of the OPMHS had been involved in the treatment decisions. Tom was not cognitively impaired, he was diagnosed with a mild depression and had been prescribed an antidepressant medication.

During his admission, the following personal problems had been identified:

- *Unresolved grief over the loss of his mother and farm life.* Tom and his mother had sold their farm and moved to a regional town 5 years previously. His mother required ongoing medical treatment for cancer and Tom had cared for her by himself until she had died 9 months ago.
- *Loneliness and limited social support.* Tom had been asked to leave his local church because a female volunteer who had been visiting him after his mother's death had interpreted a display of affection from Tom as being sexually motivated. Despite denying this was the intention, Tom continued to feel shame and embarrassment over this incident. Additionally, Tom's neighbourhood consisted of working families and, although they were friendly, there was limited social interaction and common interests with neighbours.

Tom was a keen gardener, but a small yard and water restrictions hampered this activity and there was no one with whom to share this passion.

Tom's treatment plan was aimed at addressing these issues. It consisted of support and gradual introduction into various therapeutic and social activities. These activities were:

- weekly interpersonal psychotherapy sessions for his grief and improvement of social skills
- attendance at an older men's group and a senior citizen's group (the latter was important to Tom because he enjoyed dancing and the company of women) for peer support and socialisation
- attendance at another church for spiritual needs and socialisation
- participation in a water-wise gardening cooperative that was run by the local council, and
- home visits by a mental health worker on the days he did not have any scheduled activities to establish his mental state, suicide risk, daily living skills, and to work through reactions or potential worries about scheduled activities.

Tom was also given a list of contacts to telephone if he felt suicidal and was asked to give an assurance that he would make contact.

After 3 months of interpersonal therapy and supported social interactions, Tom was able to come to better terms with his grief and build up a social support network that suited his needs. His suicidal thoughts and shameful feelings decreased and the mental health workers were able to gradually withdraw their support.

EPIDEMIOLOGY

The pattern of age-specific rates in 2005 for suicide in men and women is shown in Figure 21.1.

The following are some interesting facts and figures about suicide in older people in Australia (Australian Bureau of Statistics 2007, Caldwell et al 2004, Cantor et al 1999, de Leo et al 1999, 2001, Fairweather et al 2007, Goldney & Harrison 1998):

- Suicide rates among older people have generally declined across Australia over recent decades. In 2005, the rate of 11 suicides per 100,000 of older people was less than the 12.9 per 100,000 recorded in 1995. Possible reasons cited for this have been changes in medical prescribing habits, improved access to healthcare

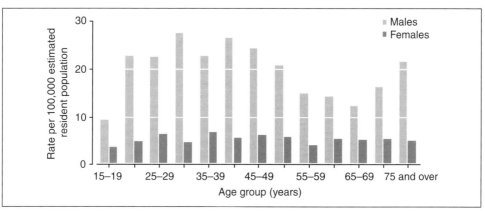

Figure 21.1 Age-specific rates in 2005 for suicide in men and women
Source: Australian Bureau of Statistics (2007).

including psychiatric services, better income support, greater acceptance of mental health problems and illnesses such as depression, and migration from countries with lower suicide rates.

- Approximately 283 older people commit suicide each year, accounting for 13.5% of all suicides in Australia. Nearly 80% of these deaths are men. However, this is thought to be an underestimate because of a high level of comorbidity issues in this age group, which may confound the cause of death, and it is sometimes difficult to know whether a death was intentional or accidental.
- Men aged 80 years of age and older have exceptionally higher rates of suicide, at just over 30 per 100,000 of population per year. The impact of poor physical and mental health resulting in dependency is thought to be a strong contributing factor to suicide for men of this age.
- In older men, for every completed suicide there are 0.9 attempts recorded and in older women for every completed suicide there are 3.1 attempts recorded. When completed suicide numbers are greater, as in the case for older men, this indicates that a suicidal act is more likely to end in death than not.
- International studies have indicated that between 2.3% and 17% of older people have recently considered suicide, and although the rates of suicidal ideation decrease with age, completion rates normally increase with age.
- Suicide rates for older people in Australia are marginally lower than suicide rates for older people in other similar English-speaking countries. The Australian suicide rate is higher than rates in the European nations of origin of the major immigrant groups, but similar to rates in other countries also recently colonised by Europeans (New Zealand, Canada and the United States).
- The suicide rate among older Aboriginal and Torres Strait Islander Australians is low. However, as a smaller number of Aboriginal and Torres Strait Islander people live to old age, it is difficult to draw clear conclusions from this. The majority of Aboriginal and Torres Strait Islander suicides are by hanging or firearms.

- Suicide rates in rural and remote areas are higher for older men with 27.7 per 100,000 of population per year compared with 22.1 in metropolitan areas. For older women, the rate is slightly higher in metropolitan areas at 6.1 per 100,000 per year compared with 4.9 in rural and remote areas.

TYPES OF SUICIDAL BEHAVIOURS

Suicidal behaviour in older people has been categorised as thoughts of hopelessness or suicidal ideation, indirect self-destructive behaviour, deliberate self-harm and completed suicide (Harwood 2002). Some very old or terminally ill people may have thoughts of hopelessness or suicidal ideation and may express statements such as 'I wish I was dead', but if questioned will vehemently deny any thought of self-harm. More serious suicidal thoughts are usually found when a person is single, has depression, physical disability, pain, sensory impairments or is institutionalised. Indirect self-destructive behaviour, sometimes known as subintentional suicide, such as failing to eat and drink or non-compliance with life-saving medication, occurs frequently in older women and in very old institutionalised people. The older person in this situation will deny that it is an act of suicide, but the likelihood of dying is increased. Deliberate self-harm differs from suicidal thoughts and indirect self-destructive behaviour because there is a definite, more determined and immediate response.

METHODS OF SUICIDE

In Australia (de Leo et al 2001), older men tend to use more violent and lethal means such as hanging, shooting and carbon monoxide poisoning (car exhaust fumes). This use of highly lethal means is thought to account in part for the higher rate of completed suicides in older men. Older women tend to use drug overdose, hanging and carbon monoxide poisoning. Drug overdoses are usually with commonly prescribed medications such as paracetamol, analgesics and antidepressants. Large-scale government policies, such as gun control laws, changing household gases to less toxic varieties and changing prescribing practices, have reduced the use of these popular methods for suicide; however, there have been compensatory rises in other methods, leading to the conclusion that limiting access to means of suicide to suicidal people who are ambivalent may be effective, but it does not change the behaviour of those people who are intent on committing suicide.

RISK FACTORS

Depression is the most common antecedent of suicide in older people. However, one does not have to be depressed to commit suicide, and being depressed does not necessarily make a person suicidal. Additionally, verbalising thoughts about suicide does not always indicate intent, but it does pay to investigate this further because it has been demonstrated that older people who have completed suicide are likely to have verbalised the thought to health workers, including their general medical practitioners. Personality profiles of older people who have completed suicide have described them as being hypochondriacal, not being open to novel or new experiences and neurotic (Conwell et al 2002). The box on the next page provides a comprehensive list of the demographic, social, clinical and historical risk factors that have been identified for suicidal behaviour in older people (Garand et al 2006, O'Connell 2005, Turvey et al 2002).

Clearly, not all of these risk factors are causal factors and the contribution of any single causative factor remains unclear, with popular opinion relying on a complex combination of multiple factors that often overlap, creating an additive effect.

SUICIDE RISK PROFILE FOR OLDER PEOPLE

Sociodemographic factors
Sociodemographic factors include:
- male gender
- unmarried, divorced or widowed
- lack of a confidant
- family discord
- interpersonal problems
- social isolation, and
- low socioeconomic status.

Clinical factors
Clinical factors include:
- poor sleep quality
- physical illness, such as cancer (particularly the first year after diagnosis), and stroke, multiple sclerosis and epilepsy
- development of a functional disability
- pain
- depressive disorder
- personality disorder (particularly with anxiety and obsessive-compulsive traits)
- early dementia
- alcohol abuse, and
- sedative or hypnotic abuse.

Historical factors
Historical factors include:
- grief, especially recent spousal bereavement
- prior suicide attempts
- a life-changing event, such as retirement and institutionalisation
- preparations for imminent death, such as making a will, paying debts and giving away possessions, and
- verbal intent statements (e.g. 'I want to die' and 'Life is not worth living').

Some of these risk factors are modifiable and treatable and therefore become important protective factors or countervailing strategies when working to lessen the likelihood of acting upon suicidal impulses. These include, but are not limited to, early identification and assertive treatment of depression, pain, anxiety, sleep disturbances and drug/alcohol abuse, encouraging an active social network, improving financial security and independence, and setting up regular appointments for ongoing care. Other protective factors found to be important for older people include concern for children, and religion.

ASSESSMENT

A comprehensive assessment is needed of the older person who is thought to be at possible risk of suicidal behaviour. Suicide assessment via direct interview of the older person is perhaps the most effective strategy for mental health workers and will provide the interviewer with a rich source of information. The interviewer should be open, pleasant and neutral (i.e. non-judgmental) and the questioning style of the interview should include a mixture of open-ended questions that allow the older person to express their concerns in whatever way they wish, and closed questions that allow the mental health worker to obtain detailed information about the person's state of mind, including their level of distress and the extent of any suicidal thoughts, plans and intent.

The interview should focus also on understanding the individual as a person, and the specific difficulties they are experiencing. So the areas for exploration include the nature of the suicidal person's problems (including duration, severity and manifestation), their coping ability and individual protective factors, and finding out what has worked in the past, and what strategies might be useful for the future. The interview should ensure that the mental health worker has a very clear idea of the suicidal person's perspective, which can then be integrated with data from clinical observations, reports from others, and knowledge of the older person's psychiatric history.

When determining the level of risk for suicide, the mental health worker cannot be reluctant in asking about suicidal thoughts and plans. Older people do not often volunteer information about their own suicidal ideation, but will usually disclose their thoughts about suicide when they are asked directly by the confident mental health worker. Asking the older person about suicide is unlikely to precipitate suicidal behaviour (Holkup et al 2003) and many older people are quite relieved to be able to unburden themselves of this information. The level of assessed risk will determine the mental health worker's response. It is important to determine:

- if there have been actual thoughts of suicide and how recent these have been
- if there is a history of previous attempts by the person themselves or someone close to them
- the level of any suicidal intent
- the ability of the person to resist these thoughts
- whether there are any mitigating factors (e.g. religious beliefs, cultural sanctions, fear of disapproval and concerns about their legacy if death is by suicide), and
- the details of the suicide plan (e.g. Are the means lethal? How available is it? Is there a chance of rescue?).

The following questions are examples of closed questions that will give the necessary information in a very direct and timely manner, but also allow for further exploration of these responses to aid in assessing the level of suicide risk.

- Have you recently had thoughts of ending your life?
- Have you thought about how you would do it?
- Have you or other people close to you tried this before?
- Is it easy for you to carry out the plan?
- Have you made preparations for doing it?
- Do you intend to carry it out?
- Can you resist the impulse to do so?
- Is there something keeping you from this course of action?

Psychological testing/scales

When the risk profile or clinical intuition is high, measuring the level of suicidal thinking by use of a rating scale can assist, particularly an inexperienced mental health worker, in the assessment process. These scales are only screening tools to supplement a well-conducted comprehensive assessment. They can make data collection more systematic. There are more than 35 suicide assessment scales available for mental health workers. The following examples are a representation of what this approach may offer.

Scale for Suicidal Ideation and Suicide Intent Scale

Both these scales were developed by Beck and associates for the measurement of suicidal ideation and intent. The Scale for Suicidal Ideation (SSI) (Beck et al 1979) is a clinician-rated instrument that contains 21 items that measure the intensity of a person's current suicidal ideation on a 3-point scale. The scale ranges from 0 (low suicidal intensity) to 2 (high suicidal intensity). The first five items are attended to first, as these are screening items and if suicidal ideation is determined at this point then the next 14 items are administered. These first 19 items are summed to give a score ranging from 0 to 38. The last two scale items document the incidence and frequency of past suicide attempts. It has been recommended that any positive response to an SSI item be followed up immediately.

The Suicide Intent Scale (SIS) (Beck et al 1974) is for use in extremely high-suicide-risk people who have recently attempted suicide. It contains 15 items that are delivered in a structured clinical interview. The SIS assesses preattempt communication patterns, the perceived likelihood of discovery/rescue during a suicide attempt, and attitudes towards living and dying.

TREATMENT
Management of acute suicidal risk

A classic danger sign that a person has decided to end their life is a sudden period of calmness and happiness after feeling down for an extended period (Mitty & Flores 2008). This often indicates that the person has made the decision and they are now feeling in control of their lives. If an older person reports suicidal ideation with a plan and ready availability of lethal means, then immediate hospitalisation will be necessary. A responsible person should remain with the suicidal older person constantly while transportation by ambulance to the nearest emergency room for psychiatric examination is arranged. Any lethal means should be made inaccessible during this time if possible. If the person refuses to go via ambulance, the police should be called and the person may have to be taken for examination under the involuntary provisions of the Mental Health Act to ensure access to a place of safety such as a hospital. Pressure on inpatient beds means that a person's length of stay may sometimes be relatively short.

A strong therapeutic relationship with the mental health workers is likely to be a protective factor against suicide in these situations. Close follow-up by the use of the telephone and scheduled appointments to monitor treatment compliance, and to sustain hope, is required in these circumstances. This should be maintained until improved mood is sustained. If an appointment is missed, the older person should be contacted immediately by someone from the support network.

Sometimes, during the course of treatment of depression in a suicidal older person, the depression starts to improve and the older person regains some energy and volition. This is a potentially dangerous time because it may herald increased risk of completed suicide.

Management of subacute suicidal risk

If the older person admits to suicidal ideation but does not have a plan in place, is not psychotic or displaying poor judgment, has few risk factors and lethal means are not available then the social support system can be activated. Whenever possible, the older person's permission must be sought to put a social safety net in place. This could include family, friends, clergy, community mental health staff, general medical practitioner and the contact details for emergency call centres if these are available.

'No suicide' or 'no harm' contracts have been used in clinical practice for the prevention of suicide. These contracts, which may be written or oral, may signal the agreement by the older person to contact an identified person (preferably someone identified previously in the discussion on a social safety net) if they intend to act upon their suicidal ideation. Professional opinions differ on the value of contracts and there is very little evidence to support this intervention strategy. Ethical issues may be raised by asking an older person to enter a contract when they are in a crisis situation (Farrow & O'Brien 2003). However, if this strategy is to be used, the contract should not be used in isolation and it should only be put in place after conducting a detailed suicide assessment and developing a comprehensive treatment plan. A drawback of a contract is that the mental health worker might perceive that the risk of suicide is lowered, whereas the risk is actually unchanged or even heightened by this misperception of risk.

Treating suicidal behaviour

Current opinion generally supports a combination of medication and psychotherapy for effective treatment of suicidal behaviour from the acute to maintenance phases. Electroconvulsive therapy also has an important role to play, particularly when older people are unremittingly suicidal. Chapters 29–31 give a comprehensive coverage of all these topics, so here only specific issues in relation to suicide in older people will be discussed.

Pharmacological therapies

If the older person has a depressive illness with suicidal ideation, this can be treated with antidepressant medication. Some information to keep in mind though when an older person is suicidal is that the choice of medications must be made judiciously to avoid the risk of lethality in overdose. The modern selective serotonin reuptake inhibitors (SSRIs) and serotonergic and noradrenergic reuptake inhibitor (SNRI) antidepressants are generally safer in this regard than the older tricyclic and monoamine oxidase inhibitor antidepressants. However, the mental health worker should further minimise risk of deliberate overdose of prescribed medication by ensuring that the older person does not have access to large quantities of medication. Additionally, the older person must be monitored for the continued presence of suicidal ideation once the somatic symptoms of depression have been alleviated by the antidepressants because this medication may enhance the older person's mental and physical capacity to carry out their plans.

Electroconvulsive therapy

Electroconvulsive therapy (ECT) is a rapid, well-tolerated and effective treatment for older people with depression and a high suicide risk. The indications for ECT include the following:
* severe suicidal intent associated with depression
* psychotic depression

- a near lethal attempt and the person continues to express suicidal ideation
- a person remains at a high risk despite medication, and
- the suicide risk is so high that the 3–6-week time lag for antidepressant medication to be effective cannot be justified.

ECT may be done on an inpatient or outpatient basis. As a treatment in the acute phase, it is extremely effective; however, longer term treatment should include anti-depressant medication and psychotherapy.

Psychotherapies

Behavioural and psychological interventions for suicidal people include interpersonal psychotherapy (IPT), cognitive behaviour therapy (CBT) and problem-solving therapy. IPT has the benefit of being able to target key areas, such as grief, role transitions, role disputes and interpersonal deficits that have been identified as risk factors for suicide in older people.

CBT can be particularly useful in opening up the narrow thinking and devaluing of options that characterise the thought processes of suicidal people. The dysfunctional beliefs and the abject feelings of helplessness and hopelessness associated with these beliefs can be challenged with CBT. Problem-solving therapy is instituted once particular problems are able to be identified and separated from the depressive symptoms. The problem is broken down into its different components and solutions, and options other than suicide are explored with the older person. These are trialled while the therapeutic support is maintained, with the goal of the older person adopting and continually developing and using effective strategies in their daily coping patterns.

THE AFTERMATH OF SUICIDE

Some people will succeed in taking their own lives despite the best efforts of the people who tried to prevent this from happening. The mental health worker should avoid assigning or accepting responsibility for the person's death. Careful documentation should reflect the steps taken to reduce suicidal risks and the responses made by the older person and their family. An unfortunate consequence of suicide can be that devastated relatives and friends feel a sense of shame, embarrassment and guilt. They may even develop more serious consequences such as somatic complaints, depression and post-traumatic stress disorder.

Suicide after-care is very similar to any other grief-related therapy, but needs to take into account that the process of grieving following the loss of a loved one through suicide may be more difficult than when a person dies of natural causes. Societal attitudes may cause the grief-stricken to receive less social support in the period following the death. The survivors of suicide are also at an increased risk of suicide themselves and appropriate monitoring strategies need to be put in place for them.

PREVENTION

At a broad level, the introduction of the National Suicide Prevention Strategy in 1999 by the Australian Government was a significant event that brought widespread attention and action for suicide prevention. Preventive strategies for older people need to have a different focus than those developed for younger people. Older people differ because they are less likely to have a history of suicidal behaviour and thinking, the act of suicide for older people is less impulsive and more determined, methods tend to be more violent, older people are more frail and therefore less likely to survive a suicide attempt, and there is usually less opportunity for rescue. The high-risk subgroups that can be targeted with prevention activities include older men, people with depressive illnesses, the recently bereaved, those with a history of suicide attempts, those with substance-use disorders, those with chronic physical illness and those who are socially isolated.

Early recognition and treatment of suicidal behaviour and depressive symptoms are important preventive strategies (Suominen et al 2004). This could be attended to by enhancing the capability of primary care, either by increasing the number of specialised health professionals within primary care settings or by providing suicide education for the primary care practitioners. Such strategies are essential because 70% of older people who completed suicide had an appointment with their primary care provider within the 30 days before death (Conwell & Duberstein 2001). These appointments may have highlighted the hopelessness about certain medical illnesses or demonstrated that older people at risk of suicide may have difficulty in recognising their need and asking for appropriate help. Or they may reflect an attempt by the older person to obtain help for their problem. The fact that older people are underrepresented in mental health services adds to this problematic issue. Nevertheless, the primary care setting remains an important context for suicide intervention and prevention.

SPECIAL TOPICS
Combined murder–suicide
Murder followed by suicide is often a seemingly inexplicable occurrence made difficult because the perpetrator is dead. Central features of this tragic phenomenon include the loss of a major element in a person's life associated with an attitude of 'If I cannot live and be happy, neither will you'. Or it may be the loss of hope in a relationship through illness and declining health for one or both partners. A single decision could be made or a pact might be formed to die together. However, it does bear consideration that the idea of a suicide pact does have to be initiated by someone, and this person could have a more domineering or persuasive personality.

Predicting or assessing for the occurrence of murder–suicide is difficult because it is such a rare event. However, like conventional suicide, the older person has often revealed their thoughts to a mental health worker. Ideally, the clinician should attempt to determine such things as the level of attachment and the belief someone has of not being able to go on without the presence of another person, the degree of feelings of rejection, the presence of obsessional thoughts, the history of past suicide attempts and any history of homicidal levels of violence (Malmquist 2006).

Assisted suicide
During 1996–97 for a period of 9 months, assisted suicide, also known as voluntary euthanasia, was legally sanctioned in the Northern Territory of Australia. After much antieuthanasia lobbying, and political and public debate, the law was overturned by Australian Commonwealth legislation. It still remains a controversial issue in Australia and elsewhere, with differences in the legal status of assisted suicide existing in jurisdictions around the world. In places where it has been legalised, assisted suicide often involves a health practitioner providing the means by which a competent person can end

their life after they have explicitly requested assistance in hastening their death (Hendin 1998). The usual people at the centre of this debate are those people with degenerative conditions or the terminally ill where there is no cure, no hope for improvement, and there is no relief for their suffering and helplessness. Outcomes for their quality of life are extremely poor. For the present, in Australia, there are no jurisdictions in which assisted suicide or voluntary euthanasia are legal.

SUMMARY

Suicide in older people is a common and tragic phenomenon that often has potentially treatable health conditions and psychosocial factors associated with it. Mental health workers can play a vital role in being diligent in the detection and the ongoing clinical management of suicidal behaviour in older people.

FURTHER READING

Simon RI, Hales RE 2006 Suicide assessment and management. American Psychiatric Publishing, Arlington VA

USEFUL WEBSITES

Australian Institute for Suicide Research and Prevention: www.griffith.edu.au/health/australian-institute-suicide-research-prevention
Australian National Depression Initiative: www.beyondblue.org.au

REFERENCES

Australian Bureau of Statistics (ABS) 2007 Suicides Australia. ABS, Canberra
Beck AT, Kovacs M, Weissman A 1979 Assessment of suicidal intention: the Scale for Suicidal Ideation. Journal of Consulting and Clinical Psychology 47(2):343–352
Beck AT, Schuyler D, Herman I 1974 Development of suicide intent scales. In: Beck AT, Resnick HLP, Lettieri DJ (eds) The prediction of suicide. The Charles Press Publishers, Bowie, MI
Caldwell TM, Jorm AF, Dear KBG 2004 Suicide and mental health in rural, remote and metropolitan areas in Australia. Medical Journal of Australia 181(7Suppl):S10–S14
Cantor C, Neulinger K, de Leo D 1999 Australian suicide trends 1964–97: youth and beyond? Medical Journal of Australia 171(3):137–141
Conwell Y, Duberstein PR 2001 Suicide in elders. Annals of the New York Academy of Science April(932):132–147
Conwell Y, Duberstein PR, Caine ED 2002 Risk factors for suicide in later life. Biological Psychiatry 52(3):193–204
de Leo D, Hickey PA, Neulinger K et al 1999 Ageing and suicide: a report to the Commonwealth Department of Health and Ageing. Australian Institute for Suicide Research and Prevention. Griffith University, Brisbane
de Leo D, Hickey PA, Neulinger K et al 2001 Ageing and suicide. Commonwealth Department of Health and Aged Care, Canberra
Fairweather AK, Anstey KJ, Rodgers B et al 2007 Age and gender differences among Australian suicide ideators. Journal of Nervous and Mental Disease 195(2):130–136
Farrow TL, O'Brien AJ 2003 No-suicide contracts and informed consent: an analysis of ethical issues. Nursing Ethics 10(2):199–207
Garand L, Mitchell AM, Dietrick A et al 2006 Suicide in older adults: nursing assessment of suicide risk. Issues in Mental Health Nursing 27(4):355–370

Goldney RD, Harrison J 1998 Suicide in the elderly: some good news. Australasian Journal on Ageing 17(2):54–55

Harwood D 2002 Suicide in older persons. In: Jacoby R, Oppenheimer C (eds) Psychiatry in the elderly. Oxford University Press, Oxford, pp. 677–682

Hendin H 1998 Suicide by death: doctors, patients, and assisted suicide. Norton, New York

Holkup PA, Hsiao-Chen J, Titler MG 2003 Evidence-based protocol. Elderly suicide—secondary prevention. Journal of Gerontological Nursing June:6–17

Malmquist CP 2006 Combined murder–suicide. In: Simon RI, Hales RE (eds) Suicide assessment and management. American Psychiatric Publishing, Arlington, VA, pp. 495–509

Mitty E, Flores S 2008 Suicide in late life. Geriatric Nursing 29(3):160–165

O'Connell H 2005 Suicide in elderly people. IPA Bulletin 2(2):1–2

Suominen K, Isometsa E, Lonnqvist J 2004 Elderly suicide attempters with depression are often diagnosed only after the attempt. International Journal of Geriatric Psychiatry 19:35–40

Turvey CL, Conwell Y, Jones MP 2002 Risk factors for late-life suicide: a prospective community-based study. American Journal of Geriatric Psychiatry 10:398–406

Chapter 22

THE OLDER PERSON WITH PSYCHOTIC SYMPTOMS

INTRODUCTION

Psychotic symptoms in older people are highly prevalent and occur in many different mental health problems, including delirium, dementia, mood disorders and psychotic disorders. Some otherwise normal older people experience hallucinations in the context of sensory impairment such as low vision or poor hearing. However, this chapter will focus on the older person with a psychotic disorder.

CASE VIGNETTE

The police liaison officer to the local health district referred Mrs GH, an 83-year-old single woman, to the older persons' mental health service (OPMHS). Mrs GH had been repeatedly telephoning the local police station over the past 4 months complaining about the behaviour of her neighbours. She claimed that her neighbours had installed a powerful electrical machine in their lounge room that they were using to send beams of radiation into her house. Mrs GH said that this radiation was causing her refrigerator to malfunction and was causing an odd sensation in her knee joints that made it difficult for her to walk. She had responded to these alleged attacks by turning off her refrigerator and by wrapping her knees in cardboard. According to the police officer, Mrs GH had angrily confronted her neighbours a few days earlier and her neighbours had lodged an official complaint with the police. The police had investigated Mrs GH's claims and found them to be baseless.

EPIDEMIOLOGY

Psychotic *symptoms* occur commonly among older people. Henderson et al (1998) surveyed 935 residents of Canberra and Queanbeyan aged 70 years and over living in the community or in supported accommodation and found that 42 (4.49%) reported hallucinations and 26 (2.78%) had delusions. Overall, the estimated prevalence of at least one psychotic symptom was 5.7% for those living in the community and 7.5% for those living in supported accommodation. People with dementia or cognitive impairment were more likely to have psychotic symptoms. When these investigators resurveyed the same people 3.6 years later, there were 35 new cases of psychotic symptoms among the 581 who did not have psychotic symptoms at baseline. Thus, the incidence (new cases) of psychotic symptoms over 3.6 years was 6.0%.

The best evidence on the prevalence of psychotic *disorders* in older people comes from a Finnish study (Perala et al 2007). Despite the emphasis given to young people with schizophrenia both in the mass media and within mental health services, the findings from this study indicate that psychotic disorders are actually more common in older people than in young or middle-aged people. The prevalence of non-affective psychotic disorders (schizophrenia, schizoaffective disorder, schizophreniform disorder, delusional disorder, brief psychotic disorder, and psychotic disorder not otherwise specified) in people aged 65 years and over was 2.32% (95% CI = 1.67–3.21), whereas the prevalence in people aged 30–44 years was 1.27% (95% CI = 0.89–1.82). In contrast, the prevalence of affective psychoses (bipolar I disorder and major depression with psychotic features) was very similar in middle-aged and older people: 0.57% (95% CI = 0.32–1.01) in people aged 65 years and over and 0.52% (95% CI = 0.32–0.87) in people aged 30–44 years.

CLINICAL FEATURES

The primary psychotic disorders such as schizophrenia are characterised by positive symptoms (hallucinations, delusions and formal thought disorder), negative symptoms (impaired volition, personality change, social impairment and communication difficulties) and cognitive impairment (principally frontal executive dysfunction). However, late-onset psychotic disorders are often characterised more by positive symptoms, rather than by negative symptoms and thought disorder.

Illusions and hallucinations

Perceptual abnormalities including illusions and hallucinations occur in normal people and in many different mental health problems. This means that the presence of these symptoms does not always mean that the person is suffering from a mental health problem. Hallucinations may be defined as perceptions without objects. In other words, the person experiences the perception in the absence of any external sensory stimulus. Hallucinations may occur in any sensory modality—vision (visual), hearing (auditory), smell (olfactory), taste (gustatory), touch (tactile) and bodily movement (kinaesthetic).

Auditory hallucinations are common in psychotic disorders. These may be complex, involving voices speaking to or about the person, or simple, including tones, clicks, buzzes or other noises. Hallucinatory music is not uncommon. Hallucinatory voices may sometimes give instructions or commands to the person. Visual hallucinations can suggest the presence of delirium, but can also occur in the Charles Bonnet syndrome in which a person with impaired eyesight (usually due to macular degeneration or glaucoma) develops visual hallucinations in the absence of cognitive impairment or symptoms of mental illness.

Hypnagogic and hypnopompic hallucinations occur when going to sleep and waking from sleep, respectively. Similar hallucinations occur in situations of sensory deprivation, including the white noise generated by heavy rain or a bathroom shower. Strong suggestion or expectation due to mental set may also lead to simple hallucinations in normal people. Hallucinations should be distinguished from illusions, in which there is a stimulus, and from visual images, which are conscious products of the imagination.

Delusions, overvalued ideas and marked preoccupations

The presence of delusions is always indicative of mental health problems, so care must be taken in their detection. Delusions are false, unshakeable beliefs of morbid origin, which are out of keeping with the person's social, cultural and educational background. By chance, some delusions turn out to be true. For instance, delusional infidelity may turn out to be true because of the high background prevalence of marital infidelity. It is sometimes difficult to distinguish delusions from unusual religious beliefs, and care should be taken when attempting to do this. The assistance of transcultural mental health workers is likely to be essential when dealing with people from other cultural or language groups.

Overvalued ideas are strongly held beliefs that dominate a person's life, but are not delusions or obsessions. Such beliefs involve non-bizarre subjects. At interview, the person with the overvalued idea will sometimes express doubt about their belief.

Delusions are said to be mood congruent when they are in keeping with the person's predominant mood. Thus, delusions of guilt, poverty and hypochondriasis are said to be mood congruent with depression, and delusions of power, beauty and boundless wealth are mood congruent with mania.

Bizarre delusions involve things that could not possibly be true, although the definition of what could not possibly be true changes with advances in science and technology. Non-bizarre delusions include things that could be true, such as being followed or being bugged. Bizarre delusions include things that could not be true, such as the neighbour beaming rays into the person's home to cause arthritis in their knees.

The content of delusions varies a lot. Delusions commonly involve themes of control, persecution, jealousy, guilt or sin, grandiosity, religion or love. Somatic delusions involve the idea that the body is diseased or changed in some way. One common type is delusional parasitosis in which the person believes that they are infested with parasites. Nihilistic delusions involve the bizarre belief that some part of the self, or some part of others or the world, no longer exists.

Partition delusions and phantom boarders are other delusions commonly seen in older people. Partition delusions refer to the belief that there are people, animals or other living things in the ceiling, beneath the floorboards or behind the walls. Some older people believe that these people or animals can move through solid walls at will. Partition delusions occur in both late-onset psychotic disorders and in dementia. The phantom boarders' delusion involves the belief that other people are living in the house. The person will refer to the other people and may take them into account when preparing meals or setting the table for dinner. In the author's experience, this delusion generally occurs in people with dementia.

Passivity phenomena and other psychotic symptoms

The main category of passivity phenomena is thought alienation, which includes thought insertion, thought withdrawal and thought broadcasting. In thought insertion the person experiences thoughts inserted into their mind by an outside agency, whereas in thought withdrawal thoughts are removed from their mind by an outside agency.

In thought broadcasting, the person is unable to contain their thoughts within their mind and has the belief that everyone else can hear their thoughts spoken aloud. Thought withdrawal is experienced by some people as thought blocking, or the sudden cessation of a train of thought.

Somatic passivity phenomena include the experience of bodily sensations generated by outside forces. It is generally considered to be a delusion of control. Such phenomena are often accompanied by hallucinatory sensations. Examples include physical sensations that the person experiences as being produced by the effects of beams of radiation or similar outside influences.

Formal thought disorder reflects abnormalities in the form rather than the content of thinking. In formal thought disorder, the person's speech and writing are less intelligible than normal to others. There may be loose or tangential associations between successive thoughts or derailing in which a thought comes off the tracks altogether. Thinking may become woolly or excessively allusive. Neologisms (new words) may be invented by the person and existing words may be given new meanings. Formal thought disorder may occur in both 'functional' disorders such as schizophrenia and in 'organic' disorders such as dementia. However, it is quite uncommon in late-onset psychotic disorders.

Disorganised thinking and behaviour are common features of psychotic disorders in young people and may persist into later life in older people with chronic psychotic disorders. However, late-onset psychotic disorders are not usually characterised by marked disorganisation of thought or behaviour in the absence of cognitive impairment.

Catatonia is an uncommon motor disturbance that may occur in psychotic disorders, mood disorders and neurological conditions. The person with catatonia may have markedly reduced or markedly increased motor behaviour. In the rigid form of catatonia the person may hold postures for hours. Catatonia needs to be distinguished from neuroleptic malignant syndrome.

Negative symptoms

Negative symptoms occur commonly in people with early-onset psychotic disorders, but are uncommon in very late onset psychotic disorders. Negative symptoms may include some or all of the following:
- blunted affect
- poverty of speech (alogia)
- poverty of content
- apathy
- ambivalence
- impaired volition (lack of willpower)
- social withdrawal, and
- psychosocial deterioration.

Negative symptoms may also be secondary to depression or to the extrapyramidal side effects of antipsychotic medication.

Cognitive impairment

People with early-onset psychotic disorders often have longstanding cognitive impairment that is an integral part of their psychotic disorder, rather than recently acquired brain damage due to dementia. Research findings suggest that this sort of cognitive impairment associated with early-onset psychosis is due to an inability to 'gate' or filter out irrelevant stimuli. This manifests as impaired attention and concentration, slowed information processing, and impaired planning and organisation. Thus, there is considerable frontal executive dysfunction.

However, when cognitive impairment occurs in late-onset psychosis, it is more likely to be due to a comorbid cognitive disorder, such as delirium or dementia.

Other symptoms

Older people with psychotic disorders commonly experience other symptoms, including depression and anxiety. They sometimes have suicidal or homicidal ideation.

PSYCHOTIC DISORDERS

A large number of different mental health problems are characterised by prominent psychotic symptoms. These include the main non-affective psychotic disorders, affective disorders with psychotic symptoms, and general medical conditions associated with psychotic symptoms. The main diagnostic categories are:

- schizophrenia
- schizoaffective disorder
- schizophreniform disorder
- delusional disorder
- brief psychotic disorder
- psychotic disorder not otherwise specified (NOS)
- bipolar I disorder
- major depressive disorder with psychotic features
- substance-induced psychotic disorder, and
- psychotic disorder due to a general medical condition.

A major challenge for the OPMHS team is to distinguish psychotic disorders with associated mild cognitive impairment from primary cognitive impairment or dementia complicated by psychotic symptoms. Often the distinction can only be made with confidence after observing the person over time with serial examination of their mental state, including serial cognitive testing.

ASSESSMENT

The domiciliary visit provides the ideal opportunity for the mental health worker to assess the older person with psychotic symptoms. Not infrequently, such people manifest their psychotic symptoms mainly at home. Neighbours, passing cars and local schoolchildren are often the objects of delusional beliefs and it is useful to examine the person while such stimuli are nearby. Persecutory beliefs may be in evidence if the mental health worker attempts to meet with the person and the health worker is refused entry to the person's residence. History may need to be obtained from family members, neighbours and the police. Many older people with persecutory delusions will have telephoned the police, often repeatedly. In our experience, the police often have excellent records of such telephone calls and these provide a good source of collateral history about the duration and content of psychotic symptoms. Other community agencies, including domiciliary nurses, social welfare agencies, home-delivered meal services, real estate agencies and local banks or post offices, may also have useful information to contribute.

History

As with most mental health problems in older people, it is crucial to establish the duration of any psychotic symptoms. This is almost always best done through the use of an informant. Psychotic symptoms have commonly been present for many years prior to coming to the attention of health workers. Family members and the police often have detailed information on duration and type of symptoms, particularly in relation to delusional beliefs.

Mental state examination

A comprehensive mental state examination (MSE) is essential. This should focus on whether psychotic phenomena such as delusions and hallucinations are present and the degree of insight, if any, the person has into these symptoms. It is important to ask the person about the impact of their symptoms on their life. Negative symptoms and cognitive symptoms must also be explored. Commonly occurring associated symptoms, including depression, anxiety and agitation, should be looked for. Suicidal and homicidal ideation must be excluded. The impact of the illness on the person's judgment and likely treatment adherence should also be investigated.

The general appearance and behaviour of the person might give clues to the likely severity and chronicity of the person's illness. Gait and posture can be affected by both the illness and its treatment.

Physical examination

A general physical examination is important in older people with psychotic symptoms. Particular issues include the following:

- Carefully look for evidence of postural hypotension. Measure blood pressure lying and standing.
- Look for extrapyramidal adverse effects such as Parkinsonism, akathisia and tardive dyskinesia, as the presence of these might be a clue to past or present treatment with antipsychotic medication.
- Weight gain, glucose intolerance and diabetes mellitus are potential adverse effects of treatment with atypical antipsychotic medications, although less common in older people than young and middle-aged people. Check height and weight and calculate body mass index (BMI = weight in kilograms divided by squared height in metres).
- Test the urine using a dipstick system to quickly check for glucosuria, proteinuria and haematuria (glucose, protein and blood in the urine).
- Look for constipation with an abdominal examination.

Laboratory investigations

It is prudent to undertake an electroencephalogram (EEG) in older people presenting for the first time with psychotic symptoms, as these are occasionally due to temporal lobe epilepsy. Screening blood tests will allow the exclusion of some intercurrent general medical conditions, including hypothyroidism and vitamin B12 deficiency, and will assess hepatic and renal function prior to starting psychotropic medication. People being commenced on clozapine require additional close monitoring of their white cell count and their cardiac status.

Neuroimaging

It is appropriate to order a brain scan, preferably a magnetic resonance imaging (MRI) brain scan, but a computed tomography (CT) brain scan will suffice. This will allow an assessment of the extent of any cerebrovascular disease and rule out normal pressure hydrocephalus and space-occupying lesions, including brain tumours and subdural and extradural haematomas.

Risk assessment

A formal risk assessment is an important component of the work-up of older people with a psychotic disorder. At a minimum, this should consider the following issues:
- suicidal ideation, plans and intent
- homicidal ideation, plans and intent
- risk of self-neglect and misadventure
- risk of falls
- vulnerability to abuse by others (financial, physical, emotional, sexual)
- non-adherence to essential medication (antipsychotics and general medical)
- financial risk (often seen in older people with persecutory ideation), and
- decisional capacity (financial, healthcare, lifestyle). See Chapter 18.

TREATMENT OUTLINE

Treatment should cover the following:
- Consider the treatment context (i.e. community treatment or hospital treatment). Issues include safety to the person and others, insight and likely treatment adherence.
- Consider whether treatment should be undertaken on a voluntary or involuntary basis. While it is preferable to manage the older person with psychotic symptoms on a voluntary basis, this is not always possible. This has been made easier with the advent of community involuntary treatment orders in many jurisdictions.
- Antipsychotic medication is usually an essential component of the treatment of older people with psychotic disorders. Carefully consider which drug and what dose.
- Treat comorbid depression and anxiety; consider both non-pharmacological and pharmacological treatments.
- Treat comorbid general medical conditions; this can be quite challenging in people with Parkinson's disease.
- Treat cognitive symptoms, as psychotic symptoms and psychotic disorders are commonly complicated by cognitive impairment, which needs assessment and treatment in its own right.
- Treat negative symptoms. Many older people with late-onset psychotic disorders do not have prominent negative symptoms, whereas older people with early-onset psychotic disorders often have prominent negative symptoms that persist into later life.

- Consider social interventions, including income support, housing assistance and home-delivered meals.
- Consider other assistance, including prepackaged medications (Webster Pak® and similar) and the use of a locked metal box to store medications between domiciliary visits.
- Consider domiciliary nursing to assist with basic activities of daily living, including showering, and the administration of medication.

Antipsychotic drugs

Although it is beyond the scope of this chapter to provide a detailed discussion of the use of antipsychotic drugs in older people, some brief observations are worthwhile. Antipsychotic drugs are potent pharmaceuticals with many significant adverse effects. They must be used judiciously in older people, particularly in frail older people. The use of antipsychotic medication in older people should occur in a setting in which regular review of the person is possible. It is important to start with a much lower dose than would be used in younger people and titrate the dose slowly according to clinical response and adverse effects. Some adverse effects, such as Parkinsonism, may occur many weeks after commencing an antipsychotic medication, and so continued surveillance is needed. Oversedation, postural hypotension and constipation are common problems, and the older person must be routinely assessed for these.

There are additional issues in older people being considered for treatment with depot antipsychotic medication or with clozapine. These issues relate mainly to the risk of adverse effects. However, in some people, these treatment options can lead to great clinical improvement so they should not be reserved only for younger people.

In residential aged care facility (RACF) people with dementia, the use of antipsychotic medication has given rise to additional concerns. In several clinical trials in people with behavioural and psychological symptoms of dementia (BPSD), there has been evidence of an increased rate of strokes and transient ischaemic attacks (TIAs). This effect seems to apply to both the newer atypical antipsychotic drugs and to the conventional agents. Most of the people affected by strokes and TIAs had pre-existing risk factors for cerebrovascular disease. Thus, caution is needed when using antipsychotic drugs, even at low doses, in this population. Communication with family members and consent from substitute decision makers is advised. See also Chapter 30.

SUMMARY

This chapter has provided a detailed account of psychotic symptoms in older people together with an approach to their assessment and management. It has emphasised that psychotic symptoms and psychotic disorders occur commonly in older people. It has provided a detailed treatment outline that includes antipsychotic medication together with a wide range of other non-pharmacological interventions.

FURTHER READING

Hassett A, Ames D, Chiu E (eds) 2005 Psychosis in the elderly. Taylor & Francis, Milton Park, UK

REFERENCES

Henderson AS, Korten AE, Levings C et al 1998 Psychotic symptoms in the elderly: a prospective study in a population sample. International Journal of Geriatric Psychiatry 13:484–492

Perala J, Suvisaari J, Saarni SI et al 2007 Lifetime prevalence of psychotic and bipolar I disorders in a general population. Archives of General Psychiatry 64:19–28

Chapter 23

THE OLDER PERSON WITH ANXIETY

INTRODUCTION

Anxiety is a universal and normal human experience. It has survival value when it leads an individual to avoid danger. Anxiety is an important component of the mammalian 'fight or flight' response and one manifestation of sympathetic nervous system arousal. A certain degree of anxiety is often associated with increased performance, but excessive anxiety is associated with reduced performance. Anxiety accompanies most general medical conditions such as heart attacks and strokes. It also accompanies most mental health problems such as depression, dementia and schizophrenia. However, anxiety can be the main feature of several anxiety disorders that are not necessarily associated with a general medical condition or another mental health problem. This chapter is about these so-called *primary* anxiety disorders. Key issues include the diverse presentation of anxiety disorders and the selection of appropriate treatment approaches for older people.

CASE VIGNETTE

An 82-year-old widower was referred by his general practitioner (GP) with a 4-week history of escalating anxiety symptoms, including feelings of panic, shortness of breath, lump in the throat, chest pain and generalised weakness and fatigue. Four months earlier, he had suffered an extensive right-sided temporoparietal stroke with left-sided hemiparesis and neglect. He had made a good recovery from his hemiparesis and neglect and had been an enthusiastic participant in an extended inpatient rehabilitation program.

However, upon returning home from hospital, he had developed a severe chest infection with associated delirium and was readmitted. He recovered well from this and once again went home only to be readmitted briefly following what was initially thought to be a transient ischaemic attack (TIA). It subsequently emerged that this was more likely to have been a panic attack. He returned home to be readmitted with a further chest infection. After a brief inpatient stay, he returned to his retirement village apartment, but had gradually become more anxious over the several months prior to referral. When seen for assessment, he was experiencing frequent panic attacks, most of which were limited-symptom attacks. He had progressively restricted his activities outside his apartment and was now avoiding all travel and rarely leaving the apartment.

EPIDEMIOLOGY

Anxiety disorders are the commonest mental disorders in older people after dementia. The 1997 National Survey of Mental Health and Wellbeing (NSMHW) (Australian Bureau of Statistics 1998) found that 3.5% of males and 5.4% of females aged 65 years and over were suffering from an anxiety disorder. This survey was limited to community-residing individuals without significant cognitive impairment and thus was likely to have underestimated the true prevalence of anxiety disorders in older people. However, the survey found that the prevalence of anxiety disorders declined with age. Table 23.1 shows the prevalence of specific anxiety disorders among people aged 65 years and over from the same survey.

CLINICAL FEATURES

Generalised anxiety disorder (GAD) is characterised by longstanding pathological anxiety. As currently defined by DSM–IV (American Psychiatric Association 2000), this anxiety must persist for at least 6 months for the diagnosis to be made. The person with GAD commonly worries or ruminates about many different things and experiences these worries as uncontrollable. Older people seem particularly prone to worry about their health and finances, or about the circumstances of their children or grandchildren. The topics of worry are often in the indeterminate future and not under the control of the person. Sometimes, the person with GAD also has free-floating anxiety (i.e. anxiety without a clear subject or focus). They usually feel nervous and unable to relax. They often feel irritable and restless and report difficulty concentrating. They are hypervigilant and startle easily. They often report increased muscle tone or tension and associated aches and pains. Not infrequently they have a fine tremor and psychomotor agitation. They commonly report marked sleep disturbance, with initial, middle and terminal insomnia and unrefreshing sleep. They often feel fatigued.

Clearly, these symptoms overlap to a considerable degree with the symptoms of major depression and may occur in many other psychiatric disorders. GAD also needs to be distinguished from what might be termed normal worry and from a variety of other conditions. These include hyperthyroidism, excessive caffeine consumption, the use of

Table 23.1 Prevalence of anxiety disorders in older people	
Disorder	**Prevalence**
Generalised anxiety disorder	2.5%
Panic disorder	0.6%
Panic disorder with agoraphobia	0.3%
Agoraphobia without a history of panic attacks	0.1%
Post-traumatic stress disorder	1.1%
Social phobia	0.5%
Obsessive-compulsive disorder	0.1%

Source: Australian Bureau of Statistics (1998).

stimulants such as pseudoephedrine and amphetamine, and alcohol or benzodiazepine withdrawal.

Panic attacks are discrete episodes of marked anxiety that typically last no more than 10 minutes. Classical panic attacks, as described in DSM–IV (American Psychiatric Association 2000), are much more commonly experienced by young and middle-aged people, but do occasionally occur in older people. The anxiety experienced in a panic attack reaches its peak intensity rapidly and physical symptoms such as shortness of breath, tachycardia, palpitations and a choking sensation occur commonly. Other likely symptoms include chest tightness, chest pain, sweating, tremor, paraesthesiae, nausea, and hot or cold flushes. The person typically catastrophises about their situation, fearing collapse, stroke or even death. This leads to frantic attempts to escape from the situation that is associated with the attack, such as a supermarket checkout queue or crowded shopping mall. Alternatively, the person is afraid that they will embarrass themselves in front of others or 'go crazy'.

When panic attacks occur both unexpectedly and frequently, in the absence of phobic avoidance but in the presence of anticipatory anxiety, *panic disorder* is diagnosed. Anticipatory anxiety refers to a persistent fear of another panic attack or fear of the consequences of a panic attack. However, it is important to emphasise that panic disorder is uncommon in older people. When classical panic attacks do occur in older people, they are often secondary to another mental health problem such as depression, psychosis, delirium or dementia.

A more common type of panic in older people is the so-called 'limited-symptom panic attack'. These episodes do not meet all the criteria for a full-blown panic attack, but nevertheless cause the older person considerable distress and may be associated with similar phobic avoidance.

'Phobic avoidance' is the term used to describe the avoidance of objects or situations that cause excessive or irrational fear. The feared objects or situations do not cause a realistic threat, although, like snakes and electrical storms, might have the potential to cause real problems in some circumstances. As already noted, such objects or situations may also be associated with panic attacks. Phobic avoidance may occur in otherwise normal older people, but when it causes marked distress, together with social or occupational dysfunction, it is likely to amount to a phobic disorder such as specific phobia (also known as simple phobia), social phobia (also known as social anxiety disorder) or agoraphobia (with or without a history of panic attacks).

Specific phobias involve the avoidance of objects (e.g. moths, spiders) or situations (e.g. flying, confined spaces). Most specific phobias come on in childhood or early adult life. Some resolve without treatment, but some persist into middle age or later life. Simple phobias are very prevalent and often do not cause significant distress or disability because the person successfully avoids the phobic stimulus (e.g. snakes, lifts). However, some cause great distress and/or disability and require treatment.

Social phobia involves the avoidance of social situations that cause marked anxiety. Such situations include public speaking, tests and examinations, eating and drinking in front of others, musical or other performances ('stage fright'), and the use of public toilets (e.g. urinals) in the presence of others. Social phobia needs to be distinguished from normal shyness and other Axis I and Axis II psychiatric disorders.

Agoraphobia is literally 'fear of the marketplace' and most commonly occurs in people who experience frequent panic attacks in the context of *panic disorder with agoraphobia*. Agoraphobia without a history of panic attacks is much less common. According to DSM–IV (American Psychiatric Association 2000), agoraphobia involves fear and avoidance of situations from which escape might be difficult or embarrassing, or in which help might not be available if a panic attack should occur. Most people with agoraphobia have much less difficulty entering feared situations if someone else accompanies them. As a consequence, they may avoid travelling alone or staying home alone. People with agoraphobia avoid crowded situations and confined spaces because escape might be difficult. Such situations commonly include public transport, lifts, tunnels and bridges. They commonly avoid situations from which it might prove embarrassing to make a hasty escape. Such situations include supermarkets, queues, restaurants and shopping malls. As time goes on, the person with agoraphobia tends to extend the number of situations they avoid until they are quite limited in where they feel they can go safely. By the time they present for treatment, they have often had symptoms for 12 years or more.

Obsessive-compulsive disorder is characterised by obsessions and compulsions. Obsessions are uncontrollable ego-dystonic thoughts, images and impulses that cause marked distress or anxiety. By 'ego-dystonic' it is meant that the person has insight into the abnormal and often bizarre nature of their symptoms while experiencing them as products of their own mind. Compulsions are repetitive behaviours that can be observable (rituals) or unobservable (mental compulsions). Compulsions are repetitive attempts to 'undo' obsessions, reduce anxiety or prevent harm. However, they provide only temporary relief from the anxiety and distress associated with the obsession. Obsessions commonly involve neatness and symmetry, pathological doubt, contamination, and sexual and aggressive themes. For instance, some people will report obsessional images of knives dripping with blood and similarly dramatic themes. These images, which are experienced 'in the mind's eye', need to be distinguished from visual illusions and hallucinations. Compulsions commonly involve checking, washing, cleaning, counting, confessing, hoarding or arranging objects in a certain pattern.

Post-traumatic stress disorder (PTSD) is a severe anxiety disorder which, according to DSM–IV (American Psychiatric Association 2000), occurs after exposure to an event in which the person experiences or witnesses actual or threatened death in themselves or others, and responds with intense fear, helplessness or horror. It occurs in about 20% of people exposed to such a traumatic event. The most characteristic symptom of PTSD is repeated intrusive reexperiencing of the traumatic event through flashbacks and dreams. This is usually associated with avoidance behaviour, hyperarousal and emotional numbness.

Avoidance behaviour involves avoiding reminders of the traumatic event, including the location of the event. Hyperarousal involves insomnia, hypervigilance, impaired concentration and a lowered startle threshold. For example, many people with PTSD startle dramatically when a car backfires. Emotional numbness may include losing interest in interpersonal relationships and a sense that they can no longer feel emotions normally. A variety of other symptoms may also occur in PTSD. These include dissociation, physical symptoms and irritability. People with PTSD may abuse alcohol, prescribed medication and illicit substances in an attempt to deal with their symptoms.

In older people, chronic PTSD has commonly resulted from wartime experiences, including combat for men and rape for women. Older refugees have often experienced torture and trauma in their countries of origin. PTSD may also arise following motor vehicle accidents and train crashes, as well as natural disasters such as earthquakes, floods and bushfires. Some victims of childhood physical and sexual abuse develop chronic

PTSD symptoms. PTSD is another condition that can be challenging to treat. Although there once was a vogue for immediate 'debriefing' of victims of traumatic events, it is now clear that this may sometimes do more harm than good. Most people recover from the effects of psychologically traumatic events without specific intervention. However, some people develop chronic and disabling symptoms that require active management.

AETIOLOGY

People vary enormously in their propensity to experience anxiety. Research suggests that the personality trait of neuroticism is powerfully associated with the risk of anxiety symptoms and anxiety disorders at all ages. Neuroticism is the tendency to get upset and remain upset following adverse life events. So it should come as no surprise to learn that adverse life events, particularly those that involve threat or loss, are strongly associated with risk of clinically significant anxiety. Although much of the tendency towards high or low neuroticism is thought to be under genetic control, no single gene of large effect has yet been discovered. Environmental factors, including early life experiences, are thought to be important in shaping the type of anxiety problem that a vulnerable individual will develop.

Even in anxiety disorders with a clear environmental precipitant, such as PTSD, genetic factors are important. Anxiety may also be secondary to other mental health problems (e.g. depression or dementia), secondary to a general medical condition (e.g. hyperthyroidism or Parkinson's disease), or secondary to drug (e.g. amphetamine) or alcohol use. Certain parts of the limbic system of the brain seem to be important for the experience of panic and anxiety. These include the amygdala, hippocampus and the nucleus coeruleus.

COMORBIDITY

Anxiety symptoms and anxiety disorders commonly occur alongside other mental and physical health problems. Approximately 30% of people with major depressive disorder have comorbid generalised anxiety disorder. When this occurs, the prognosis of the depression is much worse, with early relapse more likely. In addition, older people with one anxiety disorder commonly meet diagnostic criteria for one or more other anxiety disorders. In older people, anxiety disorders are often associated with substance (usually alcohol or benzodiazepine) abuse or dependence. When present, this needs to be treated as well.

DIFFERENTIAL DIAGNOSIS

It is sometimes difficult to distinguish anxiety disorders from depression, dementia, delirium, or the adverse effects of drugs. As previously mentioned, some general medical conditions, such as hyperthyroidism, may also mimic anxiety disorders.

ASSESSMENT

Assessment of the anxious older person involves history taking, mental state examination (MSE), physical examination and limited laboratory investigations. It may also involve the use of a rating scale. Each of these components will now be described in more detail.

History

The history is the most informative component of the assessment of the older person with a primary anxiety disorder, so it is important to do it well. It is also very useful to obtain additional information from another informant, such as a family member, community health nurse or local doctor, if the person agrees to this.

Anxiety disorders often start early in life, in adolescence or early adult life, and so a life-span perspective is important. Some anxiety disorders, such as PTSD, are precipitated by exposure to a life-threatening experience, such as combat, assault or natural disaster. It is thus important to ask the older person about these, even if they may have occurred many years earlier.

It may be necessary to take the history over more than one consultation as the older person develops greater trust and increased willingness to disclose more of their personal and developmental history.

Mental state examination

Most people with GAD will exhibit symptoms of anxiety during the clinical consultation. However, people with other anxiety disorders (e.g. panic disorder, agoraphobia, PTSD, specific phobia) may only exhibit symptoms in certain situations. Many anxious people are also depressed, and so this must be covered in the MSE. Similarly, many anxious people have dementia or delirium and these must be considered. Suicidal ideation is not restricted to depressed people, so it is important to cover this as well in the MSE of the anxious person. As anxiety is a common reaction to declining cognitive function, it is essential to test the cognitive function of the older person with prominent anxiety symptoms. However, performance on cognitive testing may be reduced by severe anxiety, so this also needs to be taken into account.

Physical examination

Anxiety symptoms frequently mimic symptoms of common cardiac, respiratory, gastrointestinal, genitourinary and neurological conditions. Anxiety may be associated with tachycardia, hypertension, hyperventilation, heightened deep tendon reflexes and sweating. However, anxiety often accompanies general medical disorders, so it is important that the older person presenting with anxiety symptoms be given a screening physical examination by their GP or by a doctor attached to the OPMHS team.

Laboratory investigations

The laboratory investigations undertaken in the work-up of the person with anxiety disorder are done primarily to eliminate causes of *secondary* anxiety. As these underlying general medical causes are more common in older people, it is important to undertake screening laboratory investigations in this age group. These should include the following:

- electrocardiogram (ECG)
- full blood examination (FBE) or full blood count (FBC)
- c-reactive protein (CRP)
- serum electrolytes
- serum glucose
- serum urea and creatinine

- liver function tests (LFTs), and
- thyroid stimulating hormone (TSH).

The mental health worker should liaise with the person's GP or with the hospital outpatient department to arrange for the blood tests and the ECG to be done. Sometimes, the GP will already have completed these tests prior to referring the person to the OPMHS and it may not be necessary to repeat them if they have been undertaken recently. Other tests, such as brain scans, electroencephalograms (EEGs) and specialised tests for phaeochromocytoma (a rare tumour that secretes noradrenaline) should be reserved for people with unusual presentations.

Rating scales

Commonly used instruments to measure anxiety in adolescents and adults are not ideal for use with many older people. Such measures usually have complex phrasing, conditional clauses and challenging response scales. Some have reversed items or use double negatives. Sinoff et al (1999) improved on this with their Short Anxiety Screening Test (SAST), which has 10 items and a 4-point response scale. However, an instrument specifically designed to measure anxiety in both normal older people and older people with mental health problems is the Geriatric Anxiety Inventory (GAI) (Pachana et al 2007). The GAI is a self-report 20-item measure with a dichotomous (agree/disagree) response scale. It minimises the use of somatic items, has simple phrasing and avoids reversed scoring (see Appendix A at the end of this chapter). The GAI can also be read aloud to the older person by a health worker or a carer. However, the GAI and other commonly used anxiety rating scales are not diagnostic instruments. This remains a clinical task. See Chapter 35.

TREATMENT PRINCIPLES
Setting

Some older people with clinically significant anxiety will not be willing or able to attend an outpatient clinic, but will be happy to receive a home visit if given appropriate notice and preparation. A multidisciplinary OPMHS team with a well-trained geropsychologist is ideally suited to this task. However, other mental health workers with appropriate training and experience should be able to undertake non-pharmacological treatment for the common anxiety disorders. Sufficient time needs to be allocated to engaging the person in the assessment and management task.

Individualised approach

Non-pharmacological methods are the treatments of choice for the anxiety disorders. The specific approaches to treatment vary from one anxiety disorder to another, but the general principles remain the same. Treatment planning should be undertaken in collaboration with the person, whose cooperation and 'ownership' of such a plan is essential to its success. Involvement of the person's family or significant others may also be critical to treatment success. If family members (or residential aged care facility (RACF) staff) have not been well briefed on the rationale and practical implementation of a treatment plan, they may well not cooperate with it and it may fail. In particular, behavioural interventions must be designed with the specific physical and human environment in mind.

Psychoeducation

People with anxiety disorders or clinically significant anxiety symptoms should be given educational instruction about the nature of anxiety and the simple measures that can be used to reduce their background level of anxiety. People are often unaware that the symptoms that they attribute to cardiac, respiratory, gastrointestinal or neurological disease are actually common symptoms of panic or anxiety. Similarly, they are often unaware that these symptoms are not usually dangerous and that these symptoms will settle spontaneously if allowed to. People should be told about the evolutionary purpose of anxiety in terms of the 'fight or flight' response of the sympathetic nervous system. They should also be told about the inverted U-shaped Yerkes-Dodson curve, which illustrates the relationship between anxiety and performance—that is, that performance improves with a little anxiety, but deteriorates with severe anxiety.

Reduced stimulant intake and increased physical activity

Many anxious older people use too much caffeine, nicotine or alcohol, and require specific advice to cease or reduce their intake of these stimulants. Conversely, many anxious people take too little exercise and get too little sleep. Physical exercise acts as a form of exposure to both interoceptive stimuli (physiological manifestations of sympathetic nervous system activity that increase during exercise, like sweating and palpitations) and exteroceptive stimuli (the setting in which the exercise takes place, such as the park, the footpath, the walking track or the gym). In addition, regular physical exercise builds stamina and is an antidote to fatigue. In an otherwise physically healthy older person, it is appropriate to recommend gradually building up to at least 30 minutes of exercise daily. If in doubt about the medical safety of advising increased physical activity, it is important to arrange for the person to be reviewed by their GP.

Sleep hygiene

Advice about sleep hygiene is also very useful for the anxious person. The sleep environment needs to be suitable for the initiation and maintenance of sleep. For most people, this means having a bedroom that is dark, an appropriate temperature and free of excessive noise. The bed itself must be comfortable and the sleeping partner, if any, should not be exhibiting disruptive behaviours. It is almost never appropriate for people with insomnia to watch television in bed. The behavioural aspects of sleep initiation also need attention. It is useful for people with insomnia to have their own standard pre-sleep routine and a set time of wakening. It is also important that people who are unable to fall asleep within 15 or 20 minutes of wanting to, get up and leave the bedroom until they feel sleepy again. Conditioned insomnia can develop through the repeated pairing of lying in bed with failure to initiate sleep. Some people need formal psychotherapy because of traumatic events that have occurred in the bedroom (e.g. childhood sexual abuse, rape or other assault, death of spouse).

Relaxation training

Training in relaxation techniques is useful in the treatment of many anxiety disorders. A variety of techniques are available. These include controlled breathing and reciprocal inhibition by visual imagery. Progressive muscular relaxation is frequently recommended to younger adults, and is an excellent technique. However, it is sometimes not very suitable for older people due to their reduced muscle bulk and the frequent presence of arthritis.

Controlled breathing is used to manage panic. The person is trained to hold their breath for 10 seconds and then to breathe in and out in 6-second cycles, thus breathing 10 times per minute. The person will need a watch or clock with a second hand to practise this technique and should do so for 10–15 minutes twice a day initially. At the first sign of emerging panic, the person should implement this technique. This approach is based on reducing hyperventilation and increasing physiological retention of carbon dioxide, thereby reducing the pH of the blood (making it more acidic) and reducing stimulation of the amygdala.

Reciprocal inhibition by visual imagery is a method of reducing the person's underlying level of anxiety and thus reducing the likelihood of breakthrough panic attacks. The person is asked to imagine a picture frame or a window frame and then to 'paint' a relaxing scene in the frame. They must put in as many sensory details as possible (e.g. the detailed visual features of the scene, and the sounds and smell of the scene). The person must then put themselves in the picture in their imagination. They then take a walk in the scene, all the while thinking how relaxing it is. When practised for 10–15 minutes twice a day, this is an effective method of reducing generalised anxiety. It is important for the person to choose a relaxing scene that has not been associated with any trauma or anxiety for them. The theory on which this technique is based is that it is impossible to be simultaneously relaxed and anxious.

Benzodiazepines

Although benzodiazepine sedatives such as diazepam and alprazolam are widely prescribed to treat anxiety symptoms and anxiety disorders in older people, they are often not effective beyond the short term. In addition, they have the potential to cause significant adverse effects in older people, including amnesia, fatigue, daytime sleepiness, disinhibition and falls. Excessive sedation may sometimes be complicated by dehydration, deep vein thrombosis and pneumonia. Furthermore, benzodiazepines are sometimes abused by older people, with escalating doses being used to obtain an effect. Thus, if benzodiazepines are to be used in older people, we recommend that they be used as a short-term expedient while other anxiety treatments are initiated.

However, this approach can be criticised, as absence of anxiety will compromise exposure techniques that rely on the natural decline in anxiety with habituation to a phobic stimulus. Benzodiazepines should generally be used for only 1 or 2 weeks. In addition, we recommend the use of particular benzodiazepines, such as oxazepam and temazepam, which are not extensively metabolised in the liver. As a general principle, lower doses should be used in older people, and they should be closely observed for adverse effects.

Antidepressants

If psychotropic medication is to be used in the management of anxiety disorders in older people, then antidepressants are the drugs of choice. There is good evidence for the anxiolytic properties of the selective serotonin reuptake inhibitors (SSRIs), as well as venlafaxine and mirtazapine. However, these drugs may initially increase anxiety and the person may need to be treated with a low-dose benzodiazepine for the first few days of treatment with an SSRI or venlafaxine. This is less likely to be necessary with mirtazapine, which is often experienced as sedating. One problem with the use of modern antidepressants in older people is their tendency to cause hyponatraemia (low serum sodium concentration), particularly in older people taking diuretics or who have cerebrovascular disease. It is prudent to check the serum sodium level before initiating antidepressants in older people, and a week or so later. It is important also to note that hyponatraemia may present with increased agitation and other mental state changes.

Behaviour therapy

The key behavioural techniques for managing phobic disorders include the exposure techniques of flooding and systematic desensitisation. Flooding involves exposing the person to the feared object or situation for real (referred to as *in vivo*). Although very effective, flooding is not commonly used in the treatment of older people. Systematic desensitisation involves exposing the person to a hierarchy of representations of the feared object or situation and then finally to the object or situation itself. Systematic desensitisation is often done initially in the imagination (referred to as *in imago*) and then *in vivo*. This is a highly effective treatment in older people with specific phobias and agoraphobia. Formal exposure interventions are best designed in consultation with an experienced geropsychologist. However, informal exposure interventions are also likely to be useful, particularly in older people with mild to moderate avoidance behaviour. One example of this, physical activity, has already been described.

Other aspects of behaviour therapy include exposure and response prevention for people with obsessive-compulsive therapy. For successful implementation in people with severe obsessive-compulsive disorder, a formally designed intervention is likely to be necessary. However, once again, informal approaches might be worthwhile in those with mild to moderate symptoms. Mental health workers are advised to consult specialised texts in relation to such techniques.

Cognitive behaviour therapy

In the cognitive component of cognitive behaviour therapy (CBT), the therapist attends to the maladaptive cognitions that are associated with anxiety symptoms. Firstly, the therapist and person identify the catastrophic cognitions and negative automatic thoughts associated with the person's panic attacks or other anxiety symptoms. Next, these maladaptive cognitions are challenged by identifying evidence that they are incorrect or exaggerated. Thirdly, alternative explanations are found and the arguments for and against these explanations are weighed. Fourthly, behavioural 'experiments' are conducted to provide further evidence that the alternative explanations are correct. Finally, the catastrophic cognitions or negative automatic thoughts are replaced with the more logical and normal explanations.

Because it requires a sophisticated and psychologically minded person, this approach is likely to have limited applicability to older people with cognitive impairment or older people with poor education. However, other components of the suite of interventions labelled CBT are likely to have wider applicability. These include relaxation training, controlled breathing and activity scheduling. Interested readers are referred to a short textbook that deals with this topic in more detail (Laidlaw et al 2003).

Although little research has been undertaken using a combination of psychological and pharmacological interventions in older people with anxiety disorders, older people with severe or chronic anxiety disorders are likely to benefit from such combination treatment. Certainly, this has been found to be the case in relation to the treatment of depression.

Treatment outlines for specific disorders are listed in the box below.

TREATMENT OUTLINES FOR SPECIFIC DISORDERS

Generalised anxiety disorder
Treatment options include:
- psychoeducation
- reduced stimulant intake
- sleep hygiene
- physical activity
- self-monitoring
- relaxation training
- worry exposure
- formal CBT, and
- antidepressant medication (SSRI/SNRI).

Panic disorder
Treatment options include:
- psychoeducation
- reduced stimulant intake
- controlled breathing
- formal CBT, and
- antidepressant medication (SSRI/SNRI).

Simple phobia
Treatment options include:
- psychoeducation
- relaxation training, and
- exposure (usually systematic desensitisation).

Social phobia
Treatment options include:
- psychoeducation
- relaxation training
- exposure
- beta-blockers (performance anxiety), and
- antidepressants (SSRI/SNRI).

Agoraphobia
Treatment options include:
- psychoeducation
- relaxation training
- treatment of panic attacks (see above), and
- exposure (usually systematic desensitisation).

Obsessive-compulsive disorder
Treatment options include:
- psychoeducation
- exposure and response prevention
- formal CBT, and
- antidepressant medication (SSRI/SNRI).

Post-traumatic stress disorder
Treatment options include:
- psychoeducation
- relaxation training
- formal CBT, and
- antidepressant medication (SSRI/SNRI).

Impediments to successful management
There are several impediments to the successful management of anxiety disorders in older people. Firstly, some older people experience and interpret their anxiety symptoms as being symptoms of a general medical condition and resist the notion that they will respond to psychological interventions. Secondly, there is a tendency by mental health workers to apply psychological treatments to young and middle-aged people and psychotropic drugs to older people. Thirdly, there is a shortage of mental health workers, particularly clinical psychologists, specifically trained in the management of anxiety disorders in older people. Finally, the management of anxiety disorders in older people with cognitive impairment is a serious challenge, as psychoeducation and treatment adherence are likely to be problematic.

TREATMENT SUMMARY: ANXIETY

Treatment should include:
- educating the person about anxiety
- reduced caffeine, nicotine and alcohol intake
- physical activity
- relaxation training
- exposure and systematic desensitisation
- other types of behaviour therapy
- formal CBT
- antidepressant medication, and
- benzodiazepines (short term only).

PREVENTION

Little is known about the primary prevention of anxiety disorders in older people. However, it is likely that efforts to reduce childhood physical and sexual abuse, together with early intervention for childhood anxiety disorders, will reduce the prevalence of anxiety disorders in middle-aged and older people. Secondary prevention of anxiety disorders in older people should involve early intervention for pathological grief, particularly following traumatic deaths. Active management of high-risk bereavements is likely to be useful. Screening high-risk populations, such as general medical outpatients, for anxiety symptoms might also pay dividends if good follow-up services are in place. There is at present too little recognition of the traumatic effects of physical illness. Although psychological debriefing following traumatic events experienced a vogue several years ago, it is now clear that debriefing is either ineffective or makes matters worse and should be avoided. However, people exposed to traumatic events are likely to benefit from humane care and support, and the early detection and treatment of a mental health problem, should it develop.

SUMMARY

Anxiety disorders occur commonly among older people and have a tendency to be chronic. However, there are effective treatments available for anxiety disorders, with the emphasis being on well-planned and executed non-pharmacological interventions.

FURTHER READING

Andrews G, Hunt C 1998 Treatments that work in anxiety disorders. eMJA. Online. Available: www.mja.com.au/public/mentalhealth/course/05andrews.pdf 3 Mar 2008
Laidlaw K, Thompson LW, Gallagher-Thompson D, Dick-Siskin L 2003 Cognitive behaviour therapy with older people. John Wiley & Sons, Chichester

REFERENCES

American Psychiatric Association 2000 Diagnostic and statistical manual of mental disorders DSM–IV–TR, 4th edn (text revision). American Psychiatric Association, Washington DC
Australian Bureau of Statistics (ABS) 1998 Mental health and wellbeing: profile of adults, Australia 1997. ABS, Canberra
Laidlaw K, Thompson LW, Gallagher-Thompson D, Dick-Siskin L 2003 Cognitive behaviour therapy with older people. John Wiley & Sons, Chichester
Pachana NA, Byrne GJ, Siddle H et al 2007 Development and validation of the Geriatric Anxiety Inventory. International Psychogeriatrics 19:103–114
Sinoff G, Ore L, Zlotogrosky D, Tamir A 1999 Short Anxiety Screening Test: a brief instrument for detecting anxiety in the elderly. International Journal of Geriatric Psychiatry 14:1062–1071

APPENDIX A: GERIATRIC ANXIETY INVENTORY

Please answer the items according to how you've felt in the last week. Tick the circle under AGREE if you mostly agree that the item describes you; tick the circle under DISAGREE if you mostly disagree that the item describes you.

		Agree	Disagree
1	I worry a lot of the time.	O	O
2	I find it difficult to make a decision.	O	O
3	I often feel jumpy.	O	O
4	I find it hard to relax.	O	O
5	I often cannot enjoy things because of my worries.	O	O
6	Little things bother me a lot.	O	O
7	I often feel like I have butterflies in my stomach.	O	O
8	I think of myself as a worrier.	O	O
9	I can't help worrying about even trivial things.	O	O
10	I often feel nervous.	O	O
11	My own thoughts often make me anxious.	O	O
12	I get an upset stomach due to my worrying.	O	O
13	I think of myself as a nervous person.	O	O
14	I always anticipate the worst will happen.	O	O
15	I often feel shaky inside.	O	O
16	I think that my worries interfere with my life.	O	O
17	My worries often overwhelm me.	O	O
18	I sometimes feel a great knot in my stomach.	O	O
19	I miss out on things because I worry too much.	O	O
20	I often feel upset.	O	O

Source: Pachana NA, Byrne GJ, Siddle H et al 2007 Development and validation of the Geriatric Anxiety Inventory. International Psychogeriatrics 19:103–114. ©Copyright 2007 The University of Queensland.

Chapter 24

THE OLDER PERSON WITH SUBSTANCE ABUSE

INTRODUCTION

Very little attention has been given to substance abuse among older people but, with the ageing population, this issue will have greater importance and prominence. Substance abuse affects a relatively small number of older people, but it has a major impact on the quality of life of the substance user and their significant others. Substance abuse exacerbates underlying illness, alters both mood and behaviour, and can result in accidents such as falls, or while doing precarious activities like driving a car (Lynskey et al 2003). With older people, it usually involves the misuse of legal (alcohol, tobacco, prescribed and over-the-counter medications), rather than illegal substances (cannabis, heroin, cocaine) (Australian Institute of Health and Welfare 2007). Therefore, it can easily be hidden and treatment for substance abuse may be overlooked, particularly when there are other acute or chronic illnesses shadowing the true picture (Culberson 2006).

In a number of ways, the issue of substance abuse is different for older people than the younger generations. Firstly, denial is a common response when an older person is asked about substance use. This response may be given because of memory problems, shame from the stigma attached to being a substance user, a desire to continue use, or perhaps it is considered as a normal behaviour for them. Secondly, the ageing body has reduced lean body mass and total body water causing higher peak blood alcohol levels; therefore, older people react more severely to the effects of some substances due to this changed physiological makeup. Moreover, older people also take more prescription medications where there is a likelihood of adverse interactions between substances, with warfarin and digoxin being good examples (Lynskey et al 2003). In order to maintain optimal health, substance abuse should be routinely screened and assessed for and, if found to be an issue, followed up with a comprehensive treatment approach.

CASE VIGNETTE

Bill is a 79-year-old returned soldier who lives alone in a sparsely furnished, tidy, but generally neglected house. His wife had divorced him many years before, but his four adult children were on reasonably amicable terms with their father. Each of the children lived with him intermittently when they themselves were experiencing financial and social difficulties; however, this was usually the last and very short-term option. Bill admitted that the heavy use of alcohol was the main cause of the breakdown of his marriage and family dysfunction. Since retiring as a watchmaker at the age of 65 years, tight financial circumstances had resulted in him not drinking as heavily, but he now experienced frequent and severe panic attacks (up to four times per week). The panic attacks resulted in a local general practitioner (GP) making a home visit to administer intramuscular (IM) diazepam and leaving prescriptions for sedative medications. Bill's son referred him to the older persons' mental health service (OPMHS), as he was not satisfied with his father's health status.

Bill relied heavily on his GP for his healthcare needs; therefore, the mental health worker developed a close working relationship with the GP. The GP was given information on controlled breathing techniques and brief interventions, and encouraged to use these strategies, rather than immediately prescribing antianxiety medication. Bill refused to participate in any therapy activities outside of his home, necessitating the mental health worker to visit regularly for about 6 months to undertake cognitive behaviour therapy (CBT).

THE SPECTRUM OF SUBSTANCE ABUSE

Drugs of abuse (e.g. alcohol, cannabis, sedative-hypnotics and opioids) have psychoactive properties, which means that they act on the central nervous system, particularly on the mind or psyche. Drugs that have non-psychoactive properties can also be misused, and these include tobacco and over-the-counter medications (e.g. analgesics, laxatives, tonics, vitamins, and cold and flu preparations). Substance use refers to any taking of a drug, whereas abuse involves some physiological, psychological and social harm. Prolonged abuse can lead to dependency and addiction, which have certain defining criteria. The *Diagnostic and Statistical Manual of Mental Disorders*, 4th edition (DSM–IV) (American Psychiatric Association 2000) provides criteria to differentiate between these terms (see Table 24.1).

Table 24.1 DSM–IV criteria for substance abuse and dependency/addiction	
Substance Abuse	**Dependency/Addiction**
Unable to fulfil role obligations at work or home	Tolerance develops
Risk of physical danger (e.g. falls, accidents, unable to operate machinery safely)	Withdrawal symptoms present
	Using larger amounts
	Using for longer periods of time
	Trying to cut down or control use
Legal problems	More time spent obtaining, using and recovering
Interpersonal problems	Changes in social, occupational and recreational activities
	Continued use despite physical and psychological dependency

EPIDEMIOLOGY

The 1997 National Survey of Mental Health and Wellbeing (Australian Bureau of Statistics 1998) established that the prevalence of substance-abuse disorders declined with age from 16.1% for 18–24-year-olds to 1.1% for those aged 65 years and older. Within that overall prevalence rate of 1.1% for older people, males recorded a rate of 2.1% compared with 0.2% for females. Older men tend to use alcohol and illegal drugs, whereas older women tend to abuse sedative-hypnotics and anxiolytics. The likelihood of using health services for a substance-abuse disorder was only 14%, whereas for affective disorders it was 56% and 28% for anxiety disorders. The decline in prevalence with increasing age is postulated as being age-related, increased mortality among those who have a lifelong history of substance abuse and less exposure and use of substances (Lynskey et al 2003).

In 2004, alcohol was the most prevalent substance used by Australians with 41% of people most likely to drink weekly and 9% consuming alcohol on a daily basis. Cannabis is the most commonly used illicit drug with 11% of people reporting to have used it in the previous 12 months; 3% of people reported the use of meth-amphetamines in the previous 12 months. Older people recorded the highest prevalence of daily drinking (17%), with a further 33% drinking weekly, and 25% less than weekly (12.2% stated they were ex-drinkers and 12.8% did not drink at the time of the survey) (Australian Institute of Health and Welfare 2007). Specific data for other drugs of concern in older people, such as prescribed narcotics and sedatives and over-the-counter medications, are not available, but anecdotal accounts point to these being reasonably problematic. Also of note is that there is an expected increase in substance abuse in older people due to the ageing of the current cohort of baby boomers (those born between 1946 and 1964), who in their youth had more widespread experiences than previous generations with legal and illegal substances such as alcohol, cannabis and narcotics (Lynskey et al 2003).

DIFFERENTIAL DIAGNOSIS

The overlay of multiple medical and psychosocial issues makes the diagnosis and treatment of substance abuse in older people a complex and often frustrating experience. Substance abuse is strongly associated with a range of problems, such as self-neglect, anxiety, depression, sleep and appetite disturbances, falls, urinary and faecal incontinence, and memory problems that may be confused with the presentation of other disorders such as dementia (O'Connell et al 2003).

RISK FACTORS

Risk factors for substance abuse include:
- family history
- previous personal history
- personality traits/disorder
- chronic illness associated with pain (opioid abuse)
- chronic insomnia (hypnotic abuse)
- chronic anxiety (anxiolytic abuse)
- caregiver overuse
- grief and loss

- isolation and loneliness, and
- depression.

SCREENING TOOLS

The use of screening tools will assist in determining if a more detailed assessment of substance abuse and related issues is required. The following screening tools have been used successfully with older populations. The first two, the CAGE questionnaire and the Alcohol Use Disorders Identification Test (AUDIT), are primarily used for the screening of alcohol abuse (Berks & McCormick 2008), whereas the Impression of Medication, Alcohol and Drug Use in Seniors (IMADUS) has a more comprehensive approach to substance abuse and screens for alcohol, prescription drugs and over-the-counter medications (see Ch 35).

CAGE questionnaire

The CAGE questionnaire (Ewing 1984) is a 4-item, easy-to-use, reliable and valid gauge of an individual's use of or potential abuse of alcohol and the effects it may be having on key life issues (see the box below). A 'yes' response to two or more of the CAGE questions is an indicator for further assessment of substance abuse, although Dekker (2002) found that a score of one or more has a sensitivity and specificity of about 80% in older people.

THE CAGE QUESTIONNAIRE

C Have you ever felt you should **c**ut down on your drinking?

A Have people **a**nnoyed you by criticising your drinking?

G Have you ever felt bad or **g**uilty about your drinking?

E Have you ever had a drink first thing in the morning to steady your nerves or get rid of a hangover (**e**ye-opener)?

Alcohol Use Disorders Identification Test (AUDIT)

The Alcohol Use Disorders Identification Test (AUDIT) (Saunders et al 1993) has a series of 10 questions for the identification of risky alcohol consumption. Each question receives a score from 0 to 4. A score of 8 or more is indicative of risky drinking patterns and the need for further assessment of alcohol dependence. It is short, easy to administer, and needs no formal training to administer.

Impression of Medication, Alcohol and Drug Use in Seniors (IMADUS)

The Impression of Medication, Alcohol and Drug Use in Seniors (IMADUS) (Shulman 2003) has 20 items and three or more 'yes' responses point to the need for a more detailed assessment. The questioning style has been designed to reduce the feelings of shame that often occur when older people are asked about substance abuse.

ASSESSMENT

The aim of undertaking a comprehensive assessment is to determine past substance-abuse patterns, current patterns, level of dependence and the substance-abuse-related problems. Asking general assessment questions that do not judge current substance-abuse behaviour is a useful, initial approach. These could be along the lines of:

- Can you tell me how you use the substance?
- Has your use of this substance caused any kinds of problems for you?
- Have you ever been concerned about your substance use?
- What benefit for you is there in using the substance?

It is important in the assessment to clarify what is meant, for example, by a 'drink'; translate this into standard units and then find out the type of substance, how many and how often.

History

A thorough history is essential for the assessment process. It is taken from the person themselves and, if possible, a reliable significant other as a source of corroborating and collateral information. The history would include details of their upbringing, education, employment, current social situation, significant personal relationships and atypical experiences, such as military service, childhood abuse and domestic violence. Additionally, past and current medical/psychiatric history needs to be obtained, including substance misuse by themselves and direct family members. A significant other who has known the older person for a long time may be able to give some idea about the older person's premorbid personality. Valuable insight into how the older person is managing their domestic situation can be gained from a visit to their home.

It is important to differentiate if the substance abuse has been a lifelong problem that has carried over into old age or whether it has developed in later life, perhaps in response to issues perpetuated by the ageing process, such as loss and loneliness. Interestingly, women tend to develop dependence in later life, whereas men tend to be all-of-life users. The time of onset is significant because early-onset people tend to have more psychopathology, dysfunctional social relationships and serious health problems, such as Korsakoff's psychosis where there could be permanent neuropsychological changes (Barrick & Connors 2002).

As with other disorders, determining factors that are maintaining the substance abuse is helpful. These could include such things as painful medical conditions, sleep disturbances, anxiety, depression, social disadvantage and dysfunctional interpersonal relationships. Resilience factors such as the older person's level of intelligence, education, social supports, neuroticism, general health, financial security and religiosity/spirituality also need to be assessed.

Mental state examination

The mental state examination (MSE) will assist in determining if an older person is abusing substances and alert the clinician to any comorbid conditions such as cognitive impairment, depressive illness or suicidal ideation. The cognitive ability of the older person will determine if such interventions as counselling will benefit them and whether or not they will be able to change their substance-related behaviour. The mental health worker also needs to be cognisant of the fact that substance abuse in older people is a risk factor for suicide, particularly the combination of alcohol abuse and suicidal intent.

Physical examination

A routine physical examination, including a neurological examination, is very important to exclude other pathologies or medical conditions that have been made worse by the substance abuse. During the examination, it is also worthwhile to take note of other presentations that may be the result of substance-abuse behaviour, such as personal neglect, particularly hygiene and nutritional deficiencies, needle marks, bruising from bumps and falls, evidence of head injury, signs of liver failure and peripheral neuropathy.

Laboratory investigations

Baseline and screening laboratory investigations should include a full blood count with platelets (may indicate vitamin B12 deficiency or alcohol excess), urea, serum electrolytes and folate levels (may indicate undernutrition), vitamin B12 estimation, liver function test, glucose level and thyroid function test.

MANAGEMENT

Once the person has been assessed and a diagnosis has been established, a collaborative management plan depending upon the severity of the problem can be implemented. Goals have to be defined in relation to the older person's readiness to change their substance-abuse behaviour (Sanchez-Craig 1990). The outcomes of care will be a reduction in intake/abstinence, improved quality of life and improved physical functioning. Treatment strategies for older people do differ from the younger populations. For example, the traditional leverages of unemployment or criminal sanctions do not have the same effect on older people who are experiencing different maturational needs and changes. Discussed below are general treatment guidelines and strategies that are applicable for all substance-abuse disorders, but there are highly specialised addiction treatment services that may use more refined/specific strategies.

TREATMENT

Detoxification

It is not necessary for a person to be substance free before treatment is commenced; however, if there is a risk of severe health problems, detoxification is recommended (Yost 1996). If consumption is low or of a short duration, usually only minor withdrawal symptoms, such as nausea, vomiting, anxiety, tremor and sweating, are experienced. These can be treated while the older person remains at home or on an outpatient or day-patient basis. If detoxification is done in these circumstances, it should be done under the supervision of a qualified health professional and the older person needs to be fully informed of the process. Ideally, they should have a support person who can remain with them constantly. Everyone needs to be aware of what symptoms to expect and how severe these may be. Withdrawal symptoms usually start 6–24 hours after the substance was last induced. It is usually resolved within 5 days, but the older person should be monitored for any danger signs that require urgent medical attention, such as seizures and the delirium tremens. Ongoing long-term supportive strategies such as counselling with a focus on dealing with any psychosocial issues, pharmacological agents and enhancement of social support networks may need to be instigated once detoxification has taken place.

It is worth keeping in mind that physiological changes such as liver damage may cause an older person to have serious withdrawal symptoms, even if their intake is considered small. Sudden cessation of the evening glass of sherry or a nightly sleeping tablet could induce more serious withdrawal symptoms. Such a situation commonly arises when these older people are admitted to hospital for surgical or medical procedures—staff are unaware of their substance use and the older person does not realise they may go into withdrawal. The symptoms of withdrawal may also be confused with other disorders of cognitive functioning such as delirium and dementia.

Serious withdrawal symptoms will require hospitalisation with longer term follow-up and referral to specialist addiction services. Withdrawal symptoms usually occur after a person stops the substance after regular intake. Withdrawal symptoms peak around 72 hours after cessation or, sometimes, even sooner, so it is important to establish when the substance was last used. The older person must be closely monitored for severe symptoms such as seizures, tachycardia, hypertension, hallucinations, confusion and the delirium tremens. If the older person is withdrawing from benzodiazepines, insomnia is one of the most troubling symptoms (Schweizer et al 1990). There are withdrawal scales that can assist with assessing the severity of the alcohol withdrawal syndrome, and these should be commenced as soon as possible. The withdrawal scales can also help monitor the efficacy of treatment.

The Clinical Institute Withdrawal Assessment for Alcohol Scale (CIWA–A) (Stuppaeck et al 1994) is a valid and reliable 12-item scale. Two of the scale items (vital functions and withdrawal seizures) are recorded, but not scored. This means that the total score is derived from the ratings of the remaining 10 items. Each item is rated from 1 to 6 with possible total scores ranging from 10 to 60. The developers recommend that a score less than 8 warrants a brief intervention, while a score between 8 and 20 warrants the introduction of a benzodiazepine to reduce the severity of symptoms, including seizures and the delirium tremens. For a score of greater than 20, an inpatient admission is recommended to implement a range of interventions. After successful medical treatment, regular follow-up with a brief intervention, more in-depth psychotherapy and referral to a support group is highly recommended because in the initial months after treatment there is a high risk of relapse (Barrick & Connors 2002).

Counselling

Brief interventions are effective for well-motivated older adults and are based on the premise of personal choice, individual responsibility for change, mutually agreed goals and an empathetic style of interaction. The therapy is very structured and only lasts for 5–30 minutes, with the aim of reducing or stopping consumption. Brief intervention is often based on the FRAMES method (Miller & Rollnick 1991):

- *Feedback*. Reinforce with the older person that their substance use is putting them at risk of serious consequences. Use educational information to compare actual intake with recommended limits.
- *Responsibility*. Reinforce that only the older person can change their behaviour.
- *Advice*. Provide specific recommendations in regard to reducing risk (e.g. lower dosages or abstinence).
- *Menu*. Offer a variety of ways to reduce the substance-abuse problem (e.g. keeping a diary of substance-abuse patterns, setting limits on intake, identifying and avoiding situations that may lead to taking of the substance, and pacing intake by dilution and smaller doses).

- *Empathetic counselling.* Show an understanding that the substance plays a role in the person's life. Use non-confrontational and supportive techniques, such as negotiation, rather than prescription and blame.
- *Self-efficacy.* Empower the older person through recognition and validation of their goals, strengths and use of positive affirmations.

Psychosocial treatments are excellent for exploration of substance-related problems. This is where the reasons for and the circumstances surrounding the substance use can be explored and the role the substance plays in the person's life established. Issues such as social isolation, depression, grief or loss, or interpersonal problems, can be addressed by building the older person's social network, general problem-solving ability and enhancement of motivation. This may include individual and group psychotherapy and attendance at inexpensive, self-help groups such as Alcoholics Anonymous and Narcotics Anonymous. These groups are present in many Australian cities and towns. These are non-professional, self-supporting, non-denominational, apolitical and multicultural organisations, although there is a religious theme. Each group member assists the others in dealing with their substance problem and it is based on the philosophy that each person has complete responsibility for their own recovery. These organisations have expanded their services to include family members who have been adversely affected by a person's misuse of substances. Other than that, specific family therapy may also be warranted (Barrick & Connors 2002).

Information and education

Education is a very important aspect of treatment because having a specific knowledge base reduces the sense of helplessness and expands the options for changing behaviour (National Drug and Alcohol Research Centre 2003). Educational sessions which focus on the physiological risks and harmful effects of substance abuse, healthy drinking patterns and techniques for behaviour modification would be helpful. A list of reputable organisations that publish educational substance-abuse information is provided in the 'Useful websites' section at the end of the chapter.

Pharmacotherapy

Pharmacotherapy may sometimes play a role in the management of substance abuse (Kranzler 2000). If it involves the use of benzodiazepines, oxazepam is the drug of choice for older people because it has no active metabolites and a short half-life. If anxiety or depression are major presenting psychological symptoms, these are treated with antianxiety agents and antidepressants respectively.

Disulfiram is an antidipsotropic, which alters the body's response to alcohol. Even a small amount of alcohol will cause nausea and vomiting. This medication may be occasionally prescribed for the prevention of relapse in alcohol abuse, but only for well-motivated individuals. However, contraindication with medical comorbidities such as cardiac and hepatic disease limits usefulness with older people. This medication works by inhibiting the enzyme responsible for catalysing the breakdown of acetaldehyde in the blood. The consumption of alcohol increases the acetaldehyde levels, which will cause shortness of breath, flushing, nausea and vomiting lasting for up to an hour. A dose of disulfiram lasts for at least 72 hours, making it difficult for an impulsive drinking session.

There are some drugs that can be used to support abstinence. Naltrexone may help prevent craving and relapse in alcohol abusers. It is a long-acting, orally administered antagonist of opiate effects. Acamprosate affects the NMDA receptors and works to reduce cravings for alcohol. Nutritional supplements high in the vitamin B group, particularly vitamin B1 (thiamine), are coadministered when there is evidence of dietary neglect and to counteract the depletion of vitamin B caused by heavy drinking.

Follow-up

Ongoing support while recovering from substance abuse is essential. This can occur by a case management process through a health service and by attendance at therapy sessions and support groups. The person needs constant reinforcement of the strategies that are working for them. Unfortunately, relapse is a possibility with a rate of around 50% (Barrick & Connors 2002). If relapse does occur, the person needs to go back to examining why they initially decided to change their behaviour and review their strengths and the positive changes they had made in their life before the relapse occurred. The relapse may have occurred because of external factors, such as loneliness, and countermeasures will need to be determined and put in place so the individual is protected from these in the future.

Prognosis

With treatment, many people can abstain from using substances, adopt a harm minimisation approach or only experience brief relapses that do not progress to abuse or dependence. With abstinence, there can also be marked improvement in physical and social functioning. Untreated conditions can result in liver cirrhosis, cardiomyopathy, hypertension, memory problems and sleep disturbances. Fractures and subdural haematomas can result from falls and accidents. Alcohol can be attributed to many hospitalisations and deaths (Chikritzhs & Pascal 2005).

Care for significant others

As with the treatment for other disorders and, if appropriate, the needs of significant others or caregivers have to be incorporated into the plan of care. One matter of particular note with substance abuse is codependence (Beattie 1992). This is the term used to describe the behaviour of a significant other (usually the spouse or partner) who enables

---

TREATMENT SUMMARY: SUBSTANCE ABUSE

- Screening: the CAGE questionnaire, the AUDIT or the IMADUS.
- Assessment: history, mental state examination, physical examination and laboratory investigations.
- Treatment: the CIWA–A, counselling (brief intervention, psychotherapy), information and education, and pharmacotherapy.
- Follow-up: support and case management, and support groups.

the addict to continue their behaviour by interfering with what would be the logical consequences of the substance abuse. For example, if a person is unable to attend an appointment because they are intoxicated, the significant other makes contact giving a more acceptable excuse, such as they have a heavy cold. This behaviour has encouraged irresponsibility and assisted in maintaining the addictive behaviour. Closer examination of the motivation for these actions usually reveals a person who defines their self-worth in terms of caring for others to the exclusion of their own needs for self-fulfilment through acknowledgment, love, intimacy and personal growth. Apart from family therapy, there are support organisations such as Al-anon, Alateen and Co-Dependents Anonymous that can play an important part in treatment.

PREVENTION

Since 1985 Australia has had a National Drug Strategy with the aim to prevent and reduce the uptake of harmful substance use and minimise the harmful effects of legal and illegal substances. The National Drug Strategy is overseen by the Ministerial Council on Drug Strategy (MCDS). The MCDS is responsible for developing policies and programs to reduce harm caused by substances to individuals, families and communities. Policies and decisions in regard to the status of legal and illegal substances are also under its directive. The MCDS ensures there is a national approach to management of substance use by coordinating and integrating the activities of all levels of government in Australia, particularly in the related areas of health, education and law enforcement.

SUMMARY

As the population ages, substance abuse among older people will become a prominent mental health issue. It is a problem that often goes undetected and therefore a need for more widespread screening is required. Treatment is based on a comprehensive history and assessment, and the greater the problem the more intensive the treatment. Treatment encompasses psychosocial, behavioural and pharmacological interventions. In all aspects of care for the older person with substance-abuse problems, taking an empathetic approach is fundamental.

FURTHER READING

National Drug and Alcohol Research Centre 2003 Guidelines for the treatment for alcohol problems. Commonwealth Department of Health and Ageing, Canberra
National Health and Medical Research Council (NHMRC) 2001 Australian alcohol guidelines: health risks and benefits. NHMRC, Canberra

USEFUL WEBSITES

Al-Anon and Alateen: www.al-anon.alateen.org
Alcoholics Anonymous: www.aa.org
Australian Institute of Health and Welfare: www.aihw.gov.au
Australian Drug Foundation: www.adf.org.au
Co-Dependents Anonymous: www.codependents.org
Narcotics Anonymous: www.na.org
National Centre for Education and Training on Addiction: www.nceta.flinders.edu.au

National Drug and Alcohol Research Centre: ndarc.med.unsw.edu.au
National Drug Research Institute: ndri.curtin.edu.au
National Health and Medical Research Council: www.nhmrc.gov.au
National Institute on Drug Abuse: www.nida.nih.gov
Turning Point: www.turningpoint.org.au

REFERENCES

American Psychiatric Association 2000 Diagnostic and statistical manual of mental disorders, 4th edn. American Psychiatric Publishing, Washington DC

Australian Bureau of Statistics (ABS) 1998 Mental health and wellbeing: profile of adults, Australia 1997. ABS, Canberra

Australian Institute of Health and Welfare (AIHW) 2007 Statistics on drug use in Australia 2006. Drug Statistics Series No.18. AIHW Cat. No. PHE 80. AIHW, Canberra

Barrick C, Connors GJ 2002 Relapse prevention and maintaining abstinence in older adults with alcohol-use disorders. Drugs Aging 19(8):583–594

Beattie M 1992 Codependent no more: how to stop controlling others and start caring for yourself. MJF Books, New York

Berks J, McCormick R 2008 Screening for alcohol misuse in elderly primary care patients: a systematic literature review. International Psychogeriatrics 20(6):1090–1103

Chikritzhs T, Pascal R 2005 Trends in alcohol consumption and related harms for Australians aged 65 to 74 years (the young–old), 1990–2003. National Alcohol Indicators, Bulletin No. 8. National Drug Research Institute. Curtin University of Technology, Perth

Culberson JW 2006 Alcohol use in the elderly: beyond the CAGE. Part 1: prevalence and patterns of problem drinking. Geriatrics 61:23–27

Dekker AH 2002 Alcoholism in the elderly. Program and abstracts presented at the 33rd Annual Medical–Scientific Conference, American Society of Addiction Medicine, Atlanta

Ewing JA 1984 Detecting alcoholism: the CAGE questionnaire. Journal of the American Medical Association 252:1905–1907

Kranzler H 2000 Pharmacotherapy of alcoholism: gaps in knowledge and opportunities for research. Alcohol and Alcoholism 35:537–547

Lynskey MT, Day C, Hall W 2003 Alcohol and other drug use disorders among older-aged people. Drug and Alcohol Review 22:125–133

Miller W, Rollnick S 1991 Motivational interviewing: preparing people to change addictive behavior. Guilford Press, New York

National Drug and Alcohol Research Centre 2003 Guidelines for the treatment for alcohol problems. Commonwealth Department of Health and Ageing, Canberra

O'Connell H, Chin A, Cunningham C, Lawlor B 2003 Alcohol use disorders in elderly people: redefining an age-old problem in old age. British Medical Journal 327:664–667

Sanchez-Craig M 1990 Brief didactic treatment for alcohol and drug-related problems: an approach based on client choice. British Journal of Addiction 85(2):169–177

Saunders J, Aasland O, Babor T et al 1993 Development on the Alcohol Use Disorders Identification Test (AUDIT). WHO collaborative project on early detection of person with harmful alcohol consumption: II. Addiction 88:791–804

Schweizer E, Rickels K, Case WG, Greenblatt DJ 1990 Long-term therapeutic use of benzodiazepines: II. Effects of gradual taper. Archives of General Psychiatry 47:908–915

Shulman G 2003 Senior moments: assessing older adults. Addiction Today 15(82):17–19

Stuppaeck CH, Barnas C, Falk M et al 1994 Assessment of the alcohol withdrawal syndrome: validity and reliability of the translated and modified Clinical Institute Withdrawal Assessment for Alcohol Scale (CIWA–A). Addiction 89:1287–1292

Yost D 1996 Alcohol withdrawal syndrome. American Family Physician 54(2):657–659

Chapter 25

THE OLDER PERSON WITH PERSONALITY DISORDER

INTRODUCTION

Personality disorders are characterised by deeply embedded, inflexible, maladaptive, overt traits characterised by dysfunctional personal relationships and cognitive, emotional, impulse control difficulties. These characteristics result in the older person encountering problems in perceiving and interpreting situations, having blunted or exaggerated emotional responses, ineffectual dealings with other people or a lack of restraint in challenging situations. Old age brings new stressors for people, particularly in relation to losses such as employment, social networks and health. For an older person with a personality disorder, there may be increased stress due to their difficulty in adapting to changes and new situations, rigid behaviours limiting relationship development and their propensity for damaging relationships.

Personality disorders usually manifest in adolescence or young adulthood and persist into later life. In other circumstances, the course of the person's life may have protected them from an early diagnosis of a personality disorder because it may not have been until a life-changing event occurred in old age that problems were manifested. A common example of this is the person with a dependent personality disorder who functions well within a relationship with their spouse, but when the spouse dies they can no longer cope. A personality disorder is usually diagnosed when the personality traits become exaggerated and counterproductive to the point that there is significant impairment in personal and social relationships. Personality disorders are extremely difficult to treat, they often complicate the course and treatment of other mental health disorders, and they adversely affect a person's quality of life. This chapter considers personality disorders in older people, examines prevalence rates, and explores relevant issues and developments associated with the contemporary treatments of psychotherapy and pharmacotherapy. The goal of care focuses on minimising social and functional impairment.

CASE VIGNETTE

Doris, a 68-year-old widow, lived alone in a small cottage in an inner-city suburb. She had a longstanding diagnosis of obsessive-compulsive personality disorder but her severe arthritis was limiting her physical capabilities to the extent she soon required permanent placement in a residential aged care facility (RACF). Doris had one daughter who was affected by depression and they did not have a close relationship, so it was not practical to consider the daughter as capable of supporting her mother on an ongoing basis. Doris's obsessive-compulsive behaviour was obvious in her excessive and pedantic approach to housework, which was done overnight so that no one saw her. In addition to the impact the arthritis was having on her need to tend to the housework, the anxious aspects of her obsessive-compulsive personality disorder were making her adjustment to the prospect of moving into an RACF very complicated.

Because the RACF placement was imminent and would be irrevocable, the goal was not to 'change her personality', but to help her and the immediate RACF community reach a satisfying and workable relationship. As problems and behavioural difficulties manifested, short-term interpersonal, cognitive-behavioural therapies and problem-solving approaches would be used to assist her adaptation. A care plan was devised to enable the RACF staff to assist Doris when she became overly anxious and obstreperous. Staff were also educated about ways of not upsetting Doris (e.g. respecting her need for orderliness and constantly interacting with her in a calm, empathetic and consistent manner so a trusting relationship could be developed). If such strategies were not put in place, there was a high risk that Doris would have alienated herself and made it very difficult for the RACF staff to provide the necessary care for her.

PERSONALITY

Personality is defined as a person's pattern of psychological processes, which includes motives, feelings, thoughts, behaviour patterns, and other areas of psychological functioning. It is expressed through its influences on the body, in conscious experience and through social behaviour. It is generally stable over time (Mayer 2006, cited in Segal et al 2006).

A personality trait is a characteristic of the personality which makes a person unique. To be a trait it has to be a persistent and pervasive characteristic. Each person has a number of traits which contribute to their personality. For example, a person may be described as shy and retiring, whereas another is loud and boisterous; some people are impetuous or insensitive, whereas others are more thoughtful and considerate. The list is endless (Segal et al 2006).

People have a mix of personality traits. Some are flexible and responsive, whereas others are the opposite and not very attractive. In healthily functioning individuals, the positive traits are persistent and pervasive and negative traits are only exhibited when necessary or fleetingly. However, not everyone has an adaptive personality style and with some people negative traits are more prominent. For example, they may be described as aloof, rigid, hostile, egocentric or shallow to the extent that their personality style limits their ability to function appropriately on an everyday basis. This is when a person may be said to have a personality disorder (Segal et al 2006).

EPIDEMIOLOGY

The prevalence of personality disorders in older people living in the community is reported as being between 10% and 20% (Ames & Molinari 1994), up to 33% in older outpatients (Molinari & Marmion 1993) and 61.5% in older inpatients (Molinari & Marmion 1995).

Analyses of data from the North American National Epidemiological Survey on Alcohol and Related Conditions, which studied over 43,000 individuals (Balsis et al 2007), found that older people were more likely to receive diagnoses of obsessive-compulsive and schizoid personality disorders and less likely to receive diagnoses of avoidant, dependent, antisocial, borderline and histrionic personality disorders. These authors were critical of the DSM measurement criteria arguing that it favours younger people. Personality disorders affect similar numbers of older and younger adults, with a higher prevalence of clusters A (odd and eccentric) and/or C (fearful or anxious) for older people (Kenan et al 2000).

CLINICAL FEATURES

The DSM–IV (American Psychiatric Association 2000) classifies 10 personality disorders into three clusters. The usefulness of the DSM–IV nosology for personality disorders in older people is currently being questioned (Balsis et al 2007, van Alphen 2006). It has been suggested that some of the specific DSM–IV criteria such as recklessness, impulsivity and functioning in the workplace are not appropriate for older people, and there is a proposal to develop more specific profiles. However, until firm recommendations are made, it is suggested that mental health workers who work with older people use the DSM–IV criteria albeit cautiously with this age group.

Cluster A personality disorders

Cluster A is characterised by the odd, eccentric disorders, which are marked by paranoid (suspicious, grandiose), schizotypal (schizophrenia like) and schizoid (distant, aloof) types. The core problems associated with the odd, eccentric disorders are distorted perceptions and interpretations of events or other people's motives, and an intolerance of intimacy.

Impact on the older person and their mental healthcare provision

The types of behaviour and thought patterns that characterise an older person with a paranoid personality disorder are (American Psychiatric Association 2000, Segal et al 2006):

1. There may be suspiciousness, without sufficient grounds, that they are being exploited, harmed or deceived by others. In the case of an older person, this presentation would require further investigation because of the risk of elder abuse (see Ch 18). A mental health worker will have to take precautions, such as having a second person present and careful documentation, so that they do not become the focus of such accusations.
2. There may be an unjustified preoccupation about the loyalty and trustworthiness of family, friends and associates. This characteristic will make it difficult for an older person who is becoming more dependent and will have to accept help from other people.
3. There may be a reluctance to confide in others because of unwarranted fears that information is being collected for malicious intent. This makes history taking and gathering assessment information a challenge.
4. There may be other characteristics of reading hidden meanings into benign remarks, bearing grudges, wrongly perceiving attacks on their character and

unjustified suspicions regarding the fidelity of their partner. This impedes the development of productive relationships and consequently their level of social support and interaction may be very poor. Additionally, sensory deficits and cognitive impairment may worsen these paranoid traits.

The older person with a schizotypal personality disorder is easily recognisable as being bizarre or eccentric in their behaviour and dress. These people find any type of social or interpersonal relationship very uncomfortable to the extent where they may experience severe social anxiety. Cognitive or perceptual distortions, including ideas of reference, odd beliefs, magical thinking, suspicious or paranoid ideation, are common. They are reclusive and unfriendly, making relationship development very challenging. A tendency for neglect of personal care and their home environment ensures unpopularity with neighbours and visitors. Older people with this type of personality disorder also have difficulties when poor health necessitates admission to an RACF where they have to endure close contact with staff and other residents. Conversely, their odd behaviour may engender social rejection. Hearing and vision impairments can exacerbate paranoia (American Psychiatric Association 2000, Segal et al 2006).

The essential characteristics of schizoid personality disorder are a pervasive pattern of detachment from social relationships and a restricted range of emotions. These people are seen as being aloof, cold and detached, with no desire for close relationships. They engage in solitary activities, have little or no interest in sexual experiences, derive very little pleasure from activities and are indifferent to praise or criticism. Not having any close friends also comes under the criteria for schizoid personality disorder. However, this may not be considered as a maladaptive personality trait for older people who have outlived all their friends. The same could be said for 'little or no interest in sexual experiences' where this could be related to physiological and social changes (Balsis et al 2007). Additionally, hearing, vision and mobility impairments could hinder the development and maintenance of relationships. The older person with this type of personality disorder will usually resist offers of help, particularly if it involves contact with other people. They can become distressed if their independence is threatened and find it very difficult fitting into communal living situations (American Psychiatric Association 2000, Segal et al 2006).

Cluster B personality disorders

The dramatic and impulsive behaviours make up cluster B and include antisocial (self-destructive, predatory loners), histrionic (overly emotional, demonstrative), borderline (intense, volatile attachments) and narcissistic (vain, insecure) diagnoses. The central features of the cluster B disorders are extreme fluctuations in emotions, very unstable interpersonal relationships and upsetting impulsive actions. Commonly, these people fear abandonment and become unrealistically upset over any sort of criticism whether it is real or imagined.

Impact on the older person and their mental healthcare provision

The older person with an antisocial personality disorder has a pervasive pattern of violating the rights of others. They unashamedly lie, steal, con and will even physically assault other people. Impulsivity with reckless disregard for the safety of self or others and engagement in illegal activities that end with imprisonment are other features of this disorder. A person with antisocial personality disorder can present as ingratiating and charming, but relationships tend to be shallow and exploitative. As these people age, physical decline will moderate some of the more aggressive and risk-taking behaviours. If they seek treatment, it is important to explore what their motivation is to ensure it is not exploitative, and interventions will focus on helping them to think through the consequences of their behaviour and to plan constructive behaviours (American Psychiatric Association 2000, Segal et al 2006).

The essential features of the histrionic personality disorder are being the centre of attention and open displays of inappropriate sexually seductive or provocative behaviour. Emotions shift rapidly and these are often dramatised and exaggerated. These people consider relationships to be more intimate than they really are and, if matters are not going their way, they can get very angry and frustrated. They will attempt to sexualise encounters with health workers and other people and be very flirtatious. Any relationships they develop tend to be shallow and short-lived, which is a reflection of their own shallow and self-centred nature. The person with this disorder can become very needy, childlike and demanding of other people. These people use their physical appearance to draw attention; therefore, the physical changes that take place with the ageing process can be upsetting. Inability to use their sex appeal to relate to others leads to much frustration, as they do not possess any other skills to build effective relationships.

Older women with histrionic personality disorder who are living among predominantly other women in an RACF that has mostly female staff may not display the flirtatious and sexualised behaviour. A tendency for suggestibility and being easily influenced by other people could be very problematic, particularly if cognitive impairment is present, as it could leave the older person open to abuse (American Psychiatric Association 2000, Segal et al 2006).

It has been suggested that borderline personality disorder diminishes as people age, whereas other theories suggest that it is a mortality effect, burnout and age-related changes in neurobiological substrates that impact on these behaviours or that the criterion for diagnosis does not fit older people (Devanand et al 2000). Either way, if pathological symptoms exist, they can be targeted for treatment. A central feature of borderline personality disorder is frantic efforts to avoid real or imagined abandonment. For an older person, this behaviour may translate into unjustified fears that their caregiver will abandon them or in the situation where an older person has great difficulty coming to terms with no longer being a lifelong caregiver when their children have left home. People with borderline personality disorder have a very unstable self-image or sense of self, and long patterns of unstable interpersonal relationships. Relationship interaction fluctuates from frantically seeking attention and support, to hostility and avoidance, to seeking forgiveness and support again. This pattern wears other people down; therefore, social support wanes. A commonly used defence mechanism is splitting, where everything and everyone is either 'good' or 'bad' and then this assessment abruptly changes for no sound reason. Such behaviours create a great deal of havoc, particularly in situations where there are a lot of people involved, such as in an RACF.

When young, these people are extremely impulsive and engage in self-damaging behaviours around sexual activity, spending, substance abuse and binge eating. However, with older age, these self-damaging behaviours may become less overt and intense, and may be replaced by acts of self-prescribing polypharmacy and refusing or sabotaging medical care. These people have chronic feelings of emptiness and have difficulty regulating and controlling their emotions such as anger. Suicidal behaviours, threats and self-mutilation are also prominent. They may also experience transient, stress-related paranoid ideation (American Psychiatric Association 2000, Segal et al 2006).

The older person with a narcissistic personality disorder typically has a grandiose sense of self-importance and entitlement, and is arrogant. They have fantasies of success, power, intelligence, beauty and ideal love. They believe they are special, should be admired by others and only associate with other special or high-status people. Lack of empathy is particularly noticeable and rage is often the response to negative feedback. To the narcissistic person, most people are considered unimportant and unworthy, so manipulating or taking advantage of them is seen as reasonable behaviour. This behaviour soon deters other people and the narcissistic person often ends up lonely and bitter. Ageing brings physical changes, loss of power, prestige, praise and independence, making this time of life exceptionally hard for these people to negotiate (American Psychiatric Association 2000, Segal et al 2006).

Cluster C personality disorders

The anxious and fearful behaviours, listed as cluster C, include avoidant (phobic), dependent (needy) and obsessive-compulsive (intrusive preoccupations and rituals) types. Typically, these people become extremely anxious in situations where a person would normally be expected to deal with the situation effectively.

Impact on the older person and their mental healthcare provision

The older person with an avoidant personality disorder is unwilling to get involved with people unless certain of being liked. Restraint is shown with intimate relationships because of feelings of inadequacy or for fear of being shamed and ridiculed. They perceive themselves as socially inept, inferior to other people and are very reluctant to take personal risks, and do not participate in social activities. Despite all these negative feelings, they long for relationships but usually end up isolated, lonely, anxious and frightened. However, there are circumstances where these characteristics occur for reasons other than personality deficits. For example, a widower, after many years of marriage to one person, may feel uncomfortable being single, or people with hearing, vision, mobility and continence impairments may be embarrassed to socialise. Older people with avoidant personality disorder may feel the losses associated with old age (spouse, friends, children) more intensely because they have more constricted networks to support them and have greater difficulty forming new relationships. Therapy with these individuals focuses on developing social and assertiveness skills (American Psychiatric Association 2000, Segal et al 2006).

The features of a dependent personality disorder are the older person needs others to assume responsibility for the major areas of their life. These people have difficulty making decisions, initiating activities and expressing disagreement. Older people with cognitive impairment may also exhibit these characteristics, so care must be taken in assessment. Older people with dependent personality disorder go to excessive lengths, such as doing demeaning tasks, to obtain affection and support from other people. They feel uncomfortable or helpless when they are alone. An unrealistic, fearful preoccupation of being left alone to fend for themselves is common. Consequently, they will remain in unhealthy or abusive relationships to avoid this from happening. If a relationship ends, they will go to great lengths to secure another relationship as quickly as possible. Widowhood is particularly problematic for older people with dependent personality disorder. In this situation, excessive helplessness and neediness may become very arduous and burdensome for people who are close to them, such as children, friends or healthcare workers (American Psychiatric Association 2000, Segal et al 2006).

The obsessive-compulsive personality disorder is characterised by a preoccupation with details, lists, rules and organisation. People affected by this disorder aspire to such perfectionism that it interferes with successful task completion. They become excessively devoted to work and productivity, often to the detriment of having social relationships and leisure interests. These people are reluctant to delegate tasks because they believe others cannot do the job as well as they can. They are rigid, stubborn, overconscientious, scrupulous and inflexible, particularly in matters of morality. Hoarding worthless objects and stinginess with money (as opposed to being cautious) are also characteristics. They are not affectionate and prefer intellectualisation and logic to spontaneity, creativity and happiness. These people like to do things their own way and this can be problematic in old age if they are becoming dependent and having to accept help, give up control and make changes to the way things are done. Retirement, particularly when much of their identity has been tied to their work life, can be stressful. Hoarding can also become problematic, with some older people's houses stacked with so many possessions and rubbish that they cannot move about freely and the house becomes a haven for vermin and a fire risk (American Psychiatric Association 2000, Neville 1995, Segal et al 2006).

COMORBIDITY

In 2000, Devanand et al found that 31.2% of older people with major depression or dysthymia had a comorbid personality disorder, with the most common types being obsessive-compulsive (17.1%) and avoidant (11.8%). Coolidge et al (2000) found that 61% of anxious older people had at least one personality disorder, with the most prevalent being obsessive-compulsive (39%), schizoid (39%) and avoidant (29%). Comorbid conditions such as major depression and anxiety disorders may also complicate the picture when trying to assess and treat an older person for difficulties created by their personality disorder and vice versa.

DIFFERENTIAL DIAGNOSIS

Personality disorders currently fall under the umbrella of minor mental disorders and their characteristics are somewhat reflective of the major mental disorders, such as schizophrenia and the anxiety disorders. Personality disorders also need to be distinguished from adverse medication reactions and disorders that cause a change in personality, such as dementia, major depression, acquired brain injuries, epilepsy, and neurodegenerative and endocrine disorders. A diagnosis of personality disorder is only given after a lifelong pattern of personal distress and social dysfunction.

ASSESSMENT

The onset of personality disorders can usually be traced back to adolescence or early adulthood, and this information is important in order to be able to make a diagnosis. It is for this reason that taking a detailed life history is essential. If the presentation of the older person is clouded by comorbidities, cognitive issues or a general sense of unreliability, it would pay, with the consent of the older person, to obtain corroborating evidence from another person who knows them well. It is important to determine the nature and severity of the personality disorder so that specific advice in regard to psychoeducation and behavioural strategies may be developed.

A mental state examination (MSE) would also be undertaken and these assessment processes could be augmented with a screening instrument for the presence of a personality disorder, such as the Gerontological Personality disorders Scale (GPS) (van Alphen et al 2006). The GPS consists of two subscales:

1.   the HABitual behaviour (HAB) subscale, which has seven items, and
2.   the BIOgraphical information (BIO) subscale, which has nine items.

In a preliminary study to test the reliability and validity of the instrument, the 16 items had a reasonable score (approximately 70%) for both sensitivity[1] and specificity.[2] The internal consistency was moderate for the HAB and excellent for the BIO. Participants are asked to respond to the questions by answering 'yes' or 'no'. Scores of less than 2 indicate no further personality disorder investigation is warranted, whereas a score of more than 4 can be an indication for an extensive personality disorder investigation. Specific personality disorders cannot be diagnosed with the GPS.

TREATMENT PRINCIPLES

Personality disorders are very complex and difficult to treat. Being unable to develop and maintain interpersonal relationships often leaves these people without strong social networks for support when things start to go wrong. Not having a support network adds to the workload for the mental health workers involved in providing the care. Ineffective communication patterns may lead to difficulties when the older person with a personality disorder seeks help from other health professionals, such as general medical practitioners or pharmacists. Therefore, part of the mental health worker's role could be advocating for the older person and repairing estranged relationships, and instructing the older person on how they may go about better communicating their needs so they receive appropriate support and care.

When unwell, these older people can have very poor personal boundaries and they can be very time-consuming and emotionally draining for the mental health worker and any other people coming into regular contact with them. It is important to set very strong boundaries around what the mental health worker is prepared to offer (e.g. setting a limit to the amount of time to be spent with them and the number of contact times). Because the pattern of behaviour has been embedded over their lifetime, it would be unrealistic to think it can be permanently altered, so the goal of treatment is to prevent them from getting worse, while reinforcing adaptive strategies to improve their interpersonal relationships. Any form of change can be catastrophic, so interventions must be introduced very cautiously.

Caring for an older person with a personality disorder can be very challenging due to the prominence of negative and unappealing traits. In general, and depending on the specific disorder, they can be demanding, manipulative, exasperating and can create

---

1   Sensitivity was the rate at which a prediction of personality disorder was made for a person who actually had a personality disorder.
2   Specificity was the rate at which a prediction of no personality disorder was made for a person who did not have a personality disorder.

antagonism and conflict between people through their lies and exaggerations. Acts of self-harm are distressing not only to themselves, but also to the people trying to help them. They try to foster a notion that they are more special than other people and go to great lengths to exploit situations and influence decisions so they always have the advantage. These behaviours evoke negative countertransference reactions where the mental health worker responds negatively and just wants to shun the person. Clinical supervision is invaluable when dealing with these types of reactions. Additionally, maintaining a positive attitude to the person, even when they are rejecting help, and keeping a consistent approach, are invaluable strategies (e.g. not rescuing people when they are being unnecessarily needy or helpless and also not withdrawing or rejecting the person when they are not satisfied with the care they are receiving) (Segal et al 2006).

Psychotherapies

In addition to cognitive behaviour, problem-solving and interpersonal therapies that are discussed in detail in Chapter 29, an adapted form of cognitive behaviour therapy (CBT) called schema-focused therapy (Young 1994) has been suggested as having some therapeutic value for older people with a personality disorder. However, as with most of the psychotherapies, its effectiveness requires further evaluation. This therapy has been developed to counter some of the unique, dysfunctional characteristics of personality disorders, such as the high prevalence of interpersonal problems, the rigid underlying belief systems and the avoidant behaviour patterns when coping with novel situations. It is conceptually focused on taking a very broad approach of trying to make sense of everything that is creating difficulties for the older person.

Schema-focused therapy incorporates interpersonal and experiential interventions into the traditional cognitive therapies. The concept of schema is the unifying feature. Schema is defined as the basic rules by which a person lives. They are developed very early in life. In schema-focused therapy, a subset of schemas called 'early maladaptive schemas' serve as templates for processing and defining later behaviour. These are designed to assist the person with the personality disorder to challenge and reformulate their early maladaptive schemas through a variety of behavioural experiments, cognitive restructuring and interpersonal strategies, and, if successful, will in turn be incorporated into their daily functioning.

Dialectical behaviour therapy (DBT) is a form of CBT. DBT addresses the components of biosocial theory for borderline personality disorder (BPD) (Lineham 1993, cited in Lynch et al 2007). Briefly, biosocial theory postulates that people with BPD have a biological disposition to emotional reactivity and sensitivity, and consequently experience emotions more intensely than other people, and it takes them longer to reach baseline. Secondly, their reading of environmental feedback does not validate their emotional experience and they have great difficulty in regulating their emotions when they become upset. DBT is a combination of individual therapy and skills group work that targets life-threatening behaviour (e.g. suicidality), therapy-avoidance behaviour (e.g. missing appointments) and behaviour that interferes with quality of life (poor interpersonal relationships). Skills group work covers the topics of core mindfulness, interpersonal effectiveness, emotion regulation and distress tolerance.

For a number of years, the Duke University Medical Center (USA) has been trialling modifications to DBT that have been developed to suit older people with comorbid personality disorder and depression. The initial research results are promising, with a combination of antidepressant medication and clinical management (MED) and DBT showing higher rates of remission from depression and depressive symptoms than MED alone. Similarly, in relation to BPD, there was lower interpersonal sensitivity and interpersonal aggression in the MED + DBT group than the MED group alone. Part of this research is the development of a new treatment manual for this group of people (Lynch et al 2007).

Pharmacological therapies

Pharmacological therapies can assist in treating the predominant symptoms of personality disorders, but the therapeutic value is limited. If episodic psychosis is the troubling condition, then psychotropic medications would be in order, as would be antidepressant therapy for anxiety or depressive symptoms and mood stabilisers for affective fluctuations. Benzodiazepines are usually avoided because of their addictive properties. Non-compliance with pharmacological treatments via excessive use or refusal to take medications is a typical example of the attitudes and behaviour of people with personality disorders. The presence of such attitudes and behaviour should be given careful consideration when medications are prescribed and for ongoing clinical management.

SUMMARY

The range of behaviours an older person with a personality disorder can display makes caring for them complex, challenging and emotionally draining. Through understanding the intractable nature of personality disorders, as well as the rigidity and the limited control the person has over their responses, it is hoped that an empathetic relationship can be developed with these older people. Engaging the older person therapeutically and persevering with this relationship, despite progress being very slow, should be considered a significant clinical achievement.

FURTHER READING

Segal DL, Coolidge FL, Rosowsky E 2006 Personality disorders and older adults: diagnosis, assessment, and treatment. John Wiley & Sons, Hoboken, NJ

REFERENCES

American Psychiatric Association 2000 Diagnostic and statistical manual of mental disorders, 4th edn. American Psychiatric Publishing, Washington DC

Ames A, Molinari V 1994 Prevalence of personality disorders in community living elderly. Journal of Geriatric Psychiatry and Neurology 7(3):189–194

Balsis SMA, Woods CM, Gleason MEJ, Oltmanns TF 2007 Overdiagnosis and underdiagnosis of personality disorders in older adults. American Journal of Geriatric Psychiatry 15(9):742–753

Coolidge FL, Segal DL, Hook JN, Stewart S 2000 Personality disorders and coping among anxious older adults. Journal of Anxiety Disorders 14(2):157–172

Devanand DP, Turret N, Moody BJ et al 2000 Personality disorders in elderly patients with dysthymic disorder. American Journal of Geriatric Psychiatry 8(3):188–195

Kenan MM, Kendjelic EM, Molinari VA et al 2000 Age-related differences in the frequency of personality disorders among inpatient veterans. International Journal of Geriatric Psychiatry 15(9):831–837

Lynch TR, Cheavens JS, Cukrowicz KC et al 2007 Treatment of older adults with co-morbid personality disorder and depression: a dialectical behaviour therapy approach. International Journal of Geriatric Psychiatry 22:131–143

Molinari V, Marmion J 1993 Personality disorders in geropsychiatric outpatients. Psychological Reports 73(1):256–258

Molinari V, Marmion J 1995 Relationship between affective disorders and Axis II diagnoses in geropsychiatric patients. Journal of Geriatric Psychiatry and Neurology 8:61–64

Neville C 1995 Community mental health nursing and the elderly client: a case presentation. Australian and New Zealand Journal of Mental Health Nursing 4(4):190–195

Segal DL, Coolidge FL, Rosowsky E 2006 Personality disorders and older adults: diagnosis, assessment, and treatment. John Wiley & Sons, Hoboken, NJ

van Alphen S 2006 The relevance of a geriatric sub-classification of personality disorders in the DSM–V. International Journal of Geriatric Psychiatry 21:205–209

van Alphen SPJ, Engelen GJJA, Kuin Y et al 2006 A preliminary study of the diagnostic accuracy of the Gerontological Personality disorders Scale (GPS). International Journal of Geriatric Psychiatry 21:862–868

Young JE 1994 Cognitive therapy for personality disorders: a schema-focused approach. Professional Resource Press, Sarasota, FL

Chapter 26

PREVENTION AND PROMOTION

INTRODUCTION

The aim of illness prevention and health promotion is to reduce the overall burden of mental health problems to improve the quality of life for older people. If there are family carers involved, which is often the case, these strategies will also decrease the likelihood of them also developing mental health problems. The needs of older people who are in higher acuity settings, such as residential aged care facilities (RACFs), must be considered by mental health workers. These older people experience greater rates of depression and dementia than their community-dwelling counterparts (O'Connor 2006, Rosewarne 1997). The presence of chronic physical conditions, such as cancer, cardiac problems, arthritis and stroke, increases the risk of mental health problems (Jorm 1995).

Awareness and understanding of positive mental health for older people may not rank highly on the list of priorities for a mental health worker surrounded by chronicity and working in a healthcare system focused on treating illness. However, the literature often states one of the reasons conditions such as depression, delirium and anxiety are so debilitating in the older age group is that they are underrecognised and under-treated in the first instance (Suominen et al 2004). Growth in this important area of healthcare has been stymied by negative attitudes of older people not having much longer to live ('Why bother?') and older people being seen as 'unable' or 'too set in their ways' to change their lifestyle (Cattan 2006). However, as much as other age groups, old age can be productive and fulfilling, and illness prevention and health promotion in this very dynamic area is easily influenced by innovations in drug treatments, therapeutic techniques, devices and technology.

The ageing of the population is now one of the driving forces for health promotion and illness prevention campaigns for older people. If the current prevalence rates of mental health problems affecting older people remain the same, this rate will increase proportionately as the number of older people increases. For example, in 2006, there were approximately 3 million (13%) older people in Australia and, therefore, 9.5% or 285,000 of these people had at least one long-term mental health or behavioural problem. However in 2056, with the impact of population ageing, there will be 9,840,000 (24%) people over the age of 65 years and, if 9.5% have a mental health problem, this equates to 934,800 in actual numbers (Australian Institute of Health and Welfare 2007).

A MODEL OF MENTAL HEALTH INTERVENTION

Conceptualisation of how to approach mental illness prevention and mental health promotion within mental healthcare is captured in Figure 26.1 (Mrazek & Haggerty 1994). This spectrum identifies the key components of promotion, prevention, early intervention, treatment and continuing care. The best mental health outcomes will be achievable if effort is directed in all these areas. Sometimes, the boundaries between the different areas are not as distinct as this representation. In the practice setting, interventions may cross these boundaries, as well as combining a number of the components. Mental health promotion is defined as 'any action taken to maximise mental health and wellbeing among populations and individuals' (Commonwealth Department of Health and Aged Care 2000b, p 29), and it is relevant across the whole spectrum of interventions. This means that health promotion is targeted at people when they are well, if they are at risk and when they are unwell. The aim of mental health promotion is to optimise the mental health and wellbeing of communities and therefore the individuals who are part of the community (Commonwealth Department of Health and Aged Care 2000b).

Illness prevention is defined as 'interventions that occur before the initial onset of a disorder' to prevent the development of a disorder (Mrazek & Haggerty 1994, p 23). The aim of prevention is to reduce the risk factors for mental health problems and enhance the protective factors of mental health. Although illness prevention and health promotion have clearly different aims, the interventions and outcomes are often very similar. For instance, a mental health promotion activity may very well reduce the incidence of a mental health problem. Within Figure 26.1, there are three different types of prevention interventions. The first is *universal*, which targets the general population and includes programs that promote a healthy mind. The second type, *selective*, is for subgroups or individuals who have a higher than average rate of developing a mental health problem. A bereavement support group is an example of a selective intervention.

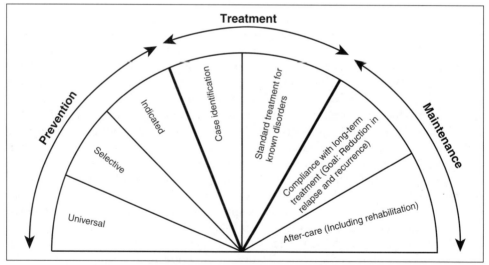

Figure 26.1 The spectrum of interventions for mental health problems
Source: Mrazek and Haggerty (1994). Reprinted with permission from the National Academies Press. ©Copyright 1994 National Academy of Sciences.

The final type, *indicated*, is directed at individuals who are high risk and may have early signs of a mental health problem. An indicated intervention could be a behaviour management program for carers of an older person with dementia (Commonwealth Department of Health and Aged Care 2000b).

PREVENTION CONCEPTS

The public health approach is a common and appropriate way of classifying preventive strategies (Jenkins 1992). 'Primary' prevention involves finding the source of the mental health problem or stopping it before it occurs, and therefore reducing its incidence. Primary prevention targets people when they are in good health and particularly if they are at risk of developing the disease at a later stage of their life. Health promotion strategies that aim to improve health, rather than prevent disease, are well situated in primary prevention.

'Secondary' prevention involves early detection and early intervention strategies and programs so that there is not any worsening of the mental health problem. The target group here is people who have an acute illness. The aim is to keep people healthy, eliminate the cause of the mental health problem, or build up resistance to the mental health problem so that the prevalence rate is reduced.

'Tertiary' prevention means ongoing treatment of the mental health problem through rehabilitation and recovery so that any long-term disabilities/complications that may follow are limited. Tertiary prevention targets chronically ill people.

How each of these concepts relates to the mental healthcare of older people in the community will now be expanded upon.

Primary prevention

The causal factors of many mental health problems are unknown, despite a considerable amount of research being undertaken (e.g. in Alzheimer's disease) (Jorm 2000). On the other hand, primary prevention can be actioned for organic brain disorders caused by poisoning (including medication reactions), infections, genetic diseases, nutritional deficiencies, injuries and systemic disorders. There have also been reasonable efforts to identify, reduce or modify risk factors for mental health problems and suicide (Suominen et al 2004).

Stress often precipitates or exacerbates a mental health problem (Norman & Malla 1993, Paykel 1994). Stressors older people have to deal with usually come about via the significant losses they endure. Some changes are positive (e.g. more leisure time for family and friends, or travel). However, negative stressful experiences through changes regarding loss such as functional decline, death of a partner and significant others, and changes in roles, financial or living status, can be very significant for the older person. Although the actual losses cannot be prevented, functional decline and quality of life may be prevented or improved (Bartels & Pratt 2009). The use of assistive technologies, bereavement counselling for loss of a partner and friends through death, and support programs for other ageing issues, all help in managing the associated stress caused by loss (White et al 2002).

These preventive strategies can be delivered on an individual or group basis. Group-based activities are helpful in reducing stress, distress, social isolation and loneliness, and increasing resilience, self-esteem and social networks (Cattan et al 2005). There have been numerous programs developed and they follow the general themes of (Cattan et al 2005, Cole 2008, Hammond 2004, Pusey & Richards 2001, Wheeler et al 1998):

- general educational programs to improve knowledge about mental health problems
- self-help groups, such as Alcoholics Anonymous, for mutual support, shared feelings, role modelling and development of coping skills, particularly leading to gaining control over one's life again
- lifestyle modification programs to improve overall mental status (e.g. 'Mind your Mind' is a dementia risk-reduction program (Alzheimer's Australia 2009))
- community participation programs (e.g. volunteering, companion programs and mentoring younger people), and
- psychoeducational and psychotherapeutic programs for enhancement of preventive behaviours (e.g. monitoring mood, increasing pleasurable activities and improving coping skills, through, for example, cognitive behavioural therapy (see Ch 29)).

Social isolation and feelings of loneliness may come about through not working, having reduced income, poorer health or grieving over loss. Loss, isolation and lack of opportunities to effectively communicate with others are associated with the development of major depression and late-onset schizophrenia (Castle 2005, Neville & Byrne 2009). Basic primary prevention strategies, such as engaging social and logistical supports, provide opportunities to improve social connections. Many people benefit from revitalised or new social connections when losses have occurred.

Another important aspect of primary prevention is programs for family carers of older people with mental health problems. Carers often experience burden when dealing with cognitive and functional decline and the behavioural disturbances that are associated with dementia or psychosis. Carer burden can lead to higher rates of mental health problems (Doran et al 2003). Maintaining good health in carers may forestall and consequently prevent early and costly institutionalisation of the older person.

Evidence base for primary prevention

One example of primary prevention is a recent Swedish study conducted by Andren and Elmstahl (2008) who set out to determine the effectiveness of a psychosocial intervention for family caregivers in delaying placement of an older person with dementia in an RACF. They had an intervention group of family carers (N = 153) and a comparable control group (N = 155). The intervention consisted of five weekly counselling sessions and a 3-month conversation group. The results showed that for the group that received the intervention, there were significant delays (6 months) in placement, and a longer time at home if the caregivers were adult children, particularly daughters.

Secondary prevention

To develop effective programs for secondary prevention, the prevalence rates of mental health problems need to be known and the characteristics of the people who suffer the particular problems. Once these people are identified, they can be screened and diagnosed, ensuring prompt treatment of the mental health problem. Such actions can shorten the length of time the older person is unwell and lessen the likelihood of long-term consequences. Another important reason for early diagnosis and treatment (e.g. of depression) is that problems associated with high doses of medication required for treatment can be prevented and more attention can be given to any pre-existing physical illness.

As the rate of older people who seek care from community mental health services is relatively low (Australian Institute of Health and Welfare 2008), it is essential that primary healthcare providers such as general practitioners (GPs) and nurses are vigilant in recognising the presence of a mental health problem. Many quick, easy-to-use screening instruments have been identified in this book (see Ch 35). The routine use of these during comprehensive assessments can assist with accurate identification of mental health problems, thereby achieving the best possible outcomes for the older person (Commonwealth Department of Health and Aged Care 2000a).

Evidence base for secondary prevention

In an Australian study, McCabe et al (2008) picked up on the issue of depression not being recognised in older people, and subsequently conducted a study to evaluate the effectiveness of a training program to enable aged care workers to better detect depression among older people in both community and RACF settings. A total of 52 aged care workers, which included personal care attendants, registered nurses and managers, underwent the training to identify and respond appropriately to the signs of depression. The registered nurses and managers were given additional training on the use of screening tools and referral processes. Outcomes were evaluated at post-test and at 6 months. At both measurement times, it was found that, for all groups, the training increased the participant's knowledge of depression and their ability to detect depression and improve the care provided to the older people.

Tertiary prevention

For older people with chronic mental health problems, tertiary prevention programs are primarily supportive and aimed at keeping them out of the RACF setting for as long as possible. This can be achieved by effectively combining the use of formal and informal services to maintain the older person's independence and reduce the burden placed on family carers. Services such as crisis response teams, respite care in all its forms, meals on wheels and home help all play an important role as part of tertiary prevention. As with all levels of prevention and promotion activities, the maintenance of protective or resilience factors, such as good physical health, supportive social networks, improved social connectedness and a sound economic status, are important, but these are particularly so with tertiary prevention (Cattan 2006).

Tertiary prevention programs focus on relapse prevention or remission maintenance. Additionally, if the program will enhance the older person's ability to exercise autonomy, it will be even better. This can be achieved by making use of residual skills to prevent the condition from worsening (e.g. simple environmental changes such as hand rails can improve quality of life and enhance autonomy). The focus on tertiary prevention does not have to be on the older person. Programs that are designed to up-skill workers who are regularly out and about in the community to identify isolated older people who lack supportive networks or those who are recently bereaved and unlikely to self-refer are examples of tertiary prevention.

Evidence base for tertiary prevention

Lyness et al (2009) established in a large North American study (N = 484) that older people from primary care medical practices who had minor and subsyndromal depression were more depressed than an equivalent, non-depressed group after 1 year of follow-up.

The researchers calculated that the older people with minor and subsyndromal depression had a seven-fold risk of developing major depression. Such results support the argument for tertiary prevention activities for this group of people, with recommendations from Lyness and colleagues that the focus should be on modifiable risks, such as psychiatric and physical functioning, and social support.

HEALTH PROMOTION

Health promotion is closely aligned with prevention and at times it is difficult to differentiate under which conceptual field an activity or strategy may fall. The link between the body, mind and soul positively compounds the effect of any health promotion program. Key areas for health promotion in any older person include the following (see also Ch 2):

- *Nutrition*. Nutrition includes knowledge of nutritional needs, having access to a variety of good-quality foods and the ability to store and prepare food. A clear association between malnutrition and loneliness, social isolation, lack of motivation and depression has been established (Baeyens 2005).
- *Exercise*. Exercise is not only important for muscle strength, flexibility and bone health, but it also has value in improving an older person's emotional outlook. Exercise has been shown to make people feel happier and improve their sense of wellbeing (Paulson 2005). It improves sleep quality, incontinence and reduces the risk for falls (Lord et al 2007) (see Ch 18).
- *Sleep*. Sleep is very important for good health. Poor sleep quality has been associated with decreased quality of life and an increased risk of depression and suicide (Rabheru 2004).
- *Proper use of medicine*. The proper use of medicine has received much attention and publicity in recent years, as older people are known to self-medicate on an ad hoc basis to the detriment of effectively managing their health (Lynskey et al 2003) (see Ch 30).
- *Safety*. Safety is an area that includes physical safety against falling by way of such things as environmental modifications. It also includes personal safety against physical, emotional and financial abuse (see Ch 18).
- *Social activities, hobbies and interests*. These are essential to preserve one's mental health. If mobility is an issue, these activities can be maintained through the use of the telephone, radio, television, pets and, increasingly, the internet (Cattan 2006).

The long-term health benefits even for older people of smoking cessation, moderate alcohol intake and reducing obesity should not be forgotten. Regular medical checkups, including visual and hearing health, should also be encouraged as health promotion activities.

SUMMARY

This chapter has highlighted the importance of illness prevention and health promotion, which are often overlooked when caring for older people. The commonly accepted concepts of primary, secondary and tertiary prevention have been utilised. In turn, each of these concepts was elaborated upon to demonstrate its applicability to the mental healthcare of older people. The targeting of health promotion activities for older people has also been addressed.

FURTHER READING

Cattan M, Tilford S 2006 Mental health promotion: a lifespan approach. Open University Press, Maidenhead

USEFUL WEBSITES

Alcoholics Anonymous: www.aa.org.au

Mind your Mind (a dementia risk-reduction program): www.goforyourlife.vic.gov.au/hav/articles.nsf/pages/Mind_your_Mind?open

REFERENCES

Alzheimer's Australia 2009 Mind your Mind (a dementia risk-reduction program). Online. Available: www.goforyourlife.vic.gov.au/hav/articles.nsf/pages/Mind_your_Mind?open 2 July 2009

Andren S, Elmstahl S 2008 Effective psychosocial intervention for family caregivers lengthens time elapsed before nursing home placement of individuals with dementia: a five-year follow-up study. International Psychogeriatrics 20:1177–1192

Australian Institute of Health and Welfare (AIHW) 2007 Older Australia at a glance, 4th edn. AIHW Cat. No. AGE 52. AIHW, Canberra

Australian Institute of Health and Welfare (AIHW) 2008 Mental health services in Australia 2005–06. Mental Health Series No. 10. AIHW Cat. No. HSE 56. AIHW, Canberra

Baeyens J-P 2005 Are your grandparents starving to death? Guardian, 7 October

Bartels SJ, Pratt SI 2009 Psychosocial rehabilitation and quality of life for older adults with serious mental illness: recent findings and future research activities. Current Opinion in Psychiatry 22(4):381–385

Castle DJ 2005 Epidemiology of late-onset schizophrenia. In: Hassett A, Ames D, Chui E (eds) Psychosis in the elderly. Taylor Francis, London

Cattan M 2006 Older people: the retirement years. In: Cattan M, Tilford S (eds) Mental health promotion: a lifespan approach. Open University Press, Maidenhead

Cattan M, White M, Bond J, Learmonth A 2005 Preventing social isolation and loneliness among older people: a systematic review of health promotion interventions. Ageing and Society 25(1):41–67

Cole M 2008 Brief interventions to prevent depression in older subjects: a systematic review of feasibility and effectiveness. American Journal of Geriatric Psychiatry 16(6):435–443

Commonwealth Department of Health and Aged Care 2000a National action plan for promotion, prevention and early intervention for mental health: a monograph. Mental Health and Special Programs Branch, Commonwealth Department of Health and Aged Care, Canberra

Commonwealth Department of Health and Aged Care 2000b Promotion, prevention and early intervention for mental health: a monograph. Mental Health and Special Programs Branch, Commonwealth Department of Health and Aged Care, Canberra

Doran T, Drever F, Whitehead M 2003 Health of young and elderly informal carers: analysis of UK census data. British Medical Journal 327:1388

Hammond C 2004 Impacts of lifelong learning upon emotional resilience, psychological and mental health: fieldwork evidence. Oxford Review of Education 30(4):551–568

Jenkins R 1992 Depression and anxiety: an overview of preventative strategies. In: Jenkins R, Newton J, Young R (eds) The prevention of depression and anxiety: the role of the primary care team. HMSO, London

Jorm AF 1995 The epidemiology of depressive states in the elderly: implications for recognition, intervention and prevention. Social Psychiatry and Psychiatric Epidemiology 30:53–59

Jorm AF 2000 Prevention and early intervention with dementia: prospects and policy implications. Dementia Forum Papers, 16–17 August 1999. Commonwealth Department of Health and Aged Care, Canberra

Lord S, Sherrington C, Menz H, Close J 2007 Falls in older people: risk factors and strategies for prevention. Cambridge University Press, Cambridge

Lyness JM, Chapman BP, McGriff J et al 2009 One-year outcomes of minor and subsyndromal depression in older primary care patients. International Psychogeriatrics 21(1):60–68

Lynskey MT, Day C, Hall W 2003 Alcohol and other drug use disorders among older-aged people. Drug and Alcohol Review 22:125–133

McCabe MP, Russo S, Mellor D et al 2008 Effectiveness of a training program for carers to recognize depression among older people. International Journal of Geriatric Psychiatry 23(12):1290–1296

Mrazek PJ, Haggerty RJ 1994 Reducing the risks for mental disorders: frontiers for preventive intervention research. National Academy Press, Washington DC

Neville CC, Byrne G 2009 Depression and suicide in older people. In: Nay R, Garratt S (eds) Older people: issues and innovations. Elsevier, Sydney

Norman RMG, Malla AK 1993 Stressful life events and schizophrenia I: a review of the research. British Journal of Psychiatry 162:161–166

O'Connor DW 2006 Do older Australians truly have low rates of anxiety and depression? A critique of the 1997 National Survey of Mental Health and Wellbeing. Australian and New Zealand Journal of Psychiatry 40(8):623–631

Paulson S 2005 The social benefits of belonging to a 'dance exercise' group for older people. Generations Review 15(4):37–41

Paykel ES 1994 Life events, social support and depression. Acta Psychiatrica Scandinavica 377:50–58

Pusey H, Richards D 2001 A systematic review of the effectiveness of psychosocial interventions for carers of people with dementia. Aging and Mental Health 5(2):107–119

Rabheru K 2004 Special issues in the management of depression in older patients. Canadian Journal of Psychiatry 49(1):41s–50s

Rosewarne R 1997 The care needs of people with dementia and challenging behaviour living in residential facilities. AGPS, Canberra

Suominen K, Isometsa E, Lonnqvist J 2004 Elderly suicide attempters with depression are often diagnosed only after the attempt. International Journal of Geriatric Psychiatry 19:35–40

Wheeler FA, Gore KM, Greenblatt B 1998 The beneficial effects of volunteering for older volunteers and the people they serve: a meta analysis. International Journal of Aging and Human Development 47(1):69–79

White H, McConnell E, Clipp E et al 2002 A randomised controlled trial of the psychosocial impact of providing internet training and access to older adults. Aging and Mental Health 6(3):213–221

Chapter 27
COMMUNITY MANAGEMENT OF ACUTELY ILL OLDER PEOPLE

INTRODUCTION

This brief chapter introduces some of the issues confronting mental health workers when dealing with acutely ill older people. Because older people have more general medical health problems than younger people, and are more prone to experience adverse effects when treated with psychotropic medication, the management of acute mental illness in the community can pose some challenges. Very little has been published on this topic, so this chapter is a distillation of the authors' experience.

LEGAL ISSUES

All mental health workers need to be familiar with the operation of the local Mental Health Act (MHA). While every effort should be made to assess and treat people as voluntary patients, using the least restrictive means, use of the involuntary provisions of the MHA is inevitable in busy acute community mental health teams, including those caring for older people. In some situations, the mental health worker will need to request the assistance of the police. Most MHAs have specific provisions for calling on the assistance of the police. It is very useful for community mental health teams to have good working relationships with the local police service. Most police services value such links, as they enhance the work of both organisations and enable challenging clientele to be appropriately managed.

MEDICAL ISSUES

Although community mental health teams are not usually responsible for providing primary healthcare to older people with mental health problems, they nevertheless are often in a good position to identify acute deteriorations in an older person's physical health. Common acute problems encountered in older people during domiciliary visits include falls and confusion. When such problems are identified, and are an immediate risk to the person's health, the community mental health team has an ethical obligation to take action. However, the management of general medical problems in older people with mental health problems will sometimes require the approval of a substitute decision maker, such as a statutory health attorney, an attorney for health matters under an enduring power, or the local guardianship authority.

WHAT CONSTITUTES AN EMERGENCY?

An emergency is any mental health problem that is immediately threatening the life of the older person or someone else, or has the potential to do so in the near future. Some clinical experience is needed to make this judgment, and inexperienced mental health workers are advised to consult with co-workers or clinical line managers if in any doubt. Other situations often treated as emergencies are those that put the person's reputation, or their legal or financial status, at severe risk.

INDICATIONS FOR HOSPITAL ADMISSION

A frequent issue for community mental health teams caring for older people is when to arrange for a hospital admission. This issue is easier to negotiate when the team is operating as an integrated hospital and community service. However, in the situation where the community team is independent of the inpatient team, more work will often be needed to arrange a hospital admission.

Almost all older people who have attempted suicide should be admitted to hospital for further assessment and treatment. Many older people with major depression complicated by psychotic symptoms, inadequate oral intake, or suicidal thoughts, should be admitted to hospital. Most older people with mania and some with hypomania should be admitted to hospital. Some older people with psychotic disorders will need hospital admission, particularly if there are risk issues, including marked disorganisation and self-neglect, poor oral intake, or suicidal or homicidal thoughts. Although people with dementia do sometimes warrant hospital admission if their dementia is complicated by severe depression or severe psychotic symptoms, many inpatient mental health units are reluctant to admit them because of the difficulty of finding accommodation for the person after the need for acute hospitalisation resolves. For this reason, and the unsuitability of many inpatient mental health units for people with cognitive impairment, it is generally best to manage people with dementia in the community rather than in hospital.

ALTERNATIVES TO HOSPITAL ADMISSION

Mobile intensive-treatment teams are often utilised with younger clientele with serious mental health problems to avoid hospitalisation or to manage the person in the community until a hospital bed becomes available. However, most of these younger people are free of serious general medical problems and some are well known to the mental health service. The use of such an approach with older people with acute mental health problems and comorbid general medical problems would be possible if the staff of such teams were appropriately experienced with the care of older people. Unfortunately, this is rarely the case, and so inpatient care under a specialised older persons' inpatient team is usually the preferred option.

ASSESSMENT OF RISK

Risk assessment is a complex but important undertaking. Several risks are routinely assessed in older people with mental health problems, including:
- suicide and other types of self-harm
- severe self-neglect, including dehydration

- homicide and other violence (victim and perpetrator)
- inappropriate sexual behaviour (victim and perpetrator)
- falls
- confusion
- environmental exposure (extreme heat or cold)
- child safety, and
- financial exploitation.

This list includes the standard mental health risks of suicide, homicide, aggressive behaviour and sexual behaviour. The latter two risks should be assessed from the perspective of the person, as both a potential perpetrator and as a potential victim. In addition, critical risks for older people are the risk of falls, confusion and dehydration. In some jurisdictions, there is now a legal requirement to assess the risk to children who might sometimes be in the care of the older person. Finally, older people are often vulnerable to financial exploitation by others, including family members, carers and vendors.

Some risks can be modified to some extent by the availability of appropriate supervision. However, it is often a mistake to rely on untrained family members or friends to carry out a suicide watch. Similarly, it is often inappropriate to assume that an older person with cognitive impairment will be able to adhere to a complex medication schedule unaided. See also Chapter 18.

MEDICAL WORK-UP IN THE COMMUNITY

The routine medical work-up of older people presenting for the first time with mental health problems has been covered in Chapter 15. For other people who are not presenting for the first time and who are experiencing a rapidly evolving deterioration in mental state or behaviour, there is often no time to undertake a considered medical assessment, particularly if the person is uncooperative. However, in more slowly evolving situations in the community, some medical work-up should be undertaken. Such situations include unexpected changes in mental state and behaviour, and unexpected adverse effects from treatment. This work-up should consist of a screening physical examination and limited laboratory investigations. In many cases, the assistance of the older person's usual general practitioner will be very helpful in completing this medical assessment.

ACUTE MANAGEMENT OF PSYCHOSIS

The acute management of an older person with psychosis is often quite challenging for the community mental health team. Ethical and legal issues commonly arise in relation to if and when to use the involuntary provisions of the MHA to transfer a person to hospital for further assessment and treatment. These can be particularly difficult to resolve when the older person has locked themselves in their home and will not answer the door. Local police often have records of telephone contacts from older people with persecutory delusions. Such records may provide valuable evidence of the older person's likely state of mind. When it is necessary to take an uncooperative older person with psychotic symptoms to hospital, it is often useful to have the police at hand or on standby. Fortunately, a show of force is often all that is needed to convince the older person to accompany mental health workers and the police to the emergency department. Rarely is it necessary to give the older person medication to effect their safe transfer to hospital. However, when this is necessary, fast dissolving oral formulations of risperidone or olanzapine, or alternatively intramuscular olanzapine or intramuscular lorazepam, are often used. The doses used depend upon the size, frailty and general condition of the person.

The older person with mania almost always needs to be hospitalised to avoid further loss of reputation and money, and to protect them against the real risk of misadventure and exposure to the elements. Medical resuscitation is commonly needed, as dehydration commonly occurs in mania and the manic older person has often neglected to take their usual medication. In cases of hypomania, the mental health worker needs to exercise their clinical judgment. Many older people with hypomania will need hospitalisation, but some may be managed in the community. See also Chapter 22.

ACUTE MANAGEMENT OF DEPRESSION

The acute management of an older person with depression depends entirely upon the severity of the depression and the situation of the person. Indications for immediate hospitalisation include suicidality, catatonia, psychosis and inadequate intake of food or fluid. Suicidality includes recent suicide attempts, and active suicidal plans or intent. Once the mental health worker has determined that the older person is actively suicidal, the person should not be left alone and urgent steps should be taken to ensure their safe transport to hospital. The assistance of emergency services, including the ambulance and the police, should be sought where necessary. In urgent situations, treatment in hospital with electroconvulsive therapy (ECT) may be life-saving. In other serious but less urgent situations, combination pharmacotherapy with an antidepressant, a mood stabiliser and an antipsychotic is likely to be needed. Occasionally, older people with psychotic depression can be managed safely in the community. However, they will still require 24 hours a day supervision, regular review and combination drug treatment. These requirements can only occasionally be met at home.

ACUTE MANAGEMENT OF DELIRIUM

Delirium is generally considered to be a medical emergency and should usually lead to the older person being transferred without delay to the nearest general hospital emergency department for assessment and treatment. Exceptions might include the situation in which an older person with dementia residing in an aged care facility develops a superimposed delirium in the context of an intercurrent illness, such as a urinary tract infection. In such circumstances, it would often be quite reasonable for the person to be assessed and treated in the aged care facility. The treatment of delirium involves providing excellent general nursing and medical care to the person, while searching for the underlying general medical condition. Once the underlying medical condition has been identified, it needs to be appropriately treated. People with agitated delirium (about one-third of all cases) generally prove the more challenging. See also Chapter 19.

ACUTE MANAGEMENT OF DEMENTIA

It is rarely necessary for older people with dementia to be treated on an emergency basis, although they are commonly sent to the emergency department of general hospitals because families and residential aged care facilities perceive that they have no alternative.

The issue that precipitates such action is generally the development of severe behavioural or psychological symptoms. Chapter 28 covers this topic.

SUMMARY

The older person with a serious and acute mental health problem can pose major challenges to the mental health worker. In most cases, such older people will need hospital admission, and this should be effected as soon as practicable. The assistance of ambulance or police personnel should be obtained when necessary. In rare cases, the older person will require treatment with psychotropic medication to safely effect their transfer to hospital.

FURTHER READING

Nassisi D, Korc B, Hahn S et al 2006 The evaluation and management of the acutely agitated elderly patient. Mt Sinai Journal of Medicine 73:976–984

Chapter 28

MANAGEMENT OF BEHAVIOUR IN DEMENTIA

INTRODUCTION

The dementia syndrome affects approximately 6.5% of older Australians and is characterised by cognitive impairment and a variety of non-cognitive clinical features, including psychological symptoms and challenging behaviours. The expression 'behavioural and psychological symptoms of dementia' (BPSD) was coined to provide an omnibus or umbrella term to describe these non-cognitive symptoms of dementia. These symptoms are also sometimes referred to as neuropsychiatric symptoms. BPSD include both psychological symptoms that are described by the older person and behaviours that are observed by others. This chapter provides an overview of BPSD and an approach to their assessment and management.

PREVALENCE

Most, if not all, people with dementia will develop BPSD at some point in their illness. In about 50% of cases, these symptoms will be clinically significant and either cause significant distress to the person with dementia or cause significant burden to carers, or both. In other cases, BPSD will be evident, but will not be a major focus of clinical attention or treatment. BPSD include psychological symptoms such as anxiety, depression, delusions and hallucinations, and challenging behaviours such as apathy, agitation, aggression and motor overactivity. The Cache County Study from the US state of Utah found that 97% of people with dementia had one or more BPSD at some point over a 5-year period. The 5-year prevalence of depression was 77%, of apathy was 71% and of anxiety was 62% (Steinberg et al 2008).

The persistence of BPSD has been investigated in the Maasbed Study from the Netherlands (Aalten et al 2005). In this study, 80.9% of people with dementia had one or more BPSD at baseline. The baseline prevalence of selected BPSD was as follows: apathy 40%; depression 35%; anxiety 21%; delusions 22%; hallucinations 10%; and agitation 19%. However, the prevalence of symptoms that persisted at each of four 6-monthly observation points over 2 years was much lower: apathy 12%; depression 2%; anxiety 1%; delusions 4%; hallucinations 2%; and agitation 0%. Thus, it is clear from this research that BPSD come and go. This has implications for uncontrolled research studies, as there is a significant risk in such studies that clinical improvement might be attributed to an intervention when it actually only reflects the natural fluctuations in BPSD prevalence over time. Thus, to be meaningful, BPSD intervention studies must have a valid control condition.

BPSD also occur in people with mild cognitive impairment (MCI) (Apostolova & Cummings 2008, Muangpaisan et al 2008) and in some people with subjective memory complaints (SMC) (Sohrabi et al 2009). In the large Cognitive Function and Ageing Study (CFAS) funded by the UK Medical Research Council (MRC) (Savva et al 2009), BPSD were found to be much more prevalent in older people with dementia than in older people without dementia, but mood symptoms, apathy, irritability and feelings of persecution were found in a significant proportion of people without dementia. Thus, the term BPSD actually refers to non-cognitive symptoms that are seen across the whole range of cognitive function in older people (not just those with dementia).

SIGNIFICANCE

BPSD are one of the risk factors for residential aged care facility (RACF) placement. In a US study, Yaffe et al (2002) found that BPSD were the fourth most important risk factor for RACF placement after living alone, having a Mini-Mental State Examination (MMSE) score of 20 or less, and having one or more activities of daily living (ADLs) dependencies. Older people with BPSD were 30% more likely than those without BPSD to be admitted to an RACF. The same study found that a Zarit Burden Interview (see Ch 35) score of 20 or greater was the most important caregiver risk factor for RACF placement. People with dementia whose caregiver reported a Zarit burden score of 20 or greater were 73% more likely to be admitted to an RACF.

There is a strong association between BPSD and carer burden, distress and depression (Black & Almeida 2004). Although there are undoubtedly emotional benefits that accrue to many carers of people with dementia as a result of their valued caregiving role, most carers report at least some sense of burden. However, burden needs to be distinguished from distress and depression, although the three phenomena are not mutually exclusive.

SYMPTOM CLUSTERS

Clinicians have long observed that certain BPSD tend to cluster together and these observations have been confirmed by research techniques, including factor analysis. In a factor analytic study conducted by the European Alzheimer's Disease Consortium (Petrovic et al 2007), four factors were identified using the Neuropsychiatric Inventory (NPI): a psychosis factor (irritability, agitation, hallucinations and anxiety); a psychomotor factor (aberrant motor behaviour and delusions); a mood lability factor (disinhibition, elation and depression); and an instinctual factor (appetite disturbance, sleep disturbance and apathy). The investigators pointed out that the association between elation, depression and disinhibition might have implications for treatment.

DIFFERENTIAL DIAGNOSIS

Challenging behaviours in people with dementia can occur for a variety of reasons, including delirium, pre-existing mental health problem (including psychosis, depression and anxiety), behavioural toxicity of prescribed medication, substance abuse or dependence, and intercurrent general medical problems (e.g. chest infection or acute coronary syndrome). Sometimes, challenging behaviours simply reflect longstanding patterns of antisocial behaviour.

Certain classes of prescribed medication are particularly prone to cause disturbed behaviour. These include sedatives, narcotic analgesics, antidepressants, antipsychotics, anticonvulsants, anti-Parkinsonian drugs, corticosteroids and chemotherapeutic agents.

AETIOLOGY

By definition, the principal aetiological factor in BPSD is thought to be the underlying dementia syndrome. However, there are substantial individual differences in the pattern and severity of BPSD that are likely to relate to other aetiological factors. Some BPSD occur more commonly in people with particular types of dementia. For example, delusions are more prevalent in dementia due to Alzheimer's disease, whereas depression is more common in dementia due to cerebrovascular disease (Lyketsos et al 2000). Behavioural disturbance occurs early in the course of the behavioural variant of fronto-temporal dementia, often before cognitive impairment is obvious.

The premorbid personality of the person with dementia is likely to influence their current behaviour. In particular, there is evidence that high levels of neuroticism are a risk factor for anxiety in people with dementia, and that high levels of agreeableness protect against agitation and irritability (Archer et al 2007).

Depression may be associated with behavioural change in someone who is unable to effectively express their distress any other way. For example, there is evidence that people with dementia and disruptive vocalisation (i.e. screaming and repetitive calling out) are more likely to be depressed than people with dementia without disruptive vocalisation (Dwyer & Byrne 2000). Pain is another powerful precipitant of challenging behaviour in people with dementia, who are often unable to articulate the source of their distress. Thus, for example, pain from arthritis or from headache might lead to psychological distress that manifests as one or more BPSD.

Sometimes, the person with dementia responds with challenging behaviour because they have been abused or neglected by others. In institutional settings, rigid care schedules may evoke behavioural resistance to care. Poor hearing or eyesight can contribute to sensory deprivation, and in the context of cognitive impairment may lead to BPSD. BPSD can be manifestations of intercurrent general medical problems, including delirium (see Ch 19).

Genetic polymorphisms may also influence BPSD. These genetic variants are known to affect the activity of neurotransmitter transporter systems in the brain and are likely to play a part in why some people with dementia get severe BPSD and others get mild BPSD (Pritchard et al 2007, 2008).

SCALES TO MEASURE BPSD

Many scales have been developed to measure BPSD. Some of these are scales that measure single constructs, such as depression (e.g. the Cornell Scale for Depression in Dementia (CSDD)) (Alexopoulos et al 1988), whereas others are omnibus scales that measure a range of phenomena. Popular omnibus scales include the Neuropsychiatric Inventory (NPI) (Cummings et al 1994, Cummings 1997) and the Cohen-Mansfield Agitation Inventory (CMAI) (Cohen-Mansfield 1986).

The CSDD is a 19-item clinician-rated instrument that rates five classes of depressive symptoms on a 3-point response scale. The NPI is a set of 12 scales (see box below), covering 10 neuropsychiatric symptoms and two vegetative symptoms (appetite and sleep) rated by a clinician following an interview with a caregiver. The CMAI includes 29 challenging behaviours, which are usually rated by nursing personnel. The NPI employs response scales that rate the frequency and severity of each item, as well as the degree of caregiver distress caused by the symptom. The CMAI employs response scales that rate the frequency and disruptiveness of each symptom. The CSDD is commonly used in both clinical and research settings and is part of the routine data set collected in Australian RACFs. The NPI is commonly used in both clinical and research settings involving people with mild to moderate dementia, whereas the CMAI is commonly used in clinical and research settings involving people in RACF settings. See also Chapter 35.

NEUROPSYCHIATRIC INVENTORY (NPI) SYMPTOMS
(ADAPTED FROM CUMMINGS 1997)

The12 NPI symptoms are:
1. delusions
2. hallucinations
3. agitation/aggression
4. depression/dysphoria
5. anxiety
6. elation/euphoria
7. apathy/indifference
8. disinhibition
9. irritability/lability
10. aberrant motor behaviour
11. sleep, and
12. appetite and eating.

INITIAL ASSESSMENT OF BPSD

For the initial BPSD assessment:
- Establish the basis for the diagnosis of dementia. It is usually based mainly on clinical assessment of the person together with history from informants.
- Consider whether potentially reversible causes of dementia have been excluded, or identified and adequately treated.
- Identify and treat intercurrent depression and delirium.
- Undertake a physical examination or arrange for this to be done.
- Identify and treat intercurrent general medical problems (e.g. stroke, heart attack, infection and hyponatraemia). This will often involve arranging for the person with dementia to undergo some laboratory investigations. Commonly, these will include urinalysis, full blood examination and a biochemical profile; less commonly, these will include a brain scan (computed tomography (CT) or magnetic resonance imaging (MRI)), an electrocardiogram (ECG), a troponin level and a chest X-ray.

- Accurately characterise the nature and significance of the reported behavioural or neuropsychiatric problem. Obtain a detailed description of the problem. Do not accept brief descriptors of a problem, such as 'wandering' or 'aggression', as these words mean different things to different people. If there are multiple problems, establish which problem is most challenging or most distressing and focus on this initially. It is rarely possible to deal with multiple problems at the same time.
- Identify contextual issues (e.g. physical environment and behaviour of significant others).
- Review the social and occupational history of the person with dementia, including premorbid personality, education, occupation and relationship history.
- Review the psychiatric history of the person with dementia.
- Identify interventions that have already been trialled and assess the adequacy of these trials.
- Consider the location in which the further management of the person with BPSD should take place. In most instances, it is appropriate for the management plan to be implemented in the community, wherever the person lives; in rare instances, it is appropriate to consider a hospital admission.
- Investigate in detail the antecedents and consequences of the behaviour, as a prelude to behavioural management. Antecedents include all aspects of the environment and all aspects of carer behaviour that precede a target behaviour (e.g. physical aggression is commonly preceded by attempts at showering or changing clothes). Consequences include all the things that follow a target behaviour (e.g. screaming or disruptive vocalisation is commonly followed by increased staff attention).
- Determine how to chart or monitor the target symptom over time. It is often best to employ a user-defined scale such as the Goal Attainment Scale (Gordon et al 1999).
- Consider whether treatment is necessary. If treatment is necessary, consider which treatment is likely to be most appropriate to the needs of the person with dementia and which treatment is likely to be most practicable to implement.

MANAGEMENT OF BPSD

The evidence base for the management of BPSD is rather modest. There is a dearth of methodologically rigorous randomised controlled trials (RCTs) of non-pharmacological and pharmacological interventions, apart from RCTs for atypical antipsychotic medication. The RCT evidence that is available suggests modest efficacy of all interventions. Reflecting this paucity of evidence, a wide variety of psychosocial interventions and many different medications have been proposed as treatments for BPSD.

Most clinicians adopt the philosophical position that it is better to start treatment with a non-pharmacological intervention because these interventions are less likely to do harm to the person with dementia than the pharmacological interventions. However, there are some situations in which there is little alternative but to use pharmacological interventions in an attempt to manage severe and dangerous BPSD.

Non-pharmacological management

There are two main evidence-based approaches to the non-pharmacological management of BPSD. The first involves the application of behaviour management techniques to reduce the frequency of problem behaviours. The second uses caregiver training to reduce burden, distress and depression, and to increase coping. In addition to these two principal approaches, several specific interventions have been shown to temporarily modify challenging behaviour.

Behaviour management

Commonly used evidence-based behaviour management techniques include stimulus control and contingency management (Logsdon et al 2007). Stimulus control involves modifying certain stimuli that are associated with an undesirable behaviour. Consider, for instance, a person with dementia who regularly becomes combative when being showered in the morning by male personnel. The stimulus control approach might suggest changing the antecedents to this behaviour. Changing from a shower to a bath, changing from the morning to the afternoon, and changing from male carers to female carers, might all modify the behaviour of the person with dementia.

Contingency management involves modifying the consequences of an undesirable behaviour in such a way as to decrease the time the person spends exhibiting the behaviour. Consider a person with dementia who screams out much of the time. Assuming that the person is not in pain or discomfort, and has no other treatable disorder, it would be reasonable to focus on shaping the symptom of screaming. Most people who scream continually do have at least short breaks when they do not scream. Although it is natural for family members or RACF staff to go to the assistance of the person with dementia when they scream, and to take a well-earned rest when the person stops screaming, this approach is likely to increase the frequency of the screaming. It does this by 'rewarding' the screaming behaviour with the attention of others. The correct, but somewhat counterintuitive, approach is to massively reward spontaneously occurring quiet periods so that the length of time that the person with dementia spends screaming decreases. This should be combined with ignoring the screaming.

The effective implementation of a behaviour management strategy is critically dependent upon relative preservation of the implicit memory (procedural memory) of the person with dementia (Parahoo et al 2006). Implicit memory is generally well preserved in cortical dementias such as those due to Alzheimer's disease. However, the application of formal behaviour modification techniques in the home or in RACF environments does pose some challenges. These include the relative lack of well-trained geropsychologists working in these settings and the counterintuitive nature of many of the interventions. In addition, in institutional settings, all personnel on all shifts must apply the intervention according to a protocol if it is to have much chance of succeeding.

Perhaps because of these challenges, many other specific types of non-pharmacological intervention have been used in people with BPSD. These include aromatherapy, massage, individualised music, simulated presence therapy, Snoezelen®, life review, reminiscence therapy, validation therapy, doll therapy and pet therapy. The use of such interventions has been critically reviewed (O'Connor et al 2009, Opie et al 1999) and the quality of the evidence found to be modest. For some such interventions, there are Cochrane Reviews. For example, Vink et al (2004) reviewed music as an intervention in dementia and found little evidence to either support or discourage the use of music therapy.

Despite this, this type of intervention is in widespread use as part of a humane program of care, particularly in RACF settings.

Caregiver counselling and training

Individualised behaviour management training for caregivers and individual or group sessions designed to improve coping are both associated with improved caregiver psychological health (Selwood et al 2007). However, supportive therapy and group behaviour management training, although popular, do not appear to work. When administered in combination with donepezil for people with Alzheimer's disease, individual and family counselling for caregivers has been demonstrated to be effective in reducing symptoms of depression in the caregivers (Mittelman et al 2008).

Pharmacological management

Because BPSD may be due to behavioural toxicity from prescribed medications, it is important to review the older person's current medication prior to considering the prescription of further medication. It is often possible to stop one or more medications without causing the person any ill effects. The best way to check on an older person's medication is to view the actual medication containers, rather than simply rely upon a list of currently prescribed medication. For a variety of reasons, the medication the person is currently taking is not necessarily the same as the computerised list provided by their general practitioner or medical specialist.

Drugs from several different classes have been trialled in people with BPSD, including cholinesterase inhibitors, the NMDA-receptor antagonist memantine, antidepressants, anticonvulsants and antipsychotics.

The cholinesterase inhibitor drugs (donepezil, galantamine and rivastigmine) that are modestly effective for the symptomatic treatment of the cognitive symptoms of dementia have been mooted also for the treatment of BPSD. Unfortunately, the cholinesterase inhibitors seem to have limited efficacy in the treatment of BPSD (Howard et al 2007). In contrast, the NMDA-receptor antagonist memantine is associated with modest improvement in behaviour in some people with dementia (Gauthier et al 2008).

Antidepressants show moderate efficacy in the treatment of major depression in people with Alzheimer's disease. While it is likely that all modern antidepressants will have some efficacy in this situation, the best evidence is for sertraline (Lyketsos et al 2003), moclobemide and citalopram.

The anticonvulsants carbamazepine and valproate have been trialled in BPSD. Valproate has been found to be ineffective (Herrmann et al 2007). The evidence for carbamazepine is more mixed, but insufficient to recommend this drug (Konovalov et al 2008). There is little evidence for the use of benzodiazepines in BPSD.

The conventional and atypical antipsychotic drugs are modestly effective (mean effect size 0.18) for the treatment of psychotic symptoms, aggression and agitation in people with dementia (Lonergan et al 2002, Rabinowitz et al 2007, Schneider et al 1990). However, they are associated with an increased risk of cerebrovascular adverse events, including stroke and transient ischaemic attacks (TIAs). They are also associated with an increased risk of death (Schneider et al 2005). It appears that this is a class effect and occurs with both atypical and conventional antipsychotics. The most susceptible individuals have preexisting risk factors for cerebrovascular disease, including, in some cases, a history of stroke or TIA. The main implication of these observations is that clinicians should obtain informed consent (often from a substitute decision maker) before prescribing psychotropic drugs to people with dementia. They should also carefully weigh the risk–benefit ratio before prescribing antipsychotic medication. Before the patient commences antipsychotic medication, the clinician should decide upon a stopping rule (e.g. stop antipsychotic medication after 6–12 weeks to see if it is still needed). Withdrawal of antipsychotic medication from people with dementia is often quite feasible, usually leads to no adverse outcomes (Ballard et al 2008) and has been shown to reduce mortality (Ballard et al 2009).

SERVICE DELIVERY ISSUES

People with dementia vary considerably in the severity of the BPSD that they exhibit. As a consequence, a range of services is needed to meet their needs. Not all of these services are available in all locations. Older persons' mental health services (OPMHS) in some districts will be able to collaborate with other community-based service providers, particularly with the Dementia Behaviour Management Advisory Service (DBMAS), auspiced by Alzheimer's Australia.

A seven-tiered BPSD service delivery model has been developed (Brodaty et al 2003), which is illustrated in Figure 28.1. Unfortunately, at the time of writing this book,

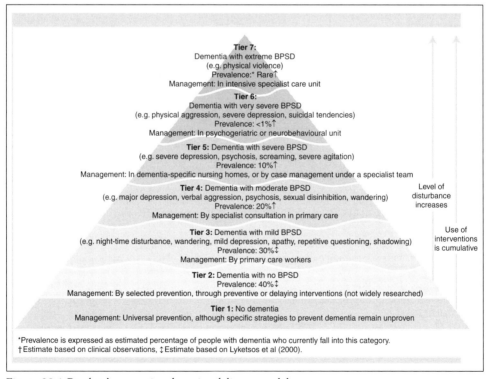

Figure 28.1 Brodaty's seven-tiered service delivery model
Source: Brodaty H, Draper BM, Low L-F 2003 Behavioural and psychological symptoms of dementia: a seven-tiered model of service delivery. Medical Journal of Australia 178(5):231–234. ©Copyright 2003 Medical Journal of Australia, reproduced with permission.

most districts in Australia do not have access to tier six and seven services. As a consequence, people with dementia complicated by severe behavioural disturbance are often managed in inappropriate settings, such as RACFs, hospital emergency departments and general psychiatric wards, by staff with inadequate training or insufficient support.

SUMMARY

BPSD are highly prevalent, and are often associated with substantial distress for the person with dementia and considerable burden for the carer. They may also lead to premature institutionalisation. Interventions include individualised behavioural management, individualised carer training and the careful use of psychotropic medications.

FURTHER READING

Bird M, Llewellyn-Jones RH, Korten A, Smithers H 2007 A controlled trial of a predominantly psychosocial approach to BPSD: treating causality. International Psychogeriatrics 19(5):874–891
Brodaty H, Draper BM, Low L-F 2003 Behavioural and psychological symptoms of dementia: a seven-tiered model of service delivery. Medical Journal of Australia 178(5):231–234
Mace NL, Rabins PV 1999 The 36-hour day, 3rd edn. Johns Hopkins University Press, Baltimore
O'Connor DW, Ames D, Gardner B, King M 2009 Psychosocial treatments of behavior symptoms in dementia: a systematic review of reports meeting quality standards. International Psychogeriatrics 21:225–240

REFERENCES

Aalten P, de Vugt ME, Jaspers N et al 2005 The course of neuropsychiatric symptoms in dementia. Part 1: findings from the two-year longitudinal Maasbed Study. International Journal of Geriatric Psychiatry 20(6):523–530
Alexopoulos GS, Abrams RC, Young RC, Shamoian CA 1988 Cornell Scale for Depression in Dementia. Biological Psychiatry 23(3):271–284
Apostolova LG, Cummings JL 2008 Neuropsychiatric manifestations in mild cognitive impairment: a systematic review of the literature. Dementia and Geriatric Cognitive Disorders 25(2):115–126
Archer N, Brown RG, Reeves SJ et al 2007 Premorbid personality and behavioral and psychological symptoms in probable Alzheimer disease. American Journal of Geriatric Psychiatry 15(3): 202–213
Ballard C, Hanney ML, Theodoulou M et al 2009 The dementia antipsychotic withdrawal trial (DART–AD): long-term follow-up of a randomised placebo-controlled trial. Lancet Neurology 8:151–157
Ballard C, Lana MM, Theodoulou M et al 2008 A randomised, blinded, placebo-controlled trial in dementia patients continuing or stopping neuroleptics (the DART–AD trial). PloS Medicine 5(4):e76
Black W, Almeida OP 2004 A systematic review of the association between the behavioral and psychological symptoms of dementia and burden of care. International Psychogeriatrics 16(3):295–315
Brodaty H, Draper BM, Low L-F 2003 Behavioural and psychological symptoms of dementia: a seven-tiered model of service delivery. Medical Journal of Australia 178(5):231–234
Cohen-Mansfield J 1986 Agitated behaviors in the elderly. II. Preliminary results in the cognitively deteriorated. Journal of the American Geriatrics Society 34(10):722–727
Cummings JL 1997 The Neuropsychiatric Inventory: assessing psychopathology in dementia patients. Neurology 48(5Suppl6):S10–S16
Cummings JL, Mega M, Gray K et al 1994 The Neuropsychiatric Inventory: comprehensive assessment of psychopathology in dementia. Neurology 44(12):2308–2314

Dwyer M, Byrne GJA 2000 Disruptive vocalisation and depression in older nursing home residents. International Psychogeriatrics 12(4):461–469

Gauthier S, Loft H, Cummings J 2008 Improvement in behavioural symptoms in patients with moderate to severe Alzheimer's disease by memantine: a pooled data analysis. International Journal of Geriatric Psychiatry 23(5):537–545

Gordon JE, Powell C, Rockwood K 1999 Goal attainment scaling as a measure of clinically important change in nursing-home patients. Age and Ageing 28:275–281

Herrmann N, Lanctot KL, Rothenburg LS, Eryavec G 2007 A placebo-controlled trial of valproate for agitation and aggression in Alzheimer's disease. Dementia and Geriatric Cognitive Disorders 23(2):116–119

Howard RJ, Juszczak E, Ballard CG et al 2007 Donepezil for the treatment of agitation in Alzheimer's disease. New England Journal of Medicine 357:1382–1392

Konovalov S, Muralee S, Tampi RR 2008 Anticonvulsants for the treatment of behavioral and psychological symptoms of dementia: a literature review. International Psychogeriatrics 20:293–308

Logsdon RG, McCurry SM, Teri L 2007 Evidence-based psychological treatments for disruptive behaviors in individuals with dementia. Psychology and Aging 22:28–36

Lonergan E, Luxenberg J, Colford JM, Birks J 2002 Haloperidol for agitation in dementia. Cochrane Database of Systematic Reviews, Issue 2. Art. No. CD002852. DOI: 10.1002/14651858.CD002852

Lyketsos CG, DelCampo L, Steinberg M et al 2003 Treating depression in Alzheimer disease: efficacy and safety of sertraline therapy, and the benefits of depression reduction: the DIADS. Archives of General Psychiatry 60:737–746

Lyketsos CG, Steinberg M, Tschanz JT et al 2000 Mental and behavioral disturbances in dementia: findings from the Cache County Study on Memory in Aging. American Journal of Psychiatry 157:708–714

Mittelman MS, Brodaty H, Wallen AS, Burns A 2008 A three-country randomized controlled trial of a psychosocial intervention for caregivers combined with pharmacological treatment for patients with Alzheimer disease: effects on caregiver depression. American Journal of Geriatric Psychiatry 16(11):893–904

Muangpaisan W, Intalapaporn S, Assantachai P 2008 Neuropsychiatric symptoms in the community-based patients with mild cognitive impairment and the influence of demographic factors. International Journal of Geriatric Psychiatry 23(7):699–703

O'Connor DW, Ames D, Gardner B, King M 2009 Psychosocial treatments of behavior symptoms in dementia: a systematic review of reports meeting quality standards. International Psychogeriatrics 21:225–240

Opie J, Rosewarne R, O'Connor DW 1999 The efficacy of psychosocial approaches to behaviour disorders in dementia: a systematic literature review. Australian and New Zealand Journal of Psychiatry 33:789–799

Parahoo K, Whall AL, Colling K, Nusbaum D 2006 Expert nurses' use of implicit memory in the care of patients with Alzheimer's disease. Journal of Advanced Nursing 54(5):563–571

Petrovic M, Hurt C, Collins D et al 2007 Clustering of behavioural and psychological symptoms in dementia (BPSD): a European Alzheimer's Disease Consortium (EADC) study. Acta Clinica Belgica 62(6):426–432

Pritchard AL, Pritchard CW, Bentham P, Lendon CL 2007 Role of serotonin transporter polymorphisms in the behavioural and psychological symptoms in probable Alzheimer disease patients. Dementia and Geriatric Cognitive Disorders 24(3):201–206

Pritchard AL, Pritchard CW, Bentham P, Lendon CL 2008 Investigation of the role of the dopamine transporter in susceptibility to behavioural and psychological symptoms of patients with probable Alzheimer's disease. Dementia and Geriatric Cognitive Disorders 26(3): 257–260

Rabinowitz J, Katz I, De Deyn PP et al 2007 Treating behavioral and psychological symptoms in patients with psychosis of Alzheimer's disease using risperidone. International Psychogeriatrics 19:227–240

Savva GM, Zaccai J, Matthews FE et al 2009 Medical Research Council Cognitive Function and Ageing Study: prevalence, correlates and course of behavioural and psychological symptoms of dementia in the population. British Journal of Psychiatry 194(3):212–219

Schneider LS, Dagerman KS, Insel P 2005 Risk of death with atypical antipsychotic drug treatment for dementia: meta-analyis of randomized placebo-controlled trials. Journal of the American Medical Association 294(15):1934–1943

Schneider LS, Pollock VE, Lyness SA 1990 A meta-analysis of controlled trials of neuroleptic treatment in dementia. Journal of the American Geriatrics Society 38(5):553–563

Selwood A, Johnston K, Katona C et al 2007 Systematic review of the effect of psychological interventions on family caregivers of people with dementia. Journal of Affective Disorders 101:75–89

Sohrabi HR, Bates KA, Rodrigues M et al 2009 The relationship between memory complaints, perceived quality of life and mental health in apolipoprotein E episilon 4 carriers and non-carriers. Journal of Alzheimer's Disease 17(1):69–79

Steinberg M, Shao H, Zandi P et al 2008 Point and 5-year period prevalence of neuropsychiatric symptoms in dementia: the Cache County Study. International Journal of Geriatric Psychiatry 23(2):170–177

Vink AC, Birks JS, Bruinsma MS, Scholten RJ 2004 Music therapy for people with dementia. Cochrane Database of Systematic Reviews, Issue 4. Art. No. CD003477. DOI: 10.1002/14651858.CD003477.pub2

Yaffe K, Fox P, Newcomer R et al 2002 Patient and caregiver characteristics and nursing home placement in patients with dementia. Journal of the American Medical Association 287:2090–2097

Chapter 29

PSYCHOTHERAPEUTIC TREATMENT

INTRODUCTION

This chapter provides information on what is known about the commonly used strategies for psychotherapeutic treatment for older people. Some of the symptoms of the mental disorders that affect older people, such as thoughts of hopelessness and negativity, the inability to enjoy pleasurable activities, anxiety and low energy levels, can be addressed with psychotherapeutic treatments alone. However, when other symptoms such as psychotic or suicidal thoughts, appetite and sleep disturbances are evident, a combination of psychotherapeutic and pharmacological treatments may be the best course of action. Psychotherapeutic treatments are important adjunctive therapies for older people, particularly when they are required to take many medications for serious medical conditions.

SPECIAL ISSUES CONCERNING OLDER PEOPLE

When entering a therapeutic relationship with an older person, it pays to be mindful of some characteristics the older person may bring into the relationship (see also Ch 11). With the ageing process comes more physical and perhaps cognitive problems against a backdrop of vast and different life experiences. Even with a lifetime of knowledge and experience, some older people just accept whatever therapy is offered or directed at them without a thorough understanding or enthusiasm for that option. A more prudent strategy to improve engagement and hopefully achieve success with the therapy would be to present all options, including information about the pace, format and purpose, allowing the person to choose and give support for that choice. If the person has had therapy previously, it would be worthwhile to revisit any successful approaches, but older people are quite capable of learning new approaches.

Working with older people requires knowledge of what has defined their generation (e.g. wars, economic crises, dominant religions and social practices). Many older Australians experienced as children the effects of the 1930s depression and World War II, and as adults the effects of the Vietnam War and major technological advances. Social practices and beliefs of always being stoic and that personal problems or mental illness are signs of weakness and failure pervade this generation. Personal problems are often not discussed at all, or only within the family, and certainly not with strangers or therapists whose intentions may be deemed akin to brainwashing. Ageist attitudes dictate that it is normal for older people to be unhappy, cranky and inflexible to change. Normal boundaries (see Ch 11) that are set up with younger clients in regard to such issues as physical contact and acceptance of gifts may have to be rethought with some older clients (e.g. when expressing gratitude, the older person may find it insulting if you do not accept an embrace or an offer of a cup of tea). In rural areas, the mental health workers often leave older people's houses with plant cuttings and bottles of homemade condiments. So it is a good idea to have a formal policy in place on how to deal with such circumstances.

If the therapist is younger, having credibility when the older person sees themselves as older and wiser may be an issue. This should be identified and acknowledged early in the relationship because it may interfere with continued engagement and the success of the therapy. The therapist needs to take the initiative and directly ask the older person what opinions they may hold that make it difficult for them to talk openly and easily with the therapist, and they need to establish a set of engagement rules to overcome any difficulties.

The mental health worker needs to inquire about the presence and impact of common ageing concerns, including poorer physical health, limited financial capacity, less independence, diminishing social supports, and loss of significant others and meaningful employment. Loss is a very challenging aspect of the therapeutic process in the sense that the many losses that older people experience are generally more major than what a younger person may experience, such as the loss of a lifelong partner or career. From this, the challenge for the mental health worker is to determine what a realistic level of grief reaction for the older person to these losses would be.

To overcome the barriers such as cognitive, medical and functional disabilities, the therapist may need to adjust the pace and length of the therapy sessions and where and how the therapy is delivered. For example, the content needs to match the person's educational level, and concepts may need repeating verbally and visually with the use of a whiteboard and handouts. What the older person brings into the therapeutic relationship should be capitalised upon, such as many life experiences and accomplishments that have required a range of interactions, decisions to be made and problems to be solved. Finally, when the relationship reaches the termination phase, this can be done by gradually spacing the sessions out with occasional follow-up sessions to maintain what has been achieved and prevent relapse.

Psychotherapeutic treatments can be delivered via individual or group formats. The group format may be more economical and is particularly useful for older people who have a limited social network. In a review conducted by Pinquart et al (2007), the individual format came out slightly ahead of the group format, with it being more efficacious and experiencing less dropout rates.

COGNITIVE BEHAVIOUR THERAPY

Cognitive behaviour therapy (CBT) has been shown to be successful in treating a wide variety of disorders that affect older people, such as depression, anxiety, panic attacks and sleep disturbance (Hill & Brettle 2006, Knight 2004, Laidlaw et al 2003, Pinquart et al 2007, Wilson et al 2009). The basic premise of CBT is determining how the older person perceives themselves and how they judge the effect certain experiences have had on their lives. The CBT therapist questions and challenges strongly held beliefs that may be reinforcing negative self-concepts. Through the therapeutic process, the older person is made aware of how they distort and misinterpret certain events in their lives, and then positive thoughts and behaviours are activated by altering these erroneous thought patterns. The therapy is usually time limited to 10 or so sessions. CBT is effective in the acute phase of treatment and also in the longer term by helping reduce the risk of recurrence. The usual protocols for CBT are behavioural strategies drawn from Lewinsohn's (1974) operant model and cognitive strategies from Beck et al's (1979) cognitive model.

Initially, to get a clear picture of what may be distressing the older person, baseline information is gathered about the situation(s) in which the symptoms occur, accompanying thoughts, the physiological response and behaviour patterns. An example would be:

- *Thought*. I'm getting old; I'm not suited to this environment; I can't be a burden on my family who have their own problems.
- *Physical symptoms*. These include hyperventilation and heart pounding.
- *Behaviour*. These include running to neighbours to get help, calling an ambulance, avoiding contact with family for fear of burdening them and sleep disturbance.

This information is obtained through direct questioning (e.g. 'What was happening when the panic attacks started?'), standardised self-report scales and a self-monitoring log of symptoms relating to feelings of sadness and/or anxiety. As well as this information, it is important to identify what activities have a positive influence of giving pleasure or a sense of achievement, and what barriers exist and ways to overcome these. Goals can be set to increase these activities.

Following the identification of thoughts, physical symptoms and behaviour pattern, how these factors interact with each other is examined. Next, a suitable intervention strategy is chosen from a range of CBT techniques. Some techniques work well with some problems and not with others. There may be some trial and error in these initial stages. A daily log is an integral part of the treatment process. It brings objective awareness of the symptoms the person is experiencing and how the treatment is progressing. The older person logs what the troubling situation is and the concurrent thoughts, physical symptoms and behaviour. This record then enables the therapist and the older person to identify the antecedents and consequences, as well as the effect of any intervention strategy. Physical responses such as rapid breathing, sweating and increased heart rate are easy to identify. Simple strategies such as breathing techniques, progressive muscle relaxation and antianxiety medications are effective in countering adverse physical responses.

With CBT, erroneous thoughts are challenged and the older person is taught how to reframe these thoughts as hypotheses so that their thinking processes are trained to be more rational. This is done by identifying the troubling thought, assembling the evidence that supports and does not support this thought, using skills to challenge the erroneous thoughts and developing alternative ways of thinking. Examples of questions would be: 'How do you know that your family thinks you are a burden?' and 'Does a person's age mean they have to behave in a certain manner?' The responses to the reframed questions can then be converted into simple, coping statements that are reflective of a more realistic situation, such as: 'My family is an important part of my support network. I do not know if I am a burden to them.' Realistic statements help to reduce anxious or depressive feelings. Brief, affirmative statements can be used by the person when they feel the onset of anxious or depressive feelings.

SOME OF THE FEATURES OF COGNITIVE BEHAVIOUR THERAPY

Features of cognitive behaviour therapy (CBT) include:
- The older person has the support of a health professional/therapist.
- It uses a structured framework, it focuses on present problems, and it is direct and quick and time limited.
- A number of techniques can be utilised to modify thoughts, physical symptoms and behaviour patterns.
- The simple skills and techniques such as abdominal breathing and the problem-solving process can be used on a continuing basis to maintain wellness and prevent relapse.

BEHAVIOUR THERAPY

Behaviour therapy (BT) that is suitable for older people includes techniques such as relaxation and exposure therapy, including systematic desensitisation (see Ch 23). It is effective generally with disorders such as depression and anxiety and dealing with specific symptoms such as insomnia (Engels & Vermey 1997).

BT has the goal of changing or positively influencing behaviour that is contributing negatively to the disorder. For example, a disorder such as depression can be almost self-perpetuating by negative behaviours reinforcing each other. A clinical feature of depression is loss of pleasure in previously enjoyed social activities. In this situation, the older person may not be inclined to participate in social activities, thereby decreasing such positive benefits of interpersonal relationships and physical exercise. The lack of both of these activities exacerbates the depressive illness. This behaviour can become so ingrained that it is difficult to change and the older person will require much direction and support to break the destructive cycle. The direction may be as specific as identifying pleasurable events, scheduling them and going with the older person so that their thoughts and perceptions during the experience can be explored and adapted. In addition to improving interpersonal skills and increasing physical activity, BT can be used to enhance activities of daily living and to manage incontinence. It can also be used to help manage problems related to the behavioural symptoms of dementia such as wandering and agitation.

A major task of BT is detailed and ongoing recording of observations of the behaviour, in particular:
- Why does it occur (antecedents/trigger)?
- What is the behaviour?
- Where does it occur?
- How does the person respond via their thoughts and feelings?
- When does the behaviour occur? When doesn't the behaviour occur?
- What happens after the behaviour has occurred (consequences/reinforcers)?

A simple and methodical process of A–B–C (antecedent–behaviour–consequence) allows for a very close examination of the behaviour (Teri et al 1997). This is important because often when people are at the point of seeking help it may be difficult for them to be objective and they can either overstate or understate the problem, making possible treatment plans ineffective. The A–B–C framework breaks complex behaviours down into more easily manageable parts, allowing the older person to exercise some control over what is happening. It is a process that appeals to a wide range of cognitive abilities because treatment plans can start off with very simple steps, be applied to usual daily activities and be built up over time. Positive reinforcements can be given for any progress and, since the process started with a detailed assessment, the outcomes are measurable and these can be demonstrated to the older person (see also Ch 28).

PSYCHODYNAMIC THERAPY

Psychodynamic therapy involves the psychological processes by delving into past unresolved conflicts for the purpose of resolution so that the older person may gain some insight and relief to be able to move on with other aspects of their lives (Shiller 1992, Thompson et al 1987). Psychodynamic therapy has been found to be effective in treating late-life depression, particularly in regard to the many losses that are experienced at this time of life (Pinquart et al 2007). For example, what was lost (partner, job) could have been covering or compensating for certain vulnerabilities that were created earlier in one's life (e.g. poor ability for emotional attachments). Once the vulnerabilities are exposed, these can lead to depression or other mental health problems.

Other than loss, some of the major psychodynamic issues arise from narcissistic, obsessional and dependent personality traits. Examples of these issues could be an older man with narcissistic traits whose self-worth is determined by a successful career and forced retirement crushes this ideal causing a serious depression. Or the older person with dependent traits, which developed from childhood insecurities, loses their spouse and finds being alone intolerable. This void is then filled with alcohol or excessive medical visits (Ardern 2002). Other common issues are fear of the future and worry about death. These issues are dealt with in therapy by building self-esteem, becoming more self-reliant and viewing old age as a rewarding experience with something to look forward to (Slater 1995). Brief or time-limited psychodynamic therapies are a popular option with older people.

SUPPORTIVE PSYCHOTHERAPY

Supportive psychotherapy is often used for older people who are very unstable psychologically (Newton & Jacobowitz 1999), although it has been used with reasonable effectiveness for anxiety symptoms in older people (Barrowclough et al 2001). It is sometimes necessary for an older person to undergo supportive psychotherapy before undertaking the other types of therapy that require a person to be reasonably 'well' to process discussion points and undertake more complex activities. The purpose of supportive psychotherapy is to strengthen the sense of self or 'ego' when it has been battered by such things as significant losses.

A qualified and experienced therapist primarily uses transference to counter negative views, provide a sense of security and belonging, and allow close identification so the older person feels they are being understood (Newton & Jacobowitz 1999). The fundamental strategies underlying supportive psychotherapy begin with asking the question: Why has the older person presented at this particular time with this particular problem? (Misch 2000). From this basis, the therapist identifies key problems and likely interventions, while appreciating that with more knowledge and understanding about the older person, these summations will change over time. An older person will need supportive psychotherapy because they are functioning ineffectually. Sometimes, in these situations, to counter stressors, the therapist may need to take on parental characteristics like comforting, praising and advising, while balancing these with limit setting when destructive behaviours manifest.

As with most psychotherapy, it is an important strategy to increase coping skills and the use of adaptive defence mechanisms, such as rationalisation, humour and sublimation. This is achieved through education and practice. Role modelling by the therapist can also be part of supportive psychotherapy. This can occur with the therapist judiciously self-disclosing how they themselves cope on good days and bad days. The therapist also assists the older person to make connections between thoughts and feelings, between behaviour and responses, and between events and subsequent thoughts and feelings. This will greatly enhance an older person's ability to function with everyday life. Additional strategies that are continually incorporated into supportive psychotherapy sessions are bolstering the older person's self-esteem, combating feelings of hopelessness, focusing on everyday functioning, encouraging activity and support networks, and educating the older person about their mental health problem and its treatment.

PROBLEM-SOLVING THERAPY

Problem-solving therapy (D'Zurilla & Nezu 1999) aims to provide a systematic approach to develop or enhance the older person's ability to solve problems. There are usually six steps involved:

1. *Problem orientation.* This is where the older person is asked to identify what they perceive their problems as being and to view these problems as being solvable. If the problem is obviously unsolvable (e.g. death of a loved one or some form of chronic illness), it is reoriented into aspects that are able to be solved, such as strategies to honour the dead person or ways to manage the chronic illness.
2. *Problem definition.* In this step, the older person is taught how to define the problem in concrete and operational terms, rather than unachievable, intractable, uncontrollable ways. For example, if a grieving person says, 'I am too old to find happiness again', this could be better defined as, 'I have to make sure I make the effort to socialise with others'.
3. *Brainstorming.* This step involves brainstorming around five to ten possible solutions. The solutions are not evaluated at this stage, and the therapist needs to be aware that depressed people, in particular, are likely to discard the solution, even before giving it careful consideration, due to their negative belief systems.
4. *Decision making.* After possible solutions are generated, the next step is decision making. All the pros and cons of each solution are debated in terms of whether they are realistic, acceptable and feasible, and the best possible solution is decided upon.
5. *Implementation.* This step involves the development and enactment of an implementation plan for the selected solution.
6. *Verification.* This step is where the success or failure of the plan is discussed. The process is taught to the older person over approximately 6 weeks (1 week for each step) and then the sessions can continue for another 6 or so weeks where all of the steps are applied to specific problems.

LIFE REVIEW AND REMINISCENCE THERAPY

Although closely aligned, life review and reminiscence therapy are different. Originally conceptualised by Butler (1963), life review has developed to take on a more focused, structured and active approach of resolving past tensions or dealing with a current problem by looking back on one's life to examine how certain issues were dealt with in the past, what was done well and can be done again, and what wasn't done so well and how those mistakes can be avoided. McDougall et al (1997) found that life review was useful with depressed older people.

Reminiscence, on the other hand, is a less structured, recollection of the past, often utilising prompts such as memorabilia, photos or journals. It is designed not to be intrusive, but to subtly encourage the older person to talk and then be willing to listen to others. It is useful in finding common ground and for the initial stages of developing a trusting relationship. Further benefits of reminiscence therapy have been postulated as enabling older people to highlight positive aspects of their lives, which in turn enhances their self-esteem and ability to recognise their individuality and identity. Reminiscence therapy has been shown to have a large effect in treating depression in older people (Pinquart et al 2007), whereas there are mixed results for its benefits for older people with dementia (Spector et al 2003, Watt & Cappeliez 2000).

The use of both these therapies has to be carefully assessed because some older people have past events in their lives they may not want to, or they may find difficult to, revisit (e.g. if they were a prisoner of war, a refugee or victim of a crime). Such issues require great sensitivity on behalf of the healthcare worker because it may not be helpful for any emotional pain to be repressed or ignored. Additionally, it is worthwhile to keep in mind that there are some people who are present and future focused, and do not see any value in reminiscing.

INTERPERSONAL THERAPY

Interpersonal therapy has its focus on changing or accepting current interpersonal behaviours by the development of insight and skills, so relationships are improved and reactions to interpersonal events are moderated (Hinrichsen & Clougherty 2006). It does not have the direct focus of other therapies such as CBT, nor is it the open-ended exploration of the older person's thoughts and feelings. With interpersonal therapy, the therapist actively works on revealing difficulties that the older person may not be consciously aware of, but which are the underlying cause of their distress. Only one or two specific issues are chosen at a time from the problematic areas of interpersonal conflicts (family disputes), interpersonal deficits (social isolation, unable to accept care and support), relationship loss (spouse, family members, friends) and role changes (retirement, caregiver). Once again, this is a time-limited therapy, with up to 20 sessions being the usual course of treatment.

PSYCHOEDUCATION

The aim of psychoeducation is to improve the long-term outcome of treatment by strengthening the older person's self-efficacy and self-management skills. It has proven effectiveness in the treatment of depression (Pinquart et al 2007). Psychoeducation usually involves face-to-face sessions that last for 60 minutes or so. Prevention plans are specifically tailored to the individual. The plans usually contain self-reporting of early symptoms or warning signs of deterioration, stress management techniques, a regular scheme of social and recreational activities, nutrition, exercise and sleep regimes, management of medication side effects and adverse reactions, and a hierarchy of contacts for mild to severe crisis situations. Telephone/internet contact may also be included to replace or supplement the face-to-face contact. Goals are usually set with associated achievement plans. The symptoms are monitored and discussed with adjustments made to the plans along the way and positive reinforcement given to encourage compliance with the prevention plan. Some examples of psychoeducation programs are: relapse-prevention programs for people with addictions; self-management programs for those who have a chronic disease; medication adherence for people who have compliance problems; and social reactivation for people who experience loneliness.

FAMILY THERAPY

When engaging with an older person, family is often involved and family issues could be the cause of the older person's distress. Family therapy is usually required when a family is struggling to adjust to a crisis. Common crises occur when an older person becomes seriously ill and death is imminent, or when determining which family members are to take on a caregiving role or whether placement of the older person in permanent care is required. At the outset of family therapy, it is important to understand what role each person plays in the family and what subsystems exist to undertake particular tasks (e.g. decision making). Knowledge of a family's intrinsic and extrinsic rules on how family business is conducted, such as who is the spokesperson, provides valuable insights for conducting family therapy (Qualls 2000). The clinical interaction focuses on each individual's patterns of interaction, alliance and communication with other family members. Interventions for family therapy focus on strengthening positive patterns that already exist and finding alternatives for failing or impeding patterns.

If it is clinically prudent to involve family members, seeking information and involving them in the treatment process can be a very sensitive and complex matter. Often families have old, unresolved conflicts or painful secrets that may surface and need to be worked through and put into perspective before dealing with present issues. Care must be taken with interpretation of past events and unresolved grievances, as this has a major influence on the type of involvement of each family member. If a lot of family conflict is present, the therapist must be cognisant of not taking any sides and remaining neutral (Asen 2002).

COUNSELLING AND CRISIS INTERVENTION

Counselling and crisis intervention are skills used regularly by mental health workers and, although loosely related to psychotherapies, they are not considered therapies as such. Counselling is entered into voluntarily. It is an intervention that is responsive to the older person's individual needs, allows people to express their own feelings, and requires flexible, unimposing responses from the health worker with the intention of assisting with psychological and behavioural changes. The process of counselling is not age-specific, but it has its place in the mental healthcare of older people who often have to endure ageist attitudes and a significant amount of loss and associated bereavement. Counselling involves setting up a therapeutic relationship that is confidential, non-directive and non-judgmental, and the counsellor displays unconditional positive regard, empathetic understanding and genuineness. The communication skills of active and attentive listening, paraphrasing and questioning are used to assist the older person with self-expression and to aid interpretation (Scrutton 1997).

Crisis intervention is a short-term interaction that aims to provide immediate and intense support for the older person to lessen the impact of the crisis, to mobilise their resources in dealing with the crisis, and to return them as close as possible to their previous level of functioning. According to Burgess (1998), ensuring a safe environment is the first action. The older person is then allowed to ventilate about what has happened to them and then reassurance is given that they reacted in the best way they could. After this, the older person can be given the opportunity to examine the circumstances surrounding the crisis and how such things may be dealt with in the future. Ongoing issues can be dealt with by supportive interventions such as counselling and support groups.

SUMMARY

Psychotherapeutic interventions can be beneficial as an alternative to, or adjunct to, pharmacological interventions. Some older people prefer non-pharmacological treatments, while other older people have serious coexistent medical conditions that limit the use of medications. A variety of therapies have been described in this chapter in order to help the mental health worker find an intervention that suits the older person's cognitive ability and their preference.

FURTHER READING

Duffy M 1999 Handbook of counselling and psychotherapy with older adults. John Wiley & Sons, New York
Knight BG 2004 Psychotherapy with older adults. Sage, Thousand Oaks, CA
Laidlaw K, Thompson LW, Dick-Siskin L, Gallagher-Thompson D 2003 Cognitive behaviour therapy with older people. Wiley, Chichester
Slater R 1995 The psychology of growing old: looking forward. Open University Press, Buckingham

REFERENCES

Asen EK 2002 Family therapy with ageing families. In: Jacoby R, Oppenheimer C (eds) Psychiatry in the elderly. Oxford University Press, Oxford
Ardern M 2002 Dynamic psychotherapy with older persons. In: Jacoby R, Oppenheimer C (eds) Psychiatry in the elderly. Oxford University Press, Oxford
Barrowclough C, King P, Colville J et al 2001 A randomized trial of the effectiveness of cognitive-behavioral therapy and supportive counselling for anxiety symptoms in older adults. Journal of Consulting and Clinical Psychology 69(5):756–762
Beck AT, Kovacs M, Weissman A 1979 Assessment of suicidal intention: the Scale for Suicidal Ideation. Journal of Consulting and Clinical Psychology 47(2):343–352
Burgess AW 1998 Advanced practice psychiatric nursing. Appleton & Lange, Stamford, CT
Butler R 1963 The life review: an interpretation of reminiscence in the aged. Psychiatry 26:65–76
D'Zurilla TJ, Nezu AM 1999 Problem solving therapy: a social competence approach to clinical intervention, 2nd edn. Springer Publishing, New York
Engels GI, Vermey M 1997 Efficacy of nonmedical treatments of depression in elders: a quantitative analysis. Journal of Clinical Geropsychology 3:17–35
Hill A, Brettle A 2006 Counselling older people: what can we learn from research evidence? Journal of Social Work Practice 20(3):281–297

Hinrichsen GA, Clougherty KF 2006 Interpersonal psychotherapy for depressed older adults. American Psychological Association, Washington DC

Knight BG 2004 Psychotherapy with older adults. Sage, Thousand Oaks, CA

Laidlaw K, Thompson LW, Dick-Siskin L, Gallagher-Thompson D 2003 Cognitive behaviour therapy with older people. John Wiley & Sons, Chichester

Lewinsohn PM 1974 A behavioural approach to depression. In: Friedman RJ, Katz NM (eds) The psychology of depression: contemporary theory and research. Winston-Wiley, Washington DC

McDougall GJ, Blixen CE, Suen L-J 1997 The process and outcome of life review psychotherapy with depressed homebound older adults. Nursing Research 46(5):277–283

Misch DA 2000 Basic strategies of dynamic supportive therapy. Journal of Psychotherapy Practice and Research 9(4):173–189

Newton NA, Jacobowitz J 1999 Transferential and countertransferential processes in therapy with older adults. In: Duffy M (ed) Handbook of counselling and psychotherapy with older adults. John Wiley & Sons, New York

Pinquart M, Duberstein PR, Lyness JM 2007 Effects of psychotherapy and other behavioural interventions on clinically depressed older adults: a meta-analysis. Aging and Mental Health 11(6):645–657

Qualls SH 2000 Therapy with aging families: rationale, opportunities and challenges. Aging and Mental Health 4(3):191–199

Scrutton S 1997 Counselling: maintaining mental health in older age. In: Norman IJ, Redfern SJ (eds) Mental health care for elderly people. Churchill Livingstone, London

Shiller A 1992 Psychotherapy with elderly patients: experiences from a psychiatric psychotherapeutic consultation service. Psychosomatics. Medicine and Psychoanalysis 38(4):371–380

Slater R 1995 The psychology of growing old: looking forward. Open University Press, Buckingham

Spector A, Orrell M, Davies S, Woods RT 2003 Reminiscence therapy for dementia: Cochrane Review. The Cochrane Library Issue 3, Oxford

Teri L, Logsdon RG, Uomoto J, McCurry SM 1997 Behavioral treatment of depression in dementia patients: a controlled clinical trial. Journal of Gerontology 52B:159–166

Thompson LW, Gallagher D, Breckenridge JS 1987 Comparative effectiveness of psychotherapies for depressed elders. Journal of Consulting and Clinical Psychology 55(3):385–390

Watt LM, Cappeliez P 2000 Integrative and instrumental reminiscence therapies for depression in older adults: intervention strategies and treatment effectiveness. Aging and Mental Health 4(2):166–177

Wilson K, Mottram PG, Vassilas C 2009 Psychotherapeutic treatments for older depressed people (review). Cochrane Collaboration

Chapter 30
PHARMACOLOGICAL TREATMENT

INTRODUCTION

The introduction of effective psychotropic medications in the 1950s transformed the lives of many people with mental health problems, including many older people who would otherwise have lived out their lives in asylums. The drugs that are currently available are powerful pharmaceutical agents and all have significant potential adverse effects. This chapter introduces core concepts in clinical psychopharmacology and outlines the major classes of psychotropics used in older people in the community. It is likely to be of most interest to medical and nursing personnel, although all mental health workers do require a working familiarity with the psychotropic medications commonly used in older people.

IMPORTANT NOTE

The use of psychotropic medications to treat mental health problems in older people requires specialised knowledge and training. The material presented in this chapter should be taken as a guide only. Prescribers should consult approved product information sources for detailed information about safe prescribing. Decisions about the drug treatment of individual patients should be made by suitably qualified practitioners.

CORE CONCEPTS IN PSYCHOPHARMACOLOGY

Psychopharmacology involves the use of medication to treat mental health and behavioural problems. The conceptual model behind the use of drugs to alter states of mind is based on the idea that a person's mental state reflects, at least in part, the state of their brain neurotransmitter systems. Neurotransmitters are chemical messengers that allow brain cells to communicate with one another. Several neurotransmitters have been found to be suitable targets for drug treatment. These include acetylcholine, dopamine, gamma amino butyric acid (GABA), glutamate, noradrenaline and serotonin. It is beyond the scope of this chapter to provide detailed information about each of these neurotransmitter systems, but there are readily accessible sources of this information in specialised texts (e.g. Stahl 2006).

Effective psychotropic medications mostly employ one of three main mechanisms of action:

1. as agonists or antagonists of cell surface receptors
2. as inhibitors of regulatory enzymes, or
3. as blockers or stimulators of synaptic reuptake mechanisms.

For example, commonly used antipsychotic medications work via post-synaptic dopamine blockade, whereas commonly used antidepressant medications work via pre-synaptic inhibition of serotonin reuptake from the synapse.

'Pharmacokinetics' refers to what the body does to a drug, whereas 'pharmacodynamics' refers to what a drug does to the body. Ageing leads to pharmacokinetic and pharmacodynamic changes, and these changes need to be taken into account when prescribing psychotropic drugs to older people.

PHARMACOKINETIC AND PHARMACODYNAMIC CHANGES IN OLDER PEOPLE

There are a number of normal physiological changes with ageing that are relevant to the way the body handles drugs. Hepatic function declines slowly with advancing age so that drugs detoxified in the liver (most psychotropic drugs other than lithium) take longer to be metabolised. If the ingested drug is in its active form and it is inactivated by hepatic metabolism, then reduced hepatic function might lead to increased serum levels of the drug for a certain dose. This might lead to increased efficacy, but it might lead also to increased adverse effects. Renal function also declines slowly with advancing age so that drugs that are primarily excreted by the kidneys (e.g. lithium) will be eliminated more slowly. Thus, for any given dose, the serum level obtained will be higher and might lead to toxic effects. Other relevant pharmacokinetic factors include absorption from the gastrointestinal tract, metabolism in the gut wall, and protein binding in the bloodstream, although these do not change that much with age. With ageing, there is usually reduced total body water and an increased proportion of fat. The latter prolongs the elimination of lipophilic drugs, including most psychotropic agents. However, there are substantial individual differences in the way the body handles psychotropic drugs due mainly to genetic variation. These genetic differences are reflected in the activity of liver enzyme systems, particularly the cytochrome P450 system (CYP450).

In addition to these changes in what an older person's body does to a drug, there are changes in the ageing brain that make it more vulnerable to the effects of psychotropic medications. Older people with cerebrovascular disease or with dementia are particularly vulnerable to the effects of psychotropic drugs, and the use of much lower initial doses is prudent.

POLYPHARMACY

Polypharmacy refers to the situation in which a person is prescribed multiple potentially interacting medications. This is a common situation in older people with several chronic illnesses. Use of multiple drugs increases the risk of drug–drug interactions and of the additive effects of the adverse effects of these drugs. Sedative and anticholinergic effects due to combinations of drugs with these properties are a common problem, and often lead to confusion and falls.

In the setting of community treatment, the mental health worker should regularly review all the medications that the people under their care are taking. The assistance of a clinical pharmacist with experience in the use of psychotropic drugs in older people can be invaluable.

PRINCIPLES OF DRUG TREATMENT

Before commencing an older person on a psychotropic drug, there are several important steps that should be undertaken. These include combining information from the psychiatric history and mental state examination (MSE) to arrive at a 'provisional diagnosis' of the person's problem. In selected cases, this diagnosis might be further refined through the use of laboratory investigations and neuroimaging studies, as discussed in Chapter 15. Most of the evidence for the efficacy of drug treatment for mental health problems comes from conducting clinical trials in people with a defined mental health problem. Thus, it is important to arrive at a diagnosis before embarking on treatment with psychotropic medication. A physical examination is also important to exclude any contraindications to drug treatment. For instance, certain antipsychotic drugs might be contraindicated in older people with postural hypotension (low blood pressure on standing). It is also important to review with the person their therapeutic responses to previous treatments and any adverse effects that they have experienced in the past. A past history of response to a particular drug often provide a good indication of which drug to choose.

Drug treatment of mental health problems should take place in the context of a biopsychosocial management plan. The medications prescribed should be recorded in the clinical file and progress notes made each visit. Laboratory tests are required when using certain drugs, such as lithium and clozapine. In older people being treated on a voluntary basis, informed consent should be obtained before treatment with psychotropic medication. The person should be provided with detailed information about their diagnosis and the rationale behind drug treatment. They should be told about the common adverse effects of the drug, any uncommon serious adverse effects, and any adverse effects that might have particular significance for them. This can really only be achieved by talking with the person at some length and allowing them time to have their questions answered. It is important also to explain the likely interval to the onset of therapeutic effects and the need for laboratory monitoring, if relevant. The drug dose and dosing interval must be titrated against therapeutic and adverse effects. The drug should be stopped if it doesn't work.

DRUG ADMINISTRATION ISSUES

In older people, poor eyesight and impaired cognition may increase the potential risk of medication errors. Older people also have a high prevalence of arthritis that affects their ability to open pill bottles. Several techniques have evolved to assist older people living in the community. These include the use of home medication dispensing systems, such as the Webster Pak®, and the use of daily visits from domiciliary nurses to ensure correct administration of medications. In people with less severe difficulties, the use of a 'pill organiser', such as a Dosette® box, can help with keeping track of daily medication use. It often helps if the medication regimen has been simplified to once daily. Prescribers should also consider carefully the route of administration. It is often safer to use transdermal delivery systems (skin patches) for potentially toxic medications, such as buprenorphine (a narcotic analgesic) or rivastigmine (a cholinesterase inhibitor medication for Alzheimer's disease).

There is an important role for case managers in community older persons' mental health teams in assisting the older person with adherence to their prescribed medication. Liaison with prescribing doctors and dispensing pharmacists is essential to safe and effective use of psychotropic medication. Case managers are likely also to have an important role in monitoring people for adverse effects from medication. Mental health workers often find it useful to develop working relationships with hospital and community pharmacists. Older people are commonly on complex treatment regimens, and it can be very useful to have a clinical pharmacist review the medication that an older person is taking to look for potential problems.

ANTIDEPRESSANTS

Antidepressant drugs are widely prescribed for depressive and anxiety disorders. The best evidence is for their use in major depression and generalised anxiety disorder, although they are also commonly used in other depressive and anxiety disorders. All antidepressants have similar efficacy in major depression, with approximately 70% of people showing a treatment effect in clinical trials, although 30–40% of this is a placebo effect. The number needed to treat (NNT) (see Ch 3) is between three and four. However, the effectiveness of antidepressants depends critically upon the person's adherence to the treatment regimen. As a consequence, antidepressant *effectiveness* is usually considerably less than the level of drug *efficacy* found in clinical trials.

The main classes of antidepressants are the selective serotonin reuptake inhibitors (SSRIs), the serotonin and noradrenaline reuptake inhibitors (SNRIs), the selective noradrenaline reuptake inhibitors (also abbreviated as SNRIs), the tricyclic antidepressants (TCAs) and the monoamine oxidase inhibitors (MAOIs). There are also several newer antidepressants that are difficult to classify into one of these classes. Contemporary first-line antidepressant treatment often involves the use of an SSRI. Examples of SSRIs include fluoxetine, fluvoxamine, sertraline, paroxetine, citalopram, escitalopram and desvenlafaxine. Although there is little to choose between these drugs in terms of efficacy, they do have different adverse effect profiles and this is their main point of differentiation. Fluoxetine has a long half-life, which can be an advantage in people who adhere poorly to their prescribed medication, but can be a problem due to delayed clearance of the drug following its cessation. Fluvoxamine can cause sedation, which can be a useful property in people with prominent agitation. Paroxetine has significant anticholinergic effects, which can lead to delirium.

Although the SSRI drugs are generally safe, they do have a range of adverse effects, including:

- nervousness, anxiety and insomnia
- nausea and diarrhoea
- anorexia and weight loss
- fatigue, headache, sedation and dizziness
- rash and pruritus, and
- sexual dysfunction (reduced libido, anorgasmia and impotence).

In addition to these adverse effects, the SSRIs can all cause hyponatraemia (low serum sodium) and the risk of this seems highest in people with cerebrovascular disease who are taking diuretics (fluid tablets). Importantly, hyponatraemia may lead to agitation and apparent worsening of depression, leading the clinician to think that a higher dose of antidepressant is needed, whereas this could actually be dangerous. In addition, these drugs can sometimes cause prolongation of the QT interval on the electrocardiogram (ECG). This leads to an increased risk for cardiac arrhythmias. Thus, it is prudent to check both the serum sodium and ECG during antidepressant treatment in older people.

In primary care settings, TCA, MAOI and both types of SNRI drugs are principally used as second-line treatments for depression or anxiety. They generally have more extensive adverse effects than the SSRIs and often require dose titration. However, venlafaxine (SNRI) and mirtazapine (multiple actions) are also being used in this setting. In secondary (specialist) and tertiary (subspecialist) care settings, these second-line drugs are commonly used as the older person has often failed treatment with an SSRI in the primary care setting. Older people being treated by community mental health teams might be trialled on a drug from any of the antidepressant classes, depending upon their treatment history.

The older TCA and MAOI drugs should be prescribed with particular care as they have quite different adverse effect profiles from the modern SSRI and SNRI drugs. In particular, the TCAs and non-selective MAOI antidepressants commonly cause anticholinergic effects that are particularly problematic in older people. They also commonly cause postural hypotension (a drop in blood pressure upon standing). In addition, the MAOI drugs require the person to adhere to a tyramine-free diet.

It is anticipated that antidepressant drugs operating on the melantonergic system, such as agomelatine, will soon gain regulatory approval. These drugs may prove superior in the management of people with depression associated with sleep disturbance.

Older people with depression often take longer to recover than younger people with depression. This is likely to be mainly due to pharmacodynamic issues, although sometimes older people are not able to tolerate therapeutic doses of antidepressant medication and sometimes antidepressants are prematurely stopped in older people. Clinical trial data suggest that the onset of clinical response to antidepressant medication in older people can sometimes take 2–3 months. This potential for delayed onset of response makes it difficult for some older people to persist with their medication, as there is often an expectation of a quicker response. There is thus a psychoeducational role for case managers in relation to this important issue.

It is generally prudent to use lower starting and final doses of psychotropic medication in older people. Suggested starting and final doses for selected modern antidepressants are listed in Table 30.1. However, it is important to note that some older people can ultimately tolerate full adult doses if the dose is titrated slowly upwards with careful attention to adverse effects. Thus, the final dose in some older people might be twice as high as the usual final doses listed in Table 30.1.

The serotonin syndrome is worthy of special mention because it can be life threatening. This most commonly occurs when the person is taking more than one medication that can increase the availability of the neurotransmitter serotonin. It is characterised by a mixture of symptoms, including irritability, agitation, confusion, tremor, ataxia, increased muscular tone, hyperreflexia, nausea, vomiting, diarrhoea, fever and changes in blood pressure. Not all of these symptoms need to be present, so the syndrome should be suspected in any person who develops any of these symptoms while on more than one serotonin-enhancing drug. It sometimes also occurs in vulnerable people on a single SSRI.

Table 30.1 Dosage information on selected antidepressants in older people		
Drug	**Usual Starting Dose**	**Usual Final Dose**
Fluvoxamine	50 mg once daily	100 mg once daily
Sertraline	25 mg once daily	50 mg once daily
Citalopram	10 mg once daily	20 mg once daily
Escitalopram	5 mg once daily	10 mg once daily
Venlafaxine	75 mg once daily	150 mg once daily
Desvenlafaxine	50 mg once daily	100 mg once daily
Mirtazapine	15 mg once daily	30 mg once daily
Duloxetine	30 mg once daily	60 mg once daily

MOOD STABILISERS

Mood stabilisers are drugs used in bipolar disorder to manage both mania and depression. They are also used as augmentation agents in people with unipolar depression. It is particularly important that continuation treatment in people completing a course of electroconvulsive therapy (ECT) include an antidepressant and a mood stabiliser, as antidepressants alone are often ineffective at preventing early relapse.

The commonly used mood stabilisers are lithium carbonate, the anticonvulsants sodium valproate and carbamazepine, and the atypical antipsychotic olanzapine. Other drugs, including lamotrigine and oxcarbazepine, have also been used as mood stabilisers. Evidence is best for the use of lithium carbonate as a mood stabiliser, although this drug must be used with care in older people. It is important to use lower doses of lithium in any person with renal impairment and in all older people. For the treatment of acute mania, it is usual to prescribe sufficient lithium to achieve a serum level of around 0.8 mmol/L, whereas for prophylaxis of both depression and mania a serum level of between 0.4 and 0.6 mmol/L is often sufficient. People on lithium must take particular care to maintain an adequate intake of fluid and salt, particularly during the summer months. Older people with cognitive impairment should not generally be prescribed lithium unless their use of medication is being closely supervised. Table 30.2 lists adverse effects of lithium.

ANTIPSYCHOTICS

Antipsychotic drugs can be divided into conventional and atypical antipsychotics. All effective antipsychotic drugs have dopamine-blocking properties, although the modern atypical antipsychotic drugs also have effects on the serotonin system. The conventional antipsychotic drugs include both low-potency drugs, like chlorpromazine, and high-potency drugs, like haloperidol. Although these conventional antipsychotic drugs transformed the treatment of people with psychotic disorders when they were first introduced in the middle of the twentieth century, they have been largely superseded by the atypical antipsychotics in wealthier countries.

Table 30.2 Adverse effects of lithium	
Symptoms in Normal Use	**Symptoms of Toxicity**
Fine tremor	Ataxia
Gastrointestinal symptoms	Dysarthria
Fatigue	Coarse tremor
Polydipsia and polyuria	Marked gastrointestinal symptoms
Goitre and mild hypothyroidism	Stupor, coma and death

Although considerably more expensive than the conventional drugs, the atypical antipsychotics, such as risperidone and aripiprazole, have a better adverse effect profile and seem to benefit both the negative and positive effects of schizophrenia. They are less likely to cause extrapyramidal side effects, such as Parkinsonism, acute dystonia, akathisia and tardive dyskinesia. However, they are not free of significant adverse effects. Common adverse effects of atypical antipsychotic medications include:

- sedation
- Parkinsonism
- glucose intolerance and diabetes
- hyperlipidaemia, and
- weight gain.

When commencing antipsychotic medication in older people, it is important to start with very low doses. This is particularly important in frail older people with dementia (e.g. risperidone 0.25–0.5 mg once or twice daily, or olanzapine 2.5 mg once or twice daily). Some people are extremely sensitive to antipsychotic medication and develop severe adverse effects, particularly Parkinsonism, even on very small doses.

In Australia, subsidised treatment with atypical antipsychotics under the Pharmaceutical Benefits Scheme (PBS) is available for people with schizophrenia, bipolar disorder and dementia. However, the use of antipsychotic medication in dementia comes with a warning that this drug class is associated with an increased risk of cerebrovascular adverse effects, including stroke and transient ischaemic attacks (TIAs). It is important that this increased risk is discussed with the person or their substitute decision maker prior to initiation of treatment. It is also important that people are assessed and treated for preexisting risk factors for cerebrovascular disease, such as history of stroke or TIA, hypertension, hyperlipidaemia and atrial fibrillation. People with dementia should be treated with antipsychotic medication at the lowest effective dose and for the shortest time practicable. A 'stopping rule' should be established at the time the antipsychotic drug is first prescribed. It is generally recommended that the use of antipsychotic medication in older people with dementia be reviewed within 3 months of commencement of treatment.

Some people with chronic psychotic disorders, principally schizophrenia, require treatment with depot antipsychotic medication administered by intramuscular injection. Such people are often on involuntary treatment orders and have not adhered to oral medication. Although some older people will be on conventional depot antipsychotic medication, including fluphenazine decanoate and flupenthixol decanoate commenced years ago, most people recently commenced on depot antipsychotic medication will be on the depot risperidone microsphere preparation. However, this preparation is not approved for use in people with dementia.

Clozapine is an atypical antipsychotic drug, which is often used in people with severe treatment-resistant psychotic disorders. Clozapine has several potentially life-threatening adverse effects, which include agranulocytosis and myocarditis. To minimise the risk of these adverse effects, people on clozapine are kept under close medical scrutiny, particularly over the first few months of treatment. This includes weekly blood tests to check the white cell count and echocardiograms (ECGs) and troponin levels to check for inflammation of the heart muscle. Clozapine can be safely used in older people, although there is an increased risk of adverse effects in this age group.

It has recently come to light that both conventional (e.g. haloperidol) and atypical (e.g. risperidone) antipsychotic drugs carry with them an increased risk of both cerebrovascular disease (stroke and TIA) and sudden death. The risk of cerebrovascular disease seems to be greatest in older people with dementia, particularly those with pre-existing risk factors for stroke. Thus antipsychotic medication should be used with great care in this group. The risk of sudden death is rare but can affect people of all ages and is probably related to the long QT syndrome, a cardiac electrical abnormality.

COGNITION ENHANCERS

At present there are two classes of drugs used to enhance cognition in people with Alzheimer's disease: cholinesterase inhibitors and NMDA-receptor antagonists. The cholinesterase inhibitors include donepezil, galantamine and rivastigmine. The only NMDA-receptor antagonist that has been marketed is memantine.

The cholinesterase inhibitors inhibit the action of the enzyme acetycholinesterase, thus increasing the availability of the neurotransmitter acetylcholine in the synapse. Acetylcholine is essential for good cognitive function and its level is decreased in the brains of people with Alzheimer's disease. Increasing the availability of acetylcholine through the use of a cholinesterase inhibitor causes a modest increase in cognitive function in some people with Alzheimer's disease. There are no large independently funded head-to-head clinical trials comparing the efficacy of the cholinesterase inhibitor drugs that are currently available (donepezil, galantamine and rivastigmine). Clinical experience suggests that there is little to choose between these three drugs in terms of efficacy. All three drugs commonly cause gastrointestinal adverse effects, including reduced appetite, weight loss, nausea, vomiting, diarrhoea and abdominal pain. In most people, tolerance develops rapidly to these gastrointestinal symptoms with continued use of the drug. In some people, however, the drug cannot be tolerated and must be ceased.

Oral rivastigmine has been associated with greater gastrointestinal symptoms than donepezil or galantamine. However, rivastigmine administered by transdermal patch is associated with considerably fewer gastrointestinal symptoms than the oral preparation. Other adverse effects include muscle cramps and increased dreams. In vulnerable people, cholinesterase inhibitors can precipitate or worsen bradycardia and heart block, and exacerbate peptic ulcer disease and asthma. People with any of these three medical problems should have these problems treated before commencing treatment with a cholinesterase inhibitor.

The NMDA-receptor antagonist memantine works by a complex mechanism that protects brain cells from damage. It is associated with modest improvements in cognition in people with moderately severe Alzheimer's disease. There is some evidence that memantine might be associated with reduced agitation as well as improved cognition. Memantine has a relatively benign adverse effect profile, although it can cause transiently increased confusion in some people.

If practicable, it is best to cease drugs with anticholinergic and sedative properties prior to prescribing cognition-enhancing drugs. The PBS subsidises donepezil, galantamine, rivastigmine and memantine for people with Alzheimer's disease who meet certain eligibility criteria. As these criteria are complex, prescribers should study the PBS rules before writing a PBS prescription for any of these drugs.

SEDATIVES AND HYPNOTICS

Although sedatives and hypnotics are widely prescribed in older people, there are relatively few appropriate indications for their use in older people treated in the community. Sedative drugs are used to treat agitation or marked anxiety, and hypnotic drugs are used to help induce sleep. Appropriate clinical indications include the temporary treatment of acute anxiety or agitation, the temporary treatment of secondary insomnia, and the temporary treatment of alcohol and drug withdrawal. Sedatives are also used in some older people with hypomania and mania. Tolerance develops to many of the effects of these drugs and withdrawal effects may occur when the drug is ceased. Sedatives and hypnotics frequently cause confusion, amnesia and falls, and for this reason are often best avoided in older people.

Many sedative/hypnotic drugs belong to the benzodiazepine class of drugs. Benzodiazepines facilitate the action of gamma amino butyric acid (GABA) in the brain. Some of the more commonly prescribed drugs in this class include diazepam, oxazepam, nitrazepam, temazepam, lorazepam and alprazolam. If benzodiazepines are to be used in older people, then oxazepam and temazepam are generally preferred, as they are not converted into long-lasting active metabolites in the liver and thus have a reduced tendency to accumulate. The usual starting dose of oxazepam in older people is 7.5 mg once or twice daily and the usual starting dose of temazepam is 10 mg at night.

There are a number of newer drugs used as hypnotics. These include the so-called 'z-drugs' zopiclone and zolpidem. Zopiclone is a cyclopyrrolone derivative that works on benzodiazepine receptors, although it does not belong to the benzodiazepine class of drugs. It was originally thought to be less addictive than the benzodiazepines, although that view has altered with time. Zolpidem is an imidazopyridine that also works on the benzodiazepine receptor. Like zopiclone and the benzodiazepines, zolpidem is associated with tolerance and withdrawal symptoms and is potentially addictive. It is unclear whether zopiclone and zolpidem have any advantages over temazepam for the temporary treatment of insomnia in older people. Regardless of whether the older benzodiazepines or one of the newer 'z-drugs' is employed, it is preferable to use hypnotics for no longer than 2–3 weeks.

MENTAL HEALTH PROBLEMS NOT USUALLY TREATED WITH MEDICATION

There are several mental health problems that are not usually treated with drugs. These include uncomplicated grief reactions, adjustment disorders, personality disorders and mild cognitive impairment.

COMPLEMENTARY MEDICINE

Complementary medicines are in widespread use and many people find them quite convenient, as they do not require a doctor's prescription and often have few adverse effects. Commonly used complementary medicines include vitamins such as vitamins C and E, cognition enhancers such as Ginkgo biloba, antidepressants such as St John's wort and various types of traditional Chinese medicine. In line with their increasing popularity, there is now a growing trend towards subjecting complementary medicines to clinical trials to assess their safety and efficacy. Some complementary medicines have even been the subject of Cochrane Reviews. While it is beyond the scope of this chapter to cover all complementary medicine with putative psychotropic properties, it is worthwhile considering Ginkgo biloba and St John's wort in a little more detail.

A large number of clinical trials have been performed on the EGb761 extract of Ginkgo biloba in older people with dementia. The extract has been demonstrated to cause no more adverse effects than placebo, so it appears quite safe to use. However, the efficacy findings have been very mixed, with three out of four recent large trials having negative results. Thus, Ginkgo biloba cannot be recommended for the treatment of dementia in general or Alzheimer's disease in particular (Birks et al 2009).

Similarly, a large number of clinical trials have investigated the safety and efficacy of extracts of *Hypericum perforatum L.*, commonly known as St John's wort, for the treatment of major depression. The findings indicate that St John's wort has fewer adverse effects than conventional antidepressants. They also indicate that St John's wort is superior to placebo for the treatment of major depression and not significantly different from conventional antidepressants for this indication (Linde et al 2008). One potential issue with these data is that many of the studies were conducted in German-speaking countries where the use of St John's wort is very popular, and the findings from these countries were more strongly positive than the findings from other countries.

While St John's wort appears safe when used alone, it does have the potential to interact with many other drugs because it induces CYP3A4 enzyme activity in the liver. Drugs potentially affected by this interaction include alprazolam, amitriptyline, simvastatin, omeprazole, digoxin and paroxetine. However, prescribers should review expert opinion about these and other interactions in any person who is taking St John's wort as well as other medication.

SUMMARY

The use of psychotropic medications has transformed the lives of many people with mental health problems and allowed them to live in the community rather than in asylums. However, these drugs are potent pharmaceuticals and need to be handled carefully in older people. The use of medication should take place within a comprehensive biopsychosocial management plan.

FURTHER READING

Katona CLE 2001 Psychotropics and drug interactions in the elderly patient. International Journal of Geriatric Psychiatry 16:S86–S90

Stahl S 2006 Essential psychopharmacology: the prescriber's guide. Cambridge University Press, New York

REFERENCES

Birks J, Grimley Evans J 2009 Ginkgo biloba for cognitive impairment and dementia. Cochrane Database of Systematic Reviews, Issue 1. Art. No. CD003120. DOI:10.1002/14651858. CD003120.pub3

Linde K, Berner MM, Kriston L 2008 St John's wort for major depression. Cochrane Database of Systematic Reviews, Issue 4. Art. No. CD000448. DOI:10.1002/14651858.CD000448.pub3

Chapter 31

ELECTROCONVULSIVE THERAPY AND OTHER PHYSICAL TREATMENTS

INTRODUCTION

This chapter covers the use of electroconvulsive therapy (ECT) and other physical treatments for older people with mental health problems. While most ECT is undertaken on an inpatient basis, older persons' community mental health teams will see people who ultimately need admission to hospital for ECT and may be managing people having outpatient maintenance ECT. Other physical treatments including bright light and physical exercise are most commonly prescribed to outpatients. The chapter finishes with brief mention of some experimental treatments.

ELECTROCONVULSIVE THERAPY

Electroconvulsive therapy (ECT) is the most effective biological treatment currently available for the treatment of severe depression, and can be life-saving. However, its use has been highly stigmatised as a result of its initial use without general anaesthesia and several cinematic depictions in which it was employed in a coercive manner, including in the Academy Award winning film, *One Flew Over The Cuckoo's Nest*, starring Jack Nicholson.

ECT involves the administration of a controlled electric current to the brain via scalp electrodes. The electric current induces a short grand mal seizure similar to the grand mal seizures seen in epilepsy. It is normal practice to establish intravenous access and to pre-oxygenate the person prior to induction of anaesthesia. The person is then given a general anaesthetic consisting of an intravenous induction agent (e.g. thiopentone) and a muscle relaxant (e.g. suxamethonium). The psychiatrist then administers the brief electric current. The seizure duration is monitored using an electroencephalographic (EEG) display and printout. The anaesthetist hand ventilates the person for the duration of the anaesthesia, usually about 5 minutes. Experienced nursing personnel then care for the person in a recovery suite after each ECT treatment.

The scalp electrodes used in ECT are small metal discs. For bilateral ECT, the electrodes are placed bitemporally, whereas for unilateral ECT the electrodes are placed over the non-dominant temporal region (usually the right side) and near the vertex of the head. Electrolytic gel is usually applied to the electrodes to improve conduction. Bilateral ECT works a little faster than unilateral ECT, but causes more confusion and amnesia. Right unilateral ECT is usually preferred in older people as it is better tolerated. However, bilateral ECT is still sometimes used in older people, particularly when unilateral ECT has not been effective or when a rapid response is essential.

ECT is indicated principally for severe, treatment-resistant depression. It is often used when people are suicidal or psychotic, or when they are not eating and drinking satisfactorily. ECT is less often used in people with mania, schizoaffective disorder and schizophrenia. The efficacy of ECT in depression has been established through the use of randomised controlled trials (RCTs) comparing real ECT to 'sham' ECT. In sham ECT the procedure is exactly the same as for real ECT, but no current is delivered and no seizure induced. The available evidence suggests that ECT works well in older people. Some evidence even suggests that ECT works better in older people than in younger people. Lisanby (2007) gives a clear description of the use of ECT in older people.

In young and middle-aged people, ECT is generally administered three times per week. However, in older people there is a greater risk of post-ECT confusion. To minimise the impact of this, ECT is often administered twice a week or even once a week. People vary considerably in the number of ECT treatments needed to obtain a therapeutic response. Generally, between 6 and 12 treatments are required. Occasionally, as many as 18 treatments may be required.

Consent for electroconvulsive therapy

ECT may be administered on a voluntary basis or on an involuntary basis under the provisions of the relevant Mental Health Act. Fully informed consent is required before voluntary ECT is administered. The person must be informed about the nature of the procedure, including the use of general anaesthesia and the application of an electric current to the head. They must understand that ECT generally involves a course of treatment extending over several weeks, rather than a single treatment. They must be informed about the potential risks of the treatment and about the potential risks of not having the treatment. They must have an opportunity to ask questions and have those questions answered. It is generally best to provide the person with written material about ECT to reinforce information given orally.

The legal requirements for the administration of involuntary ECT vary considerably between jurisdictions. For example, in Queensland, application must be made to the Mental Health Tribunal, except in an emergency situation in which case approval may be granted by a medical superintendent. When involuntary ECT is being considered, it is normal practice to obtain a second opinion from another psychiatrist.

Medical work-up for electroconvulsive therapy

It is important to establish that it is medically safe to administer ECT to the older person. The medical work-up includes a detailed physical examination, screening blood tests and an electrocardiogram (ECG). In some people, respiratory function tests and a chest X-ray are indicated. Although the yield is low, it is common for psychiatrists to order a neuroimaging study (computed tomography (CT) or magnetic resonance imaging (MRI) brain scan) prior to ECT to check for rare causes of raised intracranial pressure. Common relative contraindications to ECT include uncontrolled hypertension and hyperkalaemia (often secondary to chronic renal impairment).

Maintenance electroconvulsive therapy

After a person completes a course of ECT, they are usually prescribed continuation treatment with an antidepressant and a mood stabiliser such as lithium. Those who are not treated with combination pharmacotherapy often relapse quickly. In some cases, however, the person relapses despite continuation treatment. In these cases, maintenance ECT may be considered. Maintenance ECT is usually administered on a day-patient basis, although some older people are admitted the night before the treatment. After an effective inpatient course of ECT, maintenance treatments are usually given initially on a weekly basis and over time the interval is extended. Once ECT treatments are being administered every 4–6 weeks without evidence of relapse between treatments, consideration can be given to ceasing maintenance ECT. However, some older people require regular maintenance ECT extending over months or years.

Adverse effects of electroconvulsive therapy

Administration of ECT is commonly followed by a brief period of confusion, which resolves within a few hours. In some older people, ECT may precipitate delirium. A period of temporary amnesia also commonly occurs after administration of ECT. There are also occasional reports of persisting amnesia following ECT. There have been several reviews of the cognitive effects of ECT in older people and the reader is directed to these papers for further details (Gardner & O'Connor 2008, Tielkes et al 2008). Other common adverse effects include headache and muscle pain.

It is normal practice to require the person to remain at the clinic or hospital for 4 hours after their treatment and to advise them not to drive a motor vehicle until the day following ECT.

ELECTROCONVULSIVE THERAPY (ECT) CHECKLIST

The following should all be conducted as part of ECT:
- a general medical work-up for ECT
- a physical examination, with special emphasis on the cardiovascular system and the central nervous system
- screening blood tests, including full blood count and serum biochemistry
- an electrocardiogram (ECG)
- pre-ECT cognitive testing, usually with a brief screening test such as the Mini-Mental State Examination (MMSE)
- respiratory function tests and chest X-ray, in selected cases
- a neuroimaging study (CT or MRI brain scan), in selected cases
- discussion with the anaesthetist prior to ECT if general medical problems might increase the risk of complications arising from general anaesthesia

- an explanation to the person (and where relevant their family) of the clinical rationale for ECT
- an explanation to the person (and where relevant their family) of the administration of ECT
- the informed consent for voluntary ECT
- a second psychiatric opinion if involuntary ECT is being considered
- procedures required by local Mental Health Act if involuntary ECT is being considered, and
- a prescription of ECT, including whether to administer bilateral or unilateral ECT, and the frequency of treatments.

PHYSICAL ACTIVITY

There is now considerable evidence from RCTs that physical activity, including walking and resistance training, may be effective treatment for mild to moderate depression (Sjösten & Kivelä 2006). There are some studies also that suggest that physical activity might be an effective treatment for generalised anxiety.

There is also evidence that physical activity might improve cognitive function and prevent dementia (Taaffe et al 2008). In epidemiological research, older men who walked at least 2 miles (3.2 km) a day had half the risk of developing dementia. Walking also improves cognitive performance in people with subjective cognitive complaints and mild cognitive impairment (Lautenschlager et al 2008). In the latter instance, the dose of exercise required was 50 minutes of walking three times per week.

Behavioural theory suggests that physical activity acts as a form of exposure to aspects of the environment (exteroceptive stimuli) and to physiological symptoms (interoceptive stimuli). Research in rodents indicates that physical activity is associated with increased levels of brain-derived neurotrophic factor (BDNF) and neurogenesis (development of new brain cells). Initial findings from humans suggest that similar mechanisms may be operating.

LIGHT

The day/night light cycle and associated social cues (*zeitgebers*) entrain circadian rhythms, which are important for normal sleep and mental health. Central control of circadian rhythms involves the hormone melatonin, which is secreted by the pineal gland in the brain. Melatonin secretion is activated by darkness in combination with an endogenous pacemaker in the suprachiasmatic nucleus (situated in the anterior hypothalamus). Exposure to light suppresses melatonin secretion and maximum suppression occurs with exposure to intense light (600 lux) for 1 hour or more.

Exposure to bright light has been successfully used as a treatment for mild to moderate depression in people with seasonal affective disorder. A bank of high-intensity broad-spectrum fluorescent tubes is used to mimic daylight. This treatment is in clinical use in some Northern Hemisphere countries with long dark winters, but is rarely used in this manner elsewhere. In places like Australia, where high-intensity daylight is available for most of the year, it is not necessary to use fluorescent tubes, as simply spending time outside will expose the person to higher light intensity (lux).

There are close relationships between noradrenaline, serotonin and melatonin. Noradrenergic neurons are involved in signalling the onset of darkness that activates melatonin secretion at night, and serotonin is converted into melatonin at night.

It seems reasonable to advise depressed older people to spend time each day exposed to daylight because of its beneficial effects on circadian rhythms and mood. For this effect to occur, it is not necessary for sunlight to strike the skin, merely for bright light (but not direct sunlight) to enter the eyes. This effect seems to work even in many blind people because there appear to be separate neural pathways for vision and light/dark appreciation. Given the additional beneficial properties of physical activity, including walking, on mood and cognition, many clinicians advise their depressed older people to take a walk outside each day. The other beneficial property of sunlight in older people is increased production of vitamin D. However, for this effect to occur, the sunlight needs to strike the skin.

OTHER TREATMENTS

Transcranial magnetic stimulation (TMS) is a technique for inducing small electric currents in the brain using powerful but localised magnetic fields. Although TMS is used in many types of experimental research, its clinical application has been mainly in clinical trials for depression. Its main advantage over ECT is that it is administered to the conscious person without the use of anaesthesia and causes relatively few adverse effects. While there is increasing evidence for the efficacy of TMS in depression, the effect size in clinical trials has generally been less than for ECT. In addition, concerns have been raised about the difficulty of blinding people to treatment (TMS or a control condition) and thus the validity of some outcome measures. People who fail conventional treatments for depression, including ECT, do not often respond to treatment with TMS. At present, TMS is best regarded as a research tool rather than a clinical treatment.

Electrical stimulation of the vagus nerve has been trialled in people with treatment-resistant depression. Effects have been mixed and vagal stimulation is best considered an experimental treatment.

SUMMARY

This brief chapter has provided an overview of several physical treatments that may be used in the treatment of mental health problems in older people. However, it has focused predominantly on the use of ECT, as this is the most effective treatment for severe depression. A checklist for the preparation of the older person for treatment with ECT has been provided.

REFERENCES

Gardner BK, O'Connor DW 2008 A review of the cognitive effects of electroconvulsive therapy in older adults. Journal of Electroconvulsive Therapy 24:68–80

Lautenschlager NT, Cox KL, Flicker L et al 2008 Effect of physical activity on cognitive function in older adults at risk for Alzheimer disease. A randomized trial. Journal of the American Medical Association 300:1027–1037

Lisanby SH 2007 Electroconvulsive therapy for depression. New England Journal of Medicine 357:1939–1945 (a short clinically focused review article discussing the use of ECT to treat an 82-year-old woman with recurrent depression)

Sjösten N, Kivelä S-L 2006 The effects of physical exercise on depressive symptoms among the aged: a systematic review. International Journal of Geriatric Psychiatry 21:410–418

Taaffe DR, Irie F, Masaki KH et al 2008 Physical activity, physical function, and incident dementia in elderly men: the Honolulu–Asia Aging Study. Journals of Gerontology Series A: Biological Science and Medical Science 63:529–535

Tielkes CE, Comijs HC, Verwijk E, Stek ML 2008 The effects of ECT on cognitive functioning in the elderly: a review. International Journal of Geriatric Psychiatry 23:789–795

Chapter 32

LEGAL AND ETHICAL ISSUES

INTRODUCTION

The first part of this chapter deals with the legal and ethical issues that commonly confront mental health workers dealing with older people. As the legislation dealing with these matters differs between jurisdictions, mental health workers must understand their local law. This chapter deals with the principles that usually underpin such law. The second part of this chapter introduces the reader to capacity assessment and the common situations in which this arises.

INFORMED CONSENT

Healthcare interventions administered without consent may constitute the legal torts of assault and battery. Thus, all older people must give consent to the assessment and management of their mental health problems or be treated under the involuntary provisions of the local Mental Health Act (MHA). The only exception to these principles is the rare emergency situation in which it is necessary for a mental health worker to take immediate action to save a life.

Informed consent can only be provided by a person who has the capacity to do so. Some people with serious mental health problems, such as psychotic depression or dementia, may not have the capacity to give or withhold informed consent for assessment or treatment. In such instances, the law provides for substitute decision makers to make healthcare decisions on behalf of the person. The identity of these substitute decision makers varies from jurisdiction to jurisdiction, but often includes attorneys appointed under enduring powers of attorney and guardians appointed by guardianship tribunals. In some jurisdictions, family members and close friends can act as statutory health attorneys. Mental health workers dealing with older people need to be familiar with local legislation dealing with guardianship. The interaction of the local MHA and the local guardianship legislation must also be understood. In most jurisdictions, involuntary treatment orders under the MHA take precedence over guardianship legislation.

The usual principle of informed consent is that people are fully informed about any healthcare interventions that are proposed. Such healthcare interventions include both assessment procedures and treatments. However, experts have argued about how practicable it is to fully inform people about investigations and treatments, and in practice there are guidelines about the nature of disclosures that are necessary for informed consent to be valid. Following recent legal precedents, it is generally accepted that people should be informed about the risks and benefits of the proposed intervention, and the risks and benefits of not having the proposed intervention. The person should be told about all common and serious adverse effects of any treatment. They should also be told about any adverse effect, regardless of its rarity, that could be of particular significance to that person. They should have the opportunity to discuss the proposed treatment with other people. They should have the opportunity to ask questions and have those questions answered.

The question sometimes arises about whether consent is ever implied, as opposed to explicitly given. In routine low-risk situations in people in whom there is no reason to expect lack of capacity, consent is often taken as implied. For example, if a person voluntarily attends the clinic to see a clinical psychologist for a course of cognitive behaviour therapy (CBT) for mild depression, it is generally assumed that they are consenting to the treatment. After all, if they were not consenting they could cancel the appointment or simply not attend. On the other hand, if their depression was much more severe and had not responded to conventional treatments, electroconvulsive therapy (ECT) might be recommended. Consent for ECT must be formally obtained following a careful process of information giving.

Consent can be granted orally or in writing. For most day-to-day purposes, oral consent is entirely appropriate, whereas for risky or contentious procedures written consent is prudent. However, it is worth noting that a written record of consent is not proof of informed consent, but merely evidence that consent has been sought.

INVOLUNTARY DETENTION AND TREATMENT

As many mental health problems are associated with reduced insight and poor judgment, involuntary assessment and treatment are sometimes required. The law attempts to balance the right of individuals to autonomy with their right to receive treatment. To achieve this balance, mental health legislation mandates a series of checks and balances to make it unlikely that citizens are inappropriately detained or treated, while still making it feasible for mental health workers to assess and treat people with serious mental health problems. The way MHAs in different jurisdictions achieve this balance varies.

PRIVACY AND CONFIDENTIALITY

All healthcare consumers have a right to privacy and confidentiality. Privacy refers to the right of individuals to control access to information about themselves. Confidentiality refers to the responsibility of healthcare workers to protect private information about individuals. As a result of the stigma associated with serious mental illness, including dementia, older people with mental health problems often have serious concerns about privacy and confidentiality, and every effort must be made to work collaboratively with them to obtain the information necessary for a good standard of clinical care. However, there are situations in which the safety of the person or others must take precedence over their right to privacy and confidentiality. Some public health services separate mental health records from general health records in an attempt to improve confidentiality. Unfortunately, this is not a good policy for older persons' mental health services (OPMHS) due to the high prevalence of chronic medical conditions in older people and the frequent overlap between mental health problems and conditions such as stroke and Parkinson's disease.

Mental health workers are in a privileged position in that they have access to the most private of facts about a person's life. With this comes the responsibility to avoid talking about that person in public or semi-public situations, such as lifts or hallways, in which they might be overheard. Mental health workers should also avoid recording information in the clinical record that is irrelevant to the assessment or management of the person.

BALANCING AND MANAGING RISK

The community management of older people with mental health problems entails the management of risk (see Ch 18). Part of providing care in the least restrictive way possible necessitates weighing up the risks and benefits of autonomy and independence for the older person with a mental health problem. Providing humane mental healthcare with zero risk is probably not feasible. However, most would argue that it is important for mental health workers to minimise the impact of risks imposed on older people by their mental health problems. Despite this, many would also argue that it is not appropriate to insulate older people from risk to such an extent that the scope of their lives is so restricted that their quality of life deteriorates markedly, even if their longevity is slightly increased. In an attempt to resolve this conundrum, it might be useful to do a thought experiment in which one tries to imagine what level of risk the older person would have elected to take upon themselves if they had not been experiencing a mental health problem.

GUARDIANSHIP AND ADMINISTRATION

Guardianship orders allow the state to appoint one or more guardians to make healthcare and lifestyle decisions for a person who lacks the capacity to make such decisions. Administration orders allow the state to appoint an administrator, often the Public Trustee, to make financial decisions, including the sale and purchase of real estate, for a person who lacks the capacity to make such decisions. In most jurisdictions, there is a guardianship tribunal or similar office that adjudicates such decisions.

RESEARCH PARTICIPATION

To increase knowledge about mental health problems and their treatment, it is essential for older people to participate in clinical trials and other types of research. Research participation sometimes brings benefits to the research participant, including increased clinical attention to their mental health problem and their general health. More often, however, research participation benefits others, including people who will be treated in the future. The researcher has an ethical obligation to obtain informed consent for research procedures. This obligation is even greater when the research participants have mental health problems that might reduce their capacity to understand the nature and significance of the clinical trial. Thus, substitute decision makers, including the local guardianship authority, are often asked to assist.

END-OF-LIFE ISSUES

Mental health workers commonly encounter older people who are in the last few months of their life and can expect that some of these older people will die each year. Serious physical illness sometimes precipitates changes in mental state and behaviour that prompt a mental health referral and the person dies while waiting to be seen by the OPMHS or shortly after being seen. In other people with existing mental health problems, a life-threatening physical disorder develops leading to the person's death. Sometimes, mental health workers are asked to see people in palliative care who develop intractable neuropsychiatric symptoms. Occasionally, older people with mental health problems commit suicide. Each of these situations poses particular challenges for the mental health worker.

Mental health workers in OPMHS teams will often find their own feelings about death and dying challenged. They will also find that the older person and their family do not always share the mental health worker's view about death and dying. Some older people and their families will approach mental health workers in the hope that they might help them hasten death. Legislation in most places prohibits euthanasia and assisted suicide. The doctrine of 'double effect' holds that it is ethically acceptable to use strong medication (e.g. narcotic analgesics) to humanely care for a terminally ill person, even if an unintended consequence is their death. However, the use of narcotics in the terminally ill is not usually the role of a community mental health team. In such circumstances, mental health workers should liaise with community hospice personnel in order to ensure optimal care for the older person.

People with severe dementia sometimes lose the ability to swallow, but otherwise remain in reasonably good general health. In such circumstances, some families and some residential aged care facilities (RACFs) will request or demand the insertion of a percutaneous endoscopic gastrostomy (PEG) feeding tube to maintain the person's fluid and food intake. This raises a serious ethical dilemma in which humane care must be balanced against futile extension of life. Occasionally, the guardianship authority will be asked to adjudicate.

CAPACITY

The terms capacity and competency are used to mean slightly different things in different jurisdictions. However, for the purposes of this chapter, we will assume that capacity and competency mean essentially the same thing. By way of examples, this chapter discusses capacity to make a will, capacity to make an enduring power of attorney, and capacity to consent to ECT. However, the principles illustrated can be applied more widely than these three examples. It is important to note that final determinations of legal capacity are made by the guardianship authority or by the Supreme Court in each jurisdiction. However, mental health workers are commonly called upon to provide an opinion about a person's capacity, particularly in older people who might have cognitive impairment.

Historical approaches to judging capacity

Historically, the capacity of a person to make a decision was often based on their status, their function or the possible outcome of the decision. Thus, if a person had attracted the diagnostic label of 'dementia', they might automatically be considered to lack capacity, or if they performed poorly on a test, they might be considered to lack capacity, or if they made a 'bad' decision, they might be considered to lack capacity. These three approaches to judging capacity have been superseded by a decision-specific approach to capacity assessment. That is, the capacity of a person for a particular purpose is judged, rather than their capacity overall.

Capacity of a person for a purpose

Common law understanding of capacity has now been enshrined in statute law in many jurisdictions. These statutes vary in their wording and in the application of legal principle. In Queensland statute law, for example, there is a common definition of capacity, versions of which appear in various pieces of legislation, including the Mental Health Act and the Guardianship and Administration Act. In this jurisdiction, capacity means the person is:

1. capable of understanding the nature and effect of their decisions
2. able to freely and voluntarily make decisions, and
3. able to communicate their decisions in some way.

Capacity assessment

Before undertaking a capacity assessment, the mental health worker should ensure that there has been an appropriate trigger to the assessment. The law assumes that citizens have capacity unless demonstrated otherwise, and so capacity assessments should only be undertaken when there is an appropriate trigger.

Capacity assessment always involves consideration of both the person's ability to understand, make and communicate decisions, and the nature and complexity of the decision or decisions to be made. Thus, people with limited ability due, for example, to the presence of cognitive impairment or dysphasia, might still retain the capacity to make simple decisions. While diagnosis might be a guide to likely incapacity, it should not be relied upon. For instance, some people with dementia retain capacity.

Understanding the nature and effect of decisions

There are a number of things that might impact adversely on the ability to understand. These include sensory impairment (impaired eyesight and hearing), communication disorders (aphasia, formal thought disorder), cognitive function (memory, intelligence, foresight, insight, judgment), thought content (e.g. grandiose and persecutory delusions), and marked mood changes (depression or mania).

Freely and voluntarily making decisions

Things that might interfere with the ability to freely and voluntarily make decisions include the undue influence of others and the presence of delusional beliefs. The undue influence of others could occur in dependent relationships, and as a result of intimidation, domestic violence or elder abuse. Delusional beliefs might include persecutory beliefs and delusional misidentification.

Communicating the decisions

Things that might interfere with the ability to communicate the decisions in some way include severe dysphasia and gross formal thought disorder. Severe dysphasia might be seen in stroke, frontotemporal lobar degeneration and Alzheimer's disease. Gross formal thought disorder might include 'word salad', flight of ideas and mutism. These manifestations are found in psychotic disorders, including organic psychoses.

Mental health problems that commonly affect capacity

Mental and neurological health problems that commonly affect capacity include cognitive disorders, mood disorders, psychotic disorders and language disorders. Cognitive disorders that commonly affect capacity include dementia, delirium, amnestic disorder, frontal lobe syndromes and severe intellectual impairment. Mood disorders that commonly affect capacity include major depressive disorder, particularly if it is severe and associated with suicidal or psychotic features. Mania with psychotic features also commonly affects capacity. However, it is important to note that abnormal mood may adversely affect capacity, even in the absence of psychotic features. People with schizophrenia or delusional disorder may lack capacity when the content of their psychotic symptoms is directly related to the proposed decision. In addition, when people with schizophrenia or mania have severe disorganisation of thought, they may not be able to understand or communicate their understanding. Language disorders, particularly aphasia following a dominant hemisphere stroke, often impair communication ability. Some aphasic older people are able to say 'yes' or 'no' in response to questions, but these responses may often be provided inconsistently.

Examination issues

The mental health worker undertaking a capacity assessment must complete a detailed examination of the person. A detailed history must be obtained, including contextual issues and an informant report. A detailed mental state examination (MSE) must be undertaken, looking particularly for evidence of abnormal mood and psychotic symptoms. Cognitive testing should focus on memory and executive function. The person will also need to be asked specific questions in relation to the type of capacity being assessed.

Practical matters

When planning to undertake a capacity assessment, it is important to think carefully about what you are about to do and about whether you are the right person to do it. The following are some guidelines:

- Ensure you have made adequate preparations.
- It is essential to allow sufficient time for the interview (generally more time than you might initially think).
- Interview the person alone or with the assistance of a professional interpreter. Aim to exclude family members, friends and carers wherever possible. If a carer must be present, they should remain silent throughout the examination and out of the person's line of sight.
- Briefly assess the person's hearing and eyesight.
- Assess language function, looking for the presence of foreign language use, dysphasia and marked formal thought disorder.
- As far as practicable, ensure the person knows the purpose of the interview and that the normal rules of confidentiality do not apply.
- If the examination is not occurring in response to a guardianship tribunal or Supreme Court order, obtain the person's consent; be alert to the apparent paradox that may be inherent in this. If necessary, gain the person's assent and consent from a substitute decision maker.

- Take good notes, preferably structured, contemporaneous, and in question and answer style.
- Assess the person in relation to the particular issue or issues at stake.
- If you interview anyone else, ensure that you record their identity and their reported relationship to the person. Do not be seduced by apparently genuine and concerned relatives or friends. They may have private ends to serve.
- Observe the person's behaviour.
- Document the person's mood.
- Document in detail any psychotic symptoms.
- Tailor cognitive assessment to the person's likely premorbid level of intelligence, level of education, literacy, occupational achievement, and the complexity of the task for which capacity is being assessed.
- Note both the person's test scores and their test-taking behaviour.

Cognitive testing

Formal neuropsychological testing is useful, but time-consuming and expensive. Reserve this for particularly difficult or contentious situations. When clinical cognitive testing will suffice, commence with a screening test followed by tests of memory and executive function. For example, it would be appropriate to commence testing by administering the Mini-Mental State Examination (MMSE) and follow this with a word-list learning test, such as the Hopkins Verbal Learning Test (HVLT). After this, give the person some executive function tests, such as verbal fluency (animals in 60 seconds), Trailmaking (Trails A and B) or another set-shifting test (e.g. the card-sorting test from the Behavioral Assessment of the Dysexecutive Syndrome (BADS)), motor sequencing (e.g. the Luria fist/edge/palm sequence), and similarities and differences. See Chapter 14 for more detail on clinical cognitive testing.

The report

It is important to make a clear distinction between the data you have gathered (from documents, the older person and from other informants) and your opinion about how the data should be interpreted. If you are not sure, it is best simply to indicate your uncertainty, rather than guess. It is important to identify missing data and any limitations to your report.

Testamentary capacity

Testamentary capacity refers to the capacity to make a last will and testament. This is traditionally based on the person understanding the nature and significance of making a will, together with the person's knowledge of their assets, the identity of their natural heirs, the relative merits of claims on their assets, and the absence of delusions affecting the disposition of the assets. However, modern case law has modified this approach in some jurisdictions (Peisah 2005). Nowadays, people with complex assets rarely manage them alone; they are generally assisted by accountants or other types of financial managers. Thus, they might not have detailed knowledge of all of their assets, but might know the asset classes that their advisors are investing in on their behalf, and they might know the approximate overall value of their assets.

In practice, most older people, even those with cognitive impairment, know what a will is, but the most difficult aspect of testamentary capacity for a person to meet is understanding the relative merits of the competing demands on assets by potential beneficiaries (Peisah 2005). Social judgment (or social competency) are terms that have been used to describe the person's capacity to judge the merits of competing claims on their assets. Social judgment is a complex function likely to be subsumed by brain frontal executive function, as well as by individual psychosocial factors, including their history of family relationships.

Capacity to make or revoke an enduring power of attorney

The legal rules that apply to the making or revoking of enduring powers of attorney vary by jurisdiction, and so mental health workers need to be aware of their local legislation. In practice, many older people have difficulty understanding the complex concepts underlying enduring powers of attorney and this often affects their capacity. As with testamentary capacity, a person may make an enduring power of attorney only if they understand the nature and effect of an enduring power of attorney.

An understanding of the nature and effect of an enduring power of attorney entails the person making the power of attorney understand the following things (adapted from the Queensland Office of the Adult Guardian website):

- that the person making the enduring power of attorney may specify or limit the power given to the attorney and instruct the attorney about the exercise of the power
- when the power begins
- that once the power begins, the attorney has full control over the matters specified in the power, subject to the instructions about exercising the power
- that the person may revoke the power so long as they are capable of making an enduring power of attorney
- that the power continues even if the person develops impaired capacity, and
- that if the person is not capable of revoking the power, they are also not able to effectively oversee the use of the power.

In practice, these capacity requirements are very hard to meet for people with any clinically significant degree of cognitive impairment. Capacity assessment for enduring power of attorney involves a similar approach to that recommended for testamentary capacity assessment. Because there is much less public knowledge about enduring powers of attorney than there is about wills, it is usually necessary to educate the person about what they need to know in order to have a proper understanding of the nature and effect of an enduring power of attorney. After instructing the person, the examiner must test their retention and comprehension of what they have been told.

Capacity to consent to electroconvulsive therapy

Electroconvulsive therapy (ECT) is a highly effective treatment for severe depression (see Ch 31). It is commonly used in older people who have not responded to conventional treatments with antidepressant medication and psychotherapy. However, ECT involves a series of electrical treatments under general anaesthesia. It is also somewhat stigmatised following media portrayals. Some jurisdictions have specific legislation that covers the use of ECT, and mental health workers must adhere to their local laws. Notwithstanding local legal requirements, there are a number of things the older person must be able to do in order to have capacity to consent to ECT. The person must be able to:

- understand the nature and purpose of the treatment and why it is being recommended
- understand the main risks and benefits of the treatment
- understand the alternatives to the treatment
- understand the consequences of not having the treatment
- retain the information they have been given long enough to make an effective decision, and
- make a free choice about whether to have the treatment.

It is important to note that there are many older people who need ECT and who say they are happy to have it who do not meet this standard. It is not uncommon for people with severe depression to view ECT as a deserved punishment.

SUMMARY

The first part of this chapter has summarised some of the more salient legal and ethical issues that commonly confront the mental health worker in an older persons' team. The second part of the chapter has introduced the reader to the challenging issue of capacity assessment. In dealing with the legal issues outlined in this chapter, it will sometimes be important for the mental health worker to seek advice from senior and more experienced personnel, including legal officers. Mental health workers caring for older people must have as detailed an appreciation of the operation of their local guardianship and administration legislation as they do of the local MHA.

FURTHER READING

Bloch S, Chodoff S, Green SA 1999 Psychiatric ethics, 3rd edn. Oxford University Press, Oxford
Collier B, Coyne C, Sullivan K 2005 Mental capacity. Powers of attorney and advance health directives. Federation Press, Sydney
Darzins P, Molloy DW, Strang D 2000 Who can decide? The six step capacity assessment process. Memory Australia Press, Glenside

REFERENCES

Peisah C 2005 Reflections on changes in defining testamentary capacity. International Psychogeriatrics 17:709–712
Queensland Office of the Adult Guardian 2009. Online. Available: www.justice.qld.gov.au/guardian/ag/guidelines.htm 14 June 2009

Chapter 33

DRIVING

INTRODUCTION

There is much debate about older drivers. On the one hand are safety concerns for the older person and the wider public, while on the other is the impact of not being able to drive on the older person's autonomy and freedom. In Australia, as long as one is physically and mentally fit, one can have a licence and drive. There is no age limit and only in some jurisdictions is it a mandatory requirement to undergo regular 'fitness to drive' tests after a certain age. Surprisingly, there is no evidence to support the effectiveness of mandatory tests and, even if a person's licence is revoked, it does not necessarily mean that they will not continue to drive.

OLDER DRIVERS

As the population ages, so does the average age of drivers. Within the next decade, one in four drivers in Australia will be older than 65 years (Roads and Traffic Authority 2007). A question that is often asked is: Do older drivers pose a risk to other road users? Using Australian fatal crash data, a research team based at the Monash University Accident Research Centre (Langford et al 2008) established that on a per population and per licence basis, the older the driver the less the threat to other road users and those road users external to the driver's vehicle. However, older drivers aged over 80 years do have a higher fatality rate per kilometre driven. There is some debate regarding fatalities when compared with younger age groups, as an older person is more likely to die due to their frailty.

AGE-RELATED FACTORS

Chronic illness or multiple medical conditions are common with older age and these are an identified risk for crash involvement. Many specific age-related factors for poor driving outcomes have been identified (Dubinsky et al 2000), including:
- poor visual acuity
- declining auditory acuity
- physical and mental illness symptoms
- medications (e.g. benzodiazepines)
- slower response times
- slower cognitive processing leading to slower decision making
- attention and concentration deficits

- poorer visual–spatial and executive functions (required to judge position and distance), and
- dementia.

Dementia and cataracts featured among the conditions with a moderately elevated risk of crash involvement (Charlton et al 2004). A medical assessment for both of these problems would be beneficial, particularly for eye problems, as an eye specialist may be able to rectify these.

DEMENTIA AND DRIVING

According to Griffith (2007), the issue of the ability of older drivers can be restricted to certain subgroups of older people, rather than encompassing all older drivers, and, in particular, people with dementia. Dementia and other mental health problems affect judgment, reaction time and problem solving. In 2005, Snellgrove estimated that around 162,500 older people with cognitive impairment associated with dementia were driving on Australian roads and that 107,250 road accidents were attributable to these drivers. In the same study, Snellgrove had 115 older drivers with mild cognitive impairment or early dementia complete the Maze Task (Ott et al 2003) and an on-road driving test. The results were not in favour of older people with mild cognitive impairment or early dementia continuing to hold licences to drive. It was found that 70% of the participants failed the on-road test, most broke an important road law, and the driving assessor had to physically intervene in nearly half of the cases in order to prevent an accident. The driving deficits were identified as poor planning, poor observation skills regarding other vehicles, signs and signals, an inability to monitor and control the speed of the car, poor positioning of the car, confusion regarding the pedals and gears, and a lack of anticipatory or defensive driving. Most of the study participants did not think anything was wrong with their driving.

Not surprisingly, Snellgrove recommended cognitive screening of driving ability and the use of the Maze Task, as it identified 79% of those drivers who would pass and fail the on-road test. Her recommendations extended to preventing all people with dementia, even mild dementia, from driving for their safety and the safety of the public.

This stance is not fully supported though. For example, Alzheimer's Australia (2004), in its Driving Policy Statement, acknowledge that at some stage people with dementia will have to give up driving, but to take this away upon diagnosis would discourage some people from seeking early diagnosis and treatment. There is also other evidence that older people with dementia for the most part will themselves limit or cease their driving, or are amenable to suggestion from a relative or healthcare worker (Foley et al 2000). There are no straightforward solutions to this problem, with a number of important factors to be considered before any decision is made.

INTERVENTIONS
Mandatory assessments

In some jurisdictions, there is a requirement for all older people of a certain age, usually 75 years and older, to undergo a mandatory driving assessment every year. While there may be a sound argument in relation to high-risk subgroups, such as older people with dementia, there are challenges to the position of applying it to all older people. A significant piece of research conducted by Langford et al (2008) lends a great deal of support to no mandatory assessment. These researchers compared drivers over the age of 80 years in Sydney (where there is mandatory assessment) to their counterparts in Melbourne (where there is no mandatory assessment) in relation to casualty crash involvement rates. It was found that based on population there was no significant difference in crash risk. Furthermore, based on per licence issued and time spent driving, the Sydney drivers had statistically higher casualty crash involvement than the Melbourne drivers. These results were consistent with international studies as well.

Driving cessation

When people have significant impairments, they need to be encouraged to stop driving. The encouragement may have to come from a number of independent sources, but the professionals whose opinions are normally respected by most community members would be a general medical practitioner or a local police officer. This is a very difficult decision to be made and conversation to be had, but some people take it on board, albeit reluctantly, and give up driving altogether; others will restrict their driving (e.g. only during the day, in areas well known to them and in fine weather) (Pachana & Petriwskyj 2006).

Then there is the group who will continue to drive no matter what is said to them. If confrontation is too difficult and the situation is serious, there may be the need to hide keys or disable the car and encourage substitutes (e.g. delivery services and offers of rides to visit others or to undertake activities). It would be advisable to know the local laws around mandatory reporting, legally protected reporting and what support is available through the transport department.

As this is a sensitive issue, it may not be one that an older person is willing to initiate or discuss. However, someone has to take responsibility, whether it be a family member or mental health worker, to discuss driving with the older person when it is starting to become obvious that they are not safe. The discussion could involve financial and legal arguments (e.g. the cost of running a car and the cost of legal representation if the older person is involved in a serious accident). It would be worthwhile to first acknowledge what a safe and responsible driver the older person has been and that cessation of driving would be a noble and personally costly act to ensure other people's safety. Alternative forms of transport or other options for meeting the needs of the older person have to be identified and negotiated. This in itself could become a problematic issue, particularly in Australia where many suburbs have limited public transport. This issue is compounded for older Australians in rural and remote areas who also have to contend with country roads being more difficult and riskier to drive on.

The effect of not being able to drive can be quite traumatic for an older person. What this could mean is less mobility, independence and freedom for shopping, medical appointments, and social and community interactions. Others, particularly men, could have some of their identity associated with their car and ability to drive, and taking this away from them could affect their self-esteem. For example, this could be a man's contribution to keeping him and his wife from being dependent on other people (Foley et al 2000). Not being able to drive could manifest as a significant loss and a person may need some interpersonal counselling to come to terms with the loss.

Older people driving is an issue of juggling personal and public safety with independence. A multimodal assessment involving an occupational therapist, a neuropsychologist and a specialist driver assessor would be ideal. A comprehensive and objective battery of assessments, which highlights a person's deficits, could act as a motivator for them to give up driving. Unfortunately, when such resources are not on hand, it falls into the category of an intuitive assessment based on the concerns of other people. Various forms of guidelines and screening tools are available, but this requires identifying the specific need and finding the best tool to match.

Older driver education

Education programs that focus on maintaining safe driving skills, advice on when it would be a good time to give up driving and utilising alternative transport options could be beneficial interventions as well.

SUMMARY

The decision of whether or not an older person should be allowed to drive can be a tough one. The older person's safety and the safety of others must be considered with the enormous implications of limiting the freedom and mobility of the older person. A comprehensive assessment, which highlights deficits that can and cannot be rectified, is a sensible starting point. It has to be handled sensitively because an older person's independence and self-esteem are at stake. Educational material, testing, and a thorough exploration and discussion of alternative transport arrangements, may provide a suitable resolution.

FURTHER READING

Alzheimer's Australia 2004 Driving policy statement. Online. Available: www.alzheimers.org.au/upload/DrivingPolicyStatement.pdf

REFERENCES

Alzheimer's Australia 2004 Driving policy statement. Online. Available: www.alzheimers.org.au/upload/DrivingPolicyStatement.pdf 26 Aug 2009

Charlton J, Koppel S, O'Hare M et al 2004 Influence of chronic illness on crash involvement of motor vehicle drivers. Monash University Accident Research Centre, Melbourne

Dubinsky RM, Stein AC, Lyons K 2000 Practice parameter, risk of driving and Alzheimer's disease. Report of the Quality Standards Subcommittee of the American Academy of Neurology. Neurology 54:2205–2211

Foley DJ, Masaki KH, Ross GW 2000 Driving cessation in older men with incident dementia. Journal of the American Geriatrics Society 48:928–930

Griffith G 2007 Older drivers: a review of licensing requirements and research findings. Briefing Paper No. 11/2007. Parliament of New South Wales, Sydney

Langford J, Bohensky M, Koppel S, Newstead S 2008 Do older drivers pose a risk to other road users? Traffic Injury Prevention 9(3):181–189

Ott BR, Heindel WC, Whelihan WM et al 2003 Maze test performance and reported driving ability in early dementia. Journal of Geriatric Psychiatry and Neurology 16:151–155

Pachana NA, Petriwskyj AG 2006 Assessment of insight and self-awareness in older drivers. Clinical Geropsychologist 30:23–38

Roads and Traffic Authority (RTA) 2007 RTA: licensing of older drivers discussion paper. RTA, Sydney

Snellgrove CA 2005 Cognitive screening for the safe driving competence of older people with mild cognitive impairment or early dementia. Australian Transport Safety Bureau, Canberra

Chapter 34

PALLIATIVE AND END-OF-LIFE CARE

INTRODUCTION

Among all the medical advances and increased capability to cure in the last few decades, healthcare lost its way in relation to the fact that people do die and, when they die, they usually want a peaceful and dignified death, preferably at home with their family attending. In response to this not happening, palliative and end-of-life care have become very important and topical issues, particularly in regard to the management of death when it does not come about quickly and smoothly. Palliative and end-of-life care emerged from the realm of cancer care. However, in recent years the knowledge that has been developed in cancer care has been applied in the care of other non-malignant, terminal medical conditions (Parker et al 2005). This type of care recognises that the person is going to die, but the intention is to neither hasten nor postpone death. The focus is holistic care, with the goal of maximising quality of life through support for controlling distressing symptoms such as pain, managing psychosocial stressors and attending to a person's spiritual needs. The World Health Organization (2009) offers the following definition for palliative care:

> *Palliative care improves the quality of life of patients and families who face life-threatening illness, by providing pain and symptom relief, spiritual and psychosocial support from diagnosis to the end of life and bereavement.*

Palliative care:
- provides relief from pain and other distressing symptoms
- affirms life and regards dying as a normal process
- intends neither to hasten nor postpone death
- integrates the psychological and spiritual aspects of care
- offers a support system to help people live as actively as possible until death
- offers a support system to help the family cope during the person's illness and in their own bereavement
- uses a team approach to address the needs of people and their families, including bereavement counselling, if indicated
- will enhance quality of life, and may also positively influence the course of illness, and
- is applicable early in the course of illness, in conjunction with other therapies that are intended to prolong life, such as chemotherapy or radiation therapy, and includes those investigations needed to better understand and manage distressing clinical complications.

End-of-life care refers to the care given in the last few weeks of life. Palliative and end-of-life care typically extend to include significant others and can be delivered in the older person's home. If the older person can no longer be cared for at home, it could be in a hospice, hospital or residential aged care facility (RACF).

THE ROLE OF THE MENTAL HEALTH WORKER

Zarit and Zarit (2007) assert that mental health workers are in a unique position to address palliative care and end-of-life issues. This strong position comes about through our ability to develop a therapeutic relationship. Palliative care specialists have written extensively about the primacy of the therapeutic relationship in palliative care (Canning et al 2007). By already knowing what beliefs, attitudes and values an older person holds, the mental health worker can help maintain dignity, and support decisions that are consistent with these beliefs, attitudes and values. Although mental health workers have a strong focus on psychological and emotional needs, addressing physical needs should not be overlooked and certainly come under the role of being a mental health worker. This could mean assessing physical needs and, if required, arranging for them to be met by the appropriate people.

MENTAL HEALTH ISSUES

Palliative and end-of-life care and mental health issues can be examined from two perspectives. Firstly, older people who are terminally ill often experience depressive symptoms, and chronic/terminal illness is a recognised risk factor for depression. Secondly, older people who have a chronic mental illness may require palliative/end-of-life care. This may include an older person with dementia, an older person who has taken high doses of antipsychotic medications all their life, an older person with chronic schizophrenia which has eroded personality, social skills and the ability to manage health in relation to smoking and obesity, and an older person with substance-abuse problems.

Around 30% of people receiving palliative care are reported to be depressed and many feel anxious concerning what may be the outcomes of their illness (Hotopf et al 2002). In describing the experience of getting old and sick, Clarke (2007) suggests breaking down depression into three components:

1. demoralisation, where the ongoing helplessness leads to feelings of hopelessness, diminished capacity or competence, reduced self-esteem and a reduced sense of meaning and purpose in life to the extent where there is a loss of will to live and a desire to hasten death
2. grief, where there is a deep sense of loss and sorrow, and
3. anhedonic depression, where there is a profound loss of pleasure and, therefore, loss of interest in all things and matters.

The breaking down of a diagnosis of depression into these psychological elements will assist in understanding what feelings the older person is experiencing and enable more effective targeting of interventions. The pharmacological and non-pharmacological treatment for depression is covered comprehensively in Chapter 20. Antidepressants, at levels subtherapeutic for depression, are an effective treatment for neuropathic pain and this is something a mental health worker could reasonably expect to encounter (Carr et al 2002). In addition to the standard treatments for depression, older people in a palliative/end-of-life situation require sound and timely information and to be involved as much as possible in the decision-making processes.

Grief and bereavement are normal human responses and they should be allowed to run their natural course. Grief can be felt at many and various times throughout the dying process, however long it takes. The older person who is dying can experience grief, as well as their significant others. Grief is the response to loss and the dying person can have many losses to deal with (e.g. loss of function, control, independence and eventually loss of life). Anticipatory grief is the grief that is felt at diagnosis where a person can almost predict what their future will entail. It is during this time that many decisions concerning the future can be made. Normal and uncomplicated grief involves what would be a person's expected responses to a loss, expressed physically and/or psychologically. The signs of grief are many, but usually include crying, anorexia, lack of initiative, organisational ability and energy, inability to sleep, feelings of emptiness, questioning faith systems and soul searching. Such responses are characterised and shaped by past experiences with loss and death, and social and cultural factors.

Complicated grief occurs when the grieving period is exceptionally long (>3 months), or when there are no signs that the symptoms are resolving or the symptoms are getting worse, or when the grief interferes severely with the person's daily functioning. Complicated grief requires active intervention by a mental health professional. Bereavement applies to the ones who will be left mourning after the person has died. Bereavement care can begin before the death of the person. This is usually done to try and prevent complicated grief and bereavement.

Grief and bereavement therapy are well addressed in the literature and there are some therapists who have specialised in this field (Worden 1996). There are three main principles that are followed. The first principle is to promote emotional expression via empathetic responses. Emotions can vary from intense sorrow for losses to anger for being afflicted with the disease. The second principle is based on an understanding that people who are grieving may go through stages of denial and avoidance. These are negative defence mechanisms that need to be challenged in a gradual and gentle way to enable the person to realise the gravity of the situation so they can adjust to it. The third principle is that people need time to adjust and make sense of what is happening to them. This comes about by spending the therapy time discussing, listening and thinking through the issues that are bothering or concerning them.

Some people are prepared to face their mortality and others are not. According to Abbey (2001), it is important to determine how the older person feels about dying and how they may want to die. As a younger person, they may have said things like, 'Shoot me if I get like that' (in the case of dementia or some other incurable debilitating disease). However, as people get older, this certainty about not wanting to prolong their life can become less intense, although they may not want to suffer unbearably. In the case where people are prepared to face their mortality, there may be an option to plan end-of-life care well ahead of time, usually in the months leading up to death, rather than in the last few days when it may become more of a crisis situation.

In Australia, there are options for people to make an 'advance directive', where a competent older person can stipulate who will be their substitute decision maker if they want to be resuscitated or mechanically ventilated or have any other life-prolonging device used on them. These directives protect the right of the older person to make decisions about their care in the terminal phase, and it removes some of the burden a family may have to grapple with in the face of such difficult decisions. Advice regarding advance directives can be obtained from the office of the Adult Guardian. Another option is to appoint a power of attorney for health to act on the person's behalf. Each state and territory in Australia has different legislation pertaining to these matters, and it is beyond the scope of this chapter to go into that level of detail, but it would be a sensible approach to be familiar with what options are available in the relevant jurisdiction.

THE OLDER PERSON AND FAMILY ASSESSMENT

The purpose of assessment in palliative/end-of-life care is to identify areas of concern for the older person and their family, so plans can be formulated to meet their needs. There are a number of tools available to assist with this activity and they usually cover the essential areas of diagnosis, treatment, history of illness, physical assessment, psychosocial and spiritual assessment, and capacity/competency assessment (Parker & McLeod 2002). All of these elements have been discussed in detail in other chapters in this book. One difference is that when assessing palliative/end-of-life care, anticipatory planning for death may also be included (Doran & Geary 2005). Within palliative care, family case conferences are often used as a forum to make explicit the desires of the older person. These conferences include the relevant health professionals, such as case managers, the general medical practitioner and the mental health worker. In recent times, palliative care has become a specialty, and if such a service is available and appropriate to the older person's assessed needs, it would be very beneficial to have such expertise at hand.

Palliative care and end-of-life care have many ethical dilemmas surrounding them. The older individual or a family member may seek the advice of a mental health worker in regard to strategies that may extend a person's life. Percutaneous endoscopic gastrostomy (PEG) feeding is one such example. In these situations, the mental health worker must maintain a professional approach, which can be difficult when one may have gotten to know the family very well. The rules of informed decision making come into play here by ensuring the people involved have all the available information given to them in a format that they can understand. The mental health worker must be aware of their values and biases and ensure these do not impact on the decision. Additionally, an older person may have to be assessed for delirium, depression and anxiety, as these conditions can cloud the decision-making process (Zarit & Zarit 2007).

DEATH AND DYING

Many healthcare workers find it difficult to tell a person they are dying. Hancock et al (2007) conducted a systematic review relating to truth-telling in discussing prognosis with people with progressive, advanced life-limiting illnesses and their carers. Reasons for the healthcare worker's discomfort included perceived lack of training, stress, no time to attend to the person's emotional needs, fear of a negative impact on the person, uncertainty about prognostication, requests from family members to withhold information, and a feeling of inadequacy or hopelessness regarding the unavailability of further curative treatment. However, the authors have also identified studies suggesting that people can discuss the topic without it having a negative impact on them.

In 1970, Kubler-Ross published an influential text on death and dying where she set out the stages a person goes through when they are dying. Nowadays, palliative care experts tend not to use her stages and there are many other theories regarding the responses of people who learn they are to die soon. Either way, to offer meaningful support to a dying person, it is important to know what they may be experiencing, although in some instances it is difficult to predict prognosis and therefore going through 'stages' may be problematic. Kubler-Ross is a starting point and her stages of dying are denial, anger, bargaining, depression and acceptance. A person may not experience all of the stages or go through them sequentially; however, no matter which stage, it is important to always remain accepting, supportive and non-judgmental in all interactions.

Initially, the older person may deny that they are dying and reject any attempts that may support this notion, such as preparing a will or advance directive. The next stage is anger where the person may ask questions (e.g. 'Why me?'). This anger may be displaced at other people or objects and it is important to let people know the reason behind such behaviour. In this stage, the older person may withdraw and become more dependent. Following anger is the bargaining stage where a person may attempt to change their fate by bargaining, usually with a higher being such as 'God'. From the bargaining stage, the older person may experience depression. Thoughts in relation to dying and death can come out and the mental health worker needs to be prepared to talk about these in a sensitive but matter-of-fact manner, and to call on further assistance if required. The last stage is acceptance, where the person accepts that they are dying. In this stage, they may need to be in contact with various people so that they can put their affairs in order and say goodbye.

SUMMARY

This chapter has examined an issue that many older people and mental health workers alike find difficult to address—death and dying. Compassionate care and support of death is a skill that has been lost among the many recent medical advances that have focused on cures and prolonging life. Palliative care and end-of-life care have emerged as special areas to give guidance so that older people can have peaceful and dignified deaths that respect their wishes as much as possible. It is recognised that the inherent skills of a mental health worker can play an important role in facilitating this process, particularly in regard to the management of depression and grief that older people and their caregivers can experience during the end phase of life.

FURTHER READING

Australian Palliative Residential Aged Care (APRAC) Project 2006 Guidelines for a palliative approach in residential aged care. Online. Available: www.nhmrc.gov.au/PUBLICATIONS/synopses/_files/pc29.pdf

Jeffrey D 2005 Patient-centred ethics and communication at the end of life. Radcliff Publishing, Oxford

McLeod S 2007 The psychiatry of palliative medicine: the dying mind. Radcliff Publishing, Oxford

USEFUL WEBSITES

Austin Health: www.respectingpatientchoices.org.au

CareSearch: www.caresearch.com.au

National Health and Medical Research Council: www.nhmrc.gov.au/PUBLICATIONS/synopses/_files/pc29.pdf

National Institute for Health and Clinical Excellence: www.nice.org.uk/Guidance/CG42

REFERENCES

Abbey J 2001 Assessment of palliation. In: Koch S, Garratt S (eds) Assessing older people: a practical guide for health professionals. MacLennan & Petty, Sydney

Canning D, Rosenberg JP, Yates P 2007 Therapeutic relationships in specialist palliative care nursing practice. International Journal of Palliative Nursing 13(5):222–229

Carr D, Goudas L, Lawrence D et al 2002 Management of cancer symptoms: pain, depression, and fatigue. Agency for Healthcare Research and Quality Evidence Report/Technology Assessment 61:1–5

Clarke DM 2007 Growing old and getting sick: maintaining a positive spirit at the end of life. Australian Journal of Rural Health 15:148–154

Doran M, Geary K 2005 End of life. In: Melillo KD, Houde SC (eds) Geropsychiatric and mental health nursing. Jones and Bartlett Publishers, Boston

Hancock K, Clayton JM, Parker SM et al 2007 Truth-telling in discussing prognosis in advanced life-limiting illnesses: a systematic review. Palliative Medicine 21(6):507–517

Hotopf M, Chidgey J, Addington-Hall J, Ly KL 2002 Depression in advanced disease: a systematic review Part 1. Prevalence and case finding. Palliative Medicine 16(2):81–97

Kubler-Ross E 1970 On death and dying. Tavistock, London

Parker D, Grbich C, Brown M et al 2005 A palliative approach or specialist palliative care? What happens in aged care facilities for residents with a non-cancer diagnosis. Journal of Palliative Care 21(2):80–87

Parker D, McLeod A 2002 Assessment of need. In: Clark D, Hockey J (eds) Living and dying in institutional care: nursing and residential homes. Open University Press, London

Worden JW 1996 Dealing with grief. John Wiley & Sons, New York

World Health Organization (WHO) 2009 Online. Available: www.who.int/cancer/palliative/en/ 6 Apr 2009

Zarit SH, Zarit JM 2007 Mental disorders in older adults: fundamentals of assessment and treatment. Guilford Press, New York

Chapter 35

RATING SCALES

INTRODUCTION

Throughout this book there have been references to rating scales used to assist with assessment and to monitor and evaluate treatment. The purpose of this chapter is to provide a summary of rating scales that might make up a comprehensive battery for the mental health worker to use when caring for older people. These are only suggestions, as there are many other worthwhile instruments available in the literature. The advantages of using a rating scale include:

- It provides a systematic method of assessment.
- It aids in efficiency.
- It aids the novice mental health worker, or a mental health worker who is unfamiliar with a particular area.
- It assists with evaluation and research work.
- It assists with medicolegal reports.

However, the mental health worker needs to be aware that an overreliance on rating scales can lead to sometimes missing subjective nuances. The use of rating scales is primarily to augment clinical assessment.

Some rating scales are self-report, while others require an interviewer or an informant. Some scales assess multiple domains and others assess single domains. Quite often researchers publish detailed reviews of scales and these are helpful for the clinician. For example, Neville and Byrne (2001) reviewed behaviour rating scales for older people with dementia that were suitable for use by nurses.

The rating scales chosen for this chapter are valid and reliable for use with older people in the community setting (see Table 35.1). However, if another rating scale has been identified as more appropriate for your purpose, and it has not been validated for use in the community setting, it can still be used as an indicator of functioning, rather than determining the specific cutoffs that may point to the presence or absence of a disease process. Being mindful of the nature of the workplace and workforce means that the rating scales in this chapter are brief, easy to use and require no specialist training. Before using a rating scale, it is advisable to check if permission is required and if there is a fee attached to its use.

Table 35.1 Rating scales for the assessment of older people

Global assessment
Brief Psychiatric Rating Scale (BPRS)
General Health Questionnaire (GHQ)
Psychogeriatric Assessment Scales (PAS)

Cognitive assessment
Mini-Mental State Examination (MMSE)
Standardised Mini-Mental State Examination (SMMSE)
Telephone Interview for Cognitive Status (TICS–m)

Functional assessment
Activities of Daily Living (ADL) Scale
Instrumental Activities of Daily Living (IADL) Scale

Social assessment
Older American Resources and Services (OARS) scale

Behavioural and psychological symptoms of dementia
Dementia Behavior Disturbance Scale (DBDS)
Cohen-Mansfield Agitation Inventory (CMAI)
Crichton Visual Analogue Scale (CVAS)

Depression
Geriatric Depression Scale (GDS)
Cornell Scale for Depression in Dementia (CSDD)

Suicide
Beck Depression Inventory (BDI)
Beck Hopelessness Scale (BHS)
Scale for Suicidal Ideation (SSI)
Suicide Intent Scale (SIS)

Dementia
Consortium to Establish a Registry for Alzheimer's Disease (CERAD)
   Neuropsychological Battery and Clinical Battery
Global Deterioration Scale (GDS)

Anxiety
Geriatric Anxiety Inventory (GAI)
Rating Anxiety in Dementia (RAID)

Substance abuse
CAGE questionnaire
Michigan Alcoholism Screening Test–Geriatric (MAST–G)
Impression of Medication, Alcohol, and Drug Use in Seniors (IMADUS)
Alcohol Use Disorders Identification Test (AUDIT)

Pain
Short-Form McGill Pain Questionnaire (SF–MPQ)
Abbey Pain Scale (APS)

Table 35.1 Rating scales for the assessment of older people—cont'd
Quality of life Philadelphia Geriatric Center Morale Scale (PGCMS) Manchester Short Assessment of Quality of Life (MANSA) Dementia Quality of Life (DQoL)
Carer wellbeing and burden Caregiver Well-Being Scale (CW–BS) Caregiving Hassles Scale (CHS) Burden Interview (BI)

GLOBAL ASSESSMENT

Brief Psychiatric Rating Scale (BPRS)

The Brief Psychiatric Rating Scale (BPRS) (Overall 1974) is a clinician-rated scale that provides an assessment of common psychopathological symptoms. The primary purpose of the BPRS is to allow assessment of treatment change across a comprehensive set of common symptom characteristics. The BPRS consists of 18 items and an expanded 24-item version.

General Health Questionnaire (GHQ)

The General Health Questionnaire (GHQ) (Goldberg et al 1997) detects psychological distress and consists of four subscales: somatic symptoms; anxiety and insomnia; social dysfunction; and severe depression. It can be a self-report or administered via interview. The 28-item version is recommended and it takes 10 minutes to complete.

Psychogeriatric Assessment Scales (PAS)

The Psychogeriatric Assessment Scales (PAS) (Jorm et al 1995) are a total of six scales that assess the clinical changes that occur in dementia and depression as defined by the DSM–IV (American Psychiatric Association 2000). Three of the scales assess the older person for the domains of cognitive impairment, depression and stroke. The other three scales require an informant, and assess the domains of cognitive decline, behavioural change and stroke. The scales have good internal consistency, ranging from 0.58–0.86, and test–retest reliability between 0.47 and 0.66. Validity was established with other mood and cognitive scales. A manual accompanies the scales and administration is undertaken by a clinician or other trained person. They take 10 minutes to complete.

COGNITIVE ASSESSMENT

Mini-Mental State Examination (MMSE)

The Mini-Mental State Examination (MMSE) (Folstein et al 1975) is the best known and most widely used screening test of cognitive function in older people. It is an 11-item measure that tests five areas of cognitive function: orientation; registration; attention and calculation ability; recall; and language. A score of 24 out of 30, or lower, is generally considered to be indicative of cognitive impairment. The MMSE takes 10–15 minutes to administer by an interviewer.

Standardised Mini-Mental State Examination (SMMSE)
The Standardised Mini-Mental State Examination (SMMSE) (Molloy et al 1991) is a rating of cognitive function. It is based on the MMSE with improvements in objectivity. The SMMSE has better interrater and intrarater variance scores, and more specific instructions on scoring. This scale takes 10 minutes to complete by an interviewer.

Telephone Interview for Cognitive Status (TICS–m)
The Telephone Interview for Cognitive Status (TICS–m) (Brandt et al 1988) is an interviewer-administered scale done via the telephone, eliminating the need for an in-person assessment. It takes up to 10 minutes to complete. The TICS–m is an 11-question, 17-item test, which assesses orientation, counting, recall, calculation, repetition, knowledge, the ability to follow simple commands, and verbal reasoning. Items are scored and summed, with low TICS–m scores indicative of cognitive impairment. The TICS–m can be used for follow-up after initial MMSE assessments.

FUNCTIONAL ASSESSMENT
Activities of Daily Living (ADL) Scale
The Activities of Daily Living (ADL) Scale (Katz et al 1963) assesses levels of severe physical disability through observation or interview. It is a six-item scale that measures the older person's ability to perform the six activities of bathing, dressing, toileting, transferring, continence and feeding unaided. If done via interview, it will take 5 minutes; however, through observation it will take much longer depending on the older person's level of disability.

Instrumental Activities of Daily Living (IADL) Scale
The Instrumental Activities of Daily Living (IADL) Scale (Lawton 1988) assesses the functional ability of older people to perform activities that are of central importance in their everyday lives. The eight items include the ability to use the telephone, shop, prepare food, do housekeeping, do laundry, travel, take medications and handle finances. If done via interview, it will take around 5 minutes; however, through observation it will take much longer depending on the older person's level of disability.

SOCIAL ASSESSMENT
Older American Resources and Services scale (OARS)
The Older American Resources and Services scale (OARS) (Duke University Center for the Study of Aging and Human Development 1978) is a multidimensional functional assessment questionnaire. The first part assesses level of functioning in the areas of mental health, physical health, social resources, economic resources, and activities of daily living and instrumental activities of daily living (taking medications, transferring, walking, toileting, bathing, grooming, dressing, eating,

meal preparation, shopping, money management, travelling and housekeeping). The second part of the assessment determines the extent of use of and the need for services (e.g. meal delivery, domiciliary nursing care and household services). This questionnaire is very comprehensive and will take at least 40 minutes to complete. Koenig et al (1993) have developed an 11-item version, which takes considerably less time to complete.

BEHAVIOURAL AND PSYCHOLOGICAL SYMPTOMS OF DEMENTIA

Dementia Behavior Disturbance Scale (DBDS)

The Dementia Behavior Disturbance Scale (DBDS) (Baumgarten et al 1990) has 28 items that quantify the behavioural dimension of the dementia syndrome. The items reflect specific observable behaviours considered likely to distress the caregiver, including passive behaviours that are potentially stressful to carers. It is an observer-rater or informant scale that takes 10 minutes to complete.

Cohen-Mansfield Agitation Inventory (CMAI)

The Cohen-Mansfield Agitation Inventory (CMAI) (Cohen-Mansfield & Billig 1986) measures the frequency of 29 observable behaviours characterised as 'agitation'. It is an observer-rater or informant scale that takes 10 minutes to complete.

Crichton Visual Analogue Scale (CVAS)

The Crichton Visual Analogue Scale (CVAS) (Morrison 1983) has 10 items measuring behaviour and two additional items to assess carer's anxiety and their ability to cope with the older person. Each item is rated on a 10 cm line with anchor points at each end of the line.

DEPRESSION

Geriatric Depression Scale (GDS)

The Geriatric Depression Scale (GDS) (Sheikh & Yesavage 1986) measures the severity of depression and monitors changes in depression during treatment. The 15-item scale was devised from the original 30-item GDS. It can be self-administered or interviewer administered, with the older person answering 'yes' or 'no' to questions in reference to how they felt on the day of scale administration. Scores of 0–5 are considered as not indicating depression, while scores of 6–15 indicate depression. It takes 5–10 minutes to complete.

Cornell Scale for Depression in Dementia (CSDD)

The Cornell Scale for Depression in Dementia (CSDD) (Alexopoulos et al 1988) is a 19-item clinician-rated scale for depressive symptoms in dementia. The items are rated on the basis of observation and on their presence in the last week. Suggested cutoff scores are given. It is sensitive to change, with major depression improving with treatment. Completion time is 10 minutes.

SUICIDE

Beck Depression Inventory (BDI) and the Beck Hopelessness Scale (BHS)

The Beck Depression Inventory (BDI) (Beck et al 1996) and the Beck Hopelessness Scale (BHS) (Beck et al 1974a) are instruments for the assessment of depression that also contain items that relate directly to suicidal thoughts. The BDI is a self-report with 21 items that measure the severity of depression. The second item is labelled 'pessimism' and is central to the prediction of suicide. The BHS aims to identify the possible mediating effect hopelessness has on suicidality by measuring three key components: feelings about the future; loss of motivation; and expectations. The BHS has 20 items to which the older person answers 'true' or 'false'. A score of 9 or more is predictive of suicide. Completion time for both scales is 15 minutes each.

Scale for Suicidal Ideation (SSI) and Suicide Intent Scale (SIS)

The Scale for Suicidal Ideation (SSI) (Beck et al 1979) and Suicide Intent Scale (SIS) (Beck et al 1974b) are measurements of suicidal ideation and intent. The SSI is rated by a clinician. It contains 21 items that measure the intensity of a person's current suicidal ideation. The first five items are attended to first, as these are screening items and, if suicidal ideation is determined at this point, then the next 14 items are completed. The first 19 items are summed to give a score. The last two scale items document the incidence and frequency of past suicide attempts. It has been recommended that any positive response to an SSI item be followed up immediately.

The SIS is for use in people who have recently attempted suicide. It contains 15 items that are delivered in a structured clinical interview. The SIS assesses preattempt communication patterns, the perceived likelihood of discovery/rescue during a suicide attempt, and attitudes towards living and dying. Completion time for both scales is 20 minutes each.

DEMENTIA

Consortium to Establish a Registry for Alzheimer's Disease (CERAD) Neuropsychological Battery and Clinical Battery

The Consortium to Establish a Registry for Alzheimer's Disease (CERAD) Neuropsychological Battery and Clinical Battery (Fillenbaum et al 1997) are two assessments used to evaluate dementia. The Neuropsychological Battery determines the type and severity of cognitive impairment, and the Clinical Battery determines the presence, type and severity of dementia. The test requires an informant who knows the older person reasonably well to be able to comment on cognitive changes and changes in social habits and activities of daily living. The older person is also assessed with a clock-drawing test.

Global Deterioration Scale (GDS)

The Global Deterioration Scale (GDS) (Reisberg et al 1982) is a global rating scale which is used to summarise whether an older person has cognitive impairments consistent with dementia. Individuals are rated according to a 7-point scale, with a score of 4 or higher indicative of dementia. Its completion time is 10 minutes.

ANXIETY
Geriatric Anxiety Inventory (GAI)
The Geriatric Anxiety Inventory (GAI) (Pachana et al 2007) is a 20-item self-report or clinician-administered scale that measures dimensional anxiety in elderly people. Completion time is 10 minutes.

Rating Anxiety in Dementia (RAID)
The Rating Anxiety in Dementia (RAID) (Shanker et al 1999) is a 20-item self-report or informant-rater scale. It assesses the domains of worry, apprehension and vigilance, motor tension, autonomic hyperactivity, phobias and panic attacks. The RAID can be completed within 20 minutes.

SUBSTANCE ABUSE
CAGE questionnaire
The CAGE questionnaire (Ewing 1984) is a four-item questionnaire that gauges an individual's use of or potential abuse of alcohol and the effects it may be having on key life issues. A 'yes' response to two or more of the CAGE questions is an indicator for further assessment of substance abuse. The four questions are:
1. Have you ever felt you should **c**ut down on your drinking?
2. Have people **a**nnoyed you by criticising your drinking?
3. Have you ever felt bad or **g**uilty about your drinking?
4. Have you ever had a drink first thing in the morning to steady your nerves or get rid of a hangover (**e**ye-opener)?

Michigan Alcoholism Screening Test–Geriatric (MAST–G)
The Michigan Alcoholism Screening Test–Geriatric (MAST–G) (Blow et al 1992) is a 24-item questionnaire that requires a 'yes' or 'no' response for the identification of alcohol abuse/dependence. Five or more 'yes' responses indicates that further assessment of alcohol dependence is required. There is also a shorter 10-item version, where a score of 2 or more 'yes' responses indicates the need for further assessment.

Impression of Medication, Alcohol, and Drug Use in Seniors (IMADUS)
The Impression of Medication, Alcohol, and Drug Use in Seniors (IMADUS) (Shulman 2003) assesses many types of substance abuse, not only alcohol use. The questions have been structured so that feelings of shame are minimised. There are 20 items and three or more 'yes' responses means further assessment is needed.

Alcohol Use Disorders Identification Test (AUDIT)
The Alcohol Use Disorders Identification Test (AUDIT) (Saunders et al 1993) has a series of 10 questions for the identification of risky alcohol consumption. Each question receives a score from 0 to 4. A score of 8 or more is indicative of risky drinking patterns

and the need for further assessment of alcohol dependence. It is short, easy to administer, and needs no formal training to administer.

PAIN
Short-Form McGill Pain Questionnaire (SF–MPQ)
The Short-Form McGill Pain Questionnaire (SF–MPQ) (Melzack 1987) is a widely used, conceptually based, multidimensional tool that incorporates the sensory, affective, evaluative and temporal qualities of the pain experience. The main component of the SF–MPQ consists of 15 descriptors (1–11 represent the sensory dimension of pain experience and 12–15 represent the affective dimension). Three pain scores are derived from the sum of the intensity rank values of the words chosen for sensory, affective and total descriptors. The SF–MPQ also includes the Present Pain Intensity (PPI) index of the standard MPQ and a Visual Analogue Scale (VAS) to provide overall intensity scores.

Abbey Pain Scale (APS)
The Abbey Pain Scale (APS) (Abbey et al 2004) was developed specifically for older people with end-stage dementia who are unable to respond verbally. It is a unidimensional scale, with items reflecting observable behaviours and physiological changes that are known indicators of pain. The APS measures the severity of pain from six items: vocalisation; facial expression; change in body language; behavioural change; physiological change; and physical changes. Each item has descriptive prompts to assist staff with their observations and to enhance reliability. It takes less than 1 minute to complete.

QUALITY OF LIFE
Philadelphia Geriatric Center Morale Scale (PGCMS)
The Philadelphia Geriatric Center Morale Scale (PGCMS) (Lawton 1975) has 17 items and assesses the wellbeing of older people living in institutions. It contains three sub-scales: agitation (six items), attitude towards own ageing (seven items) and lonely dissatisfaction (four items). Completion time is 15 minutes.

Manchester Short Assessment of Quality of Life (MANSA)
The Manchester Short Assessment of Quality of Life (MANSA) (Priebe et al 1999) evaluates the quality of life for older people with chronic mental illness. The MANSA rates a person's satisfaction with 12 aspects of life: number and quality of friendships; fellow residents; sex life; relationship with family; daily routine; not having paid employment; financial status; living conditions; personal safety; physical health; mental health; and life in general. Completion time is 25 minutes.

Dementia Quality of Life (DQoL)
The Dementia Quality of Life (DQoL) (Brod et al 1999) consists of 29 items, measuring five domains: positive affect; negative affect; feelings of belonging; self-esteem; and sense of aesthetics. Completion time is 30 minutes.

CARER WELLBEING AND BURDEN
Caregiver Well-Being Scale (CW–BS)
The Caregiver Well-Being Scale (CW–BS) (Tebb 1995) measures the resources and strengths of carers and can be used for screening and intervention planning. It has 45 items divided into two subscales, with strong reliability and validity scores. One sub-scale measures basic needs in the areas of physical health, esteem, expression of feelings and security. The other subscale concentrates on activities of daily living in relation to household maintenance, leisure activities, family support and functioning outside of the home. Completion time is 55 minutes.

Caregiving Hassles Scale (CHS)
The Caregiving Hassles Scale (CHS) (Kinney & Stephens 1989) is a 42-item scale designed to assess the daily hassles of caring for a family member with Alzheimer's disease, rather than the longer term events or wider caregiver responsibilities. The daily hassles are associated with helping with activities of daily living and the care recipient's cognitive status, behaviour and social network. It is a self-report or interviewer scale and takes 25 minutes to complete.

Burden Interview (BI)
The Burden Interview (BI) (Zarit et al 1980) is a 22-item, self-report or interview measure of perceived burden. The BI measures a carer's psychological health, emotional wellbeing, social and family life, finances, and degree of control over their own life. Completion time is 10 minutes.

SUMMARY
This chapter has given an overview of the value of rating scales to clinical practice. A selection of valid and reliable scales that may be used in the community mental health setting has been provided.

FURTHER READING
Burns A, Lawlor B, Craig S 2004 Assessment scales in old age psychiatry. Martin Duntz, London
McDowell I 2006 Measuring health: a guide to rating scales and questionnaires. Oxford University Press, New York

REFERENCES
Abbey J, Piller N, De Bellis A et al 2004 The Abbey Pain Scale: a 1-minute numerical indicator for people with end stage dementia. International Journal of Palliative Nursing 10(1):6–13
Alexopoulos GS, Abrams RC, Young RC, Shamoian CA 1988 Cornell Scale for Depression in Dementia. Biological Psychiatry 23:271–284
American Psychiatric Association 2000 Diagnostic and statistical manual of mental disorders, 4th edn. American Psychiatric Publishing, Washington DC
Baumgarten M, Becker R, Gauthier S 1990 Validity and reliability of the Dementia Behavior Disturbance Scale. Journal of the American Geriatrics Society 38:221–226
Beck AT, Brown G, Steer RA 1996 Beck Depression Inventory II Manual. The Psychological Corporation, San Antonio, TX

Beck AT, Kovacs M, Weissman A 1979 Assessment of suicidal intention: the Scale for Suicidal Ideation. Journal of Consulting and Clinical Psychology 47(2):343–352

Beck AT, Schuyler D, Herman I 1974b Development of suicide intent scales. In: Beck AT, Resnick HLP, Lettieri DJ (eds) The prediction of suicide. The Charles Press Publishers, Bowie, MI

Beck AT, Weissman A, Lester D, Trexler L 1974a The measurement of pessimism: the Hopelessness Scale. Journal of Consulting and Clinical Psychology 42(6):861–865

Blow FC, Brower KJ, Schulenberg JE et al 1992 The Michigan Alcoholism Screening Test–Geriatric Version (MAST–G): a new elderly specific screening instrument. Alcoholism: Clinical and Experimental Research 16:372

Brandt J, Spencer M, Folstein M 1988 The Telephone Interview for Cognitive Status. Neuropsychiatry, Neuropsychology and Behavioral Neurology 1:111–117

Brod M, Stewart A, Sands L, Qalton P 1999 Conceptualization and measurement of quality of life in dementia: the Dementia–QoL Instrument. Gerontologist 39(1):1–11

Cohen-Mansfield J, Billig N 1986 Agitated behaviors in the elderly I. A Conceptual Review Journal of the American Geriatrics Society 34:711–721

Duke University Center for the Study of Aging and Human Development 1978 Multidimensional functional assessment: the OARS methodology. Duke University Medical Center, Durham

Ewing JA 1984 Detecting alcoholism. The CAGE questionnaire. Journal of the American Medical Association 252(14):1905–1907

Fillenbaum GG, Beekly D, Edland S et al 1997 Consortium to Establish a Registry for Alzheimer's Disease (CERAD): development, database structure, and selected findings. Topics in Health Information Management 18(1):47–58

Folstein M, Folstein SE, McHugh PR 1975 'Mini-Mental State': a practical method for grading the cognitive state of patients for the clinician. Psychiatric Research 12:189–198

Goldberg DP, Gater R, Sartorius N et al 1997 The validity of two versions of the GHQ in the WHO study of mental illness in general health care. Psychological Medicine 27:191–197

Jorm AF, MacKinnon AJ, Henderson AS et al 1995 The Psychogeriatric Assessment Scales: a multidimensional alternative to categorical diagnosis of dementia and depression in the elderly. Psychological Medicine 25:447–460

Katz S, Ford AB, Moskowitz RW et al 1963 Studies of illness in the aged. The index of ADL: a standardized measure of biological and psychosocial function. Journal of the American Medical Association 185(12):914–919

Kinney JM, Stephens MAP 1989 Caregiving Hassles Scale: assessing the daily hassles of caring for a family member with dementia. Gerontologist 29(3):328–332

Koenig HG, Westlund RE, George LK et al 1993 Abbreviating the Duke Social Support Index for use in chronically ill elderly individuals. Psychosomatics 34:61–69

Lawton MP 1975 The Philadelphia Geriatric Center Morale Scale: a revision. Journal of Gerontology 30:85–89

Lawton MP 1988 Instrumental Activities of Daily Living (IADL) Scale: original observer-rater version. Psychopharmacological Bulletin 24(4):785–787

Melzack R 1987 The Short-Form McGill Pain Questionnaire. Pain 30:191–197

Molloy DW, Alemayehu E, Roberts R 1991 Reliability of a Standardised Mini-Mental State Examination compared with the traditional Mini-Mental State Examination. American Journal of Psychiatry 148:102–105

Morrison DP 1983 The Crichton Visual Analogue Scale for the assessment of behaviour in the elderly. Acta Psychiatrica Scandinavica 68:408–413

Neville CC, Byrne GJA 2001 Rating scales for disruptive behaviour in older people with dementia: which is the best for nurses to use? Australasian Journal on Ageing 20(4):166–172

Overall JE 1974 The Brief Psychiatric Rating Scale in psychopharmacology research. In: Pichot P, Olivier-Martin R (eds) Psychological measurements in psychopharmacology: modern problems in psychopharmacology, Volume 7. Karger, Basel, Switzerland, pp 67–78

Pachana NA, Byrne GJ, Siddle H et al 2007 Development and validation of the Geriatric Anxiety Inventory. International Psychogeriatrics 19(1):103–114

Priebe S, Huxley P, Knight S, Evans S 1999 Application and results of the Manchester Short Assessment of Quality of Life (MANSA). International Journal of Social Psychiatry 45:7–12

Reisberg B, Ferris SH, de Leon MJ, Crook T 1982 The Global Deterioration Scale for assessment of primary degenerative dementia. American Journal of Psychiatry 139(9):1136–1139

Saunders J, Aasland O, Babor T et al 1993 Development on the Alcohol Use Disorders Identification Test (AUDIT). WHO collaborative project on early detection of person with harmful alcohol consumption—II. Addiction 88:791–804

Shanker KK, Walker M, Frost D, Orrell MW 1999 The development of a valid and reliable scale for Rating Anxiety in Dementia (RAID). Aging and Mental Health 3(1):39–49

Sheikh RL, Yesavage JA 1986 Geriatric Depression Scale (GDS): recent evidence and development of a shorter version. Clinical Gerontologist 5:165–173

Shulman G 2003 Senior moments: assessing older adults. Addiction Today 15(82):17–19

Tebb S 1995 An aid to empowerment: a Caregiver Well-Being Scale. Health and Social Work 20(2):87–92

Zarit SH, Reever KE, Bach-Peterson J 1980 Relatives of the impaired elderly: correlates of feelings of burden. Gerontologist 20:649–655

Chapter 36

OUTCOME EVALUATION

INTRODUCTION

The demonstration of quality of care requires evaluation from a number of aspects. Outcome measurement can occur at a variety of levels (government, service and individual), and can involve participation of the older person with a mental health problem, the carer and the mental health worker. This chapter briefly examines what type of outcome evaluation data are being collected at a national level, and then goes on to the other areas of symptom reduction, quality of life, and consumer and carer satisfaction. Constantly evaluating health services and implementing the recommendations from the evaluations will ensure that high-quality and responsive services are delivered.

LARGE-SCALE OUTCOME MEASUREMENT

Continual improvement in the quality and effectiveness of the treatment of all people with a mental illness is a major objective of Australia's National Mental Health Strategy. Routine outcome measurements are undertaken to monitor the impact of services on people with mental health problems and to develop casemix systems. The National Outcomes and Casemix Collection (NOCC) comprises clinician-rated, consumer-rated and carer-rated instruments. The instruments applicable to older persons' mental health services (OPMHS) are:

- the Health of the Nation Outcome Scales (HoNOS 65+)
- the Life Skills Profile 16 (LSP–16)
- the Resource Utilisation Groups–Activities of Daily Living (RUG–ADL)
- the Mental Health Inventory (MHI)
- the Kessler–10 Plus (K–10+), and
- the Behaviour and Symptom Identification Scale 32 (BASIS–32).

People with mental health problems find benefit in routine outcome measurement and believe it leads to improvement in care (Guthrie et al 2008).

Health of the Nation Outcome Scales (HoNOS 65+)

The Health of the Nation Outcome Scales (HoNOS) (Wing et al 1996) are a British development designed to gather information from key areas of mental health and social function for the purpose of comparing mental health services and monitoring changes both within individuals and within services. Although the HoNOS were developed for the full age range, by 1999, arguments had been put forward that the scales needed to be modified to be more suitable for the assessment of older people with mental health problems. Modifications and revisions were made to capture greater rating accuracy for depression and dementia, while the essential structure of the HoNOS was maintained. This work produced the HoNOS 65+ (Burns et al 2004, HoNOS 65+ Implementation Group 2002).

HoNOS and various derivatives have been in routine use in many Australian mental health services since 2000. It appears that, in this country at least, the data are being collected, but they are only utilised in very general terms for service evaluation, rather than clinical management or service development (Andrews & Page 2005). This may be due to a number of problems with data collection, including:

1. Clinicians need to be trained in the use of the scale.
2. Clinicians do not complete all data-collection points (e.g. the start episode and the end episode).
3. Clinicians do not complete the form fully.
4. The forms get lost or misplaced. It is anticipated that online forms will help solve this problem.

Overall, as an outcome measure for inpatient and community services, it has been established that the HoNOS 65+ is acceptable to mental health workers, has satisfactory reliability, is sensitive to change, and has good concurrent validity and interrater reliability. However, it lacks content validity, construct validity, predictive validity and test–retest reliability (Cheung & Strachan 2007, Spear et al 2002, Turner 2004). The HoNOS 65+ is a global assessment tool; therefore, if some areas of assessment require other information, a more specific screening and assessment tool should be used.

The HoNOS 65+ assessment is based on clinical judgment, taking into account the most severe symptom or problem during the previous 2 weeks. Assessment information can be obtained from the older person themselves, from clinical notes, through observation and interview, or via other informants such as family carers. The scale has 12 items, with each item contributing equally to the total score. Each item is rated as: 0 = no problem; 1 = minor problem, which requires no intervention; 2 = mild problem, which would need intervention; 3 = moderate problem; and 4 = severe problem. It can be completed by any one of the mental health disciplines and administration time is between 5 and 15 minutes.

The items are as follows (HoNOS 65+ Implementation Group 2004):

1. *Behavioural disturbance.* This can be due to any cause and includes the more overt behaviours of overactivity, aggressiveness, resistance and wandering through to posturing.
2. *Non-accidental self-injury.* This item relates to suicide risk (thoughts, intent and attempts) in the reference period.
3. *Problem drinking or drug use.* This item covers cravings through to frequency and effects of intoxication, plus risk-taking behaviour.
4. *Cognitive problems.* These can be associated with any disorder and the key areas of memory, orientation and language are covered.
5. *Problems related to physical illness or disability.* These can be from any cause. The scale covers physical health, mobility, sensory impairment, falls, medication side effects, pain and injury.

6. *Problems associated with hallucinations and/or delusions or false beliefs.* This item is irrespective of diagnosis and includes delusions, hallucinations and thought disorder.

7. *Problems associated with depressive symptoms.* This item covers mood disturbance.

8. *Other mental and behavioural problems.* This item is for the most severe clinical problem not covered previously. It rates the severity, frequency, degree of control and distress of such problems as phobias, anxiety, somatoform, eating, sleeping and sexual disorders.

9. *Problems with social or supportive relationships.* These may be self-identified or noted by others. Overall, this item examines the quality and quantity of interpersonal relationships and if the older person withdraws or becomes distressed by relationships with others.

10. *Problems with activities of daily living.* This item covers activities of daily living (ADLs), including toileting, eating and dressing, as well as instrumental activities of daily living (IADLs), such as cooking, shopping and financial management. The developers of HoNOS prefer to use the term 'personal', instead of ADL, and 'domestic', instead of IADL.

11. *Overall problems with living conditions.* This item considers the degree to which the older person's living conditions impact on their intact skills and abilities. It includes assessment of any environment, be it a family home or residential aged care facility (RACF). Environmental factors include: lighting and heating; relationships with relatives, neighbours or staff; facilities available and if these are used by the older person; the degree of satisfaction with the home; and qualifications and experience of staff.

12. *Problems with work and leisure activities—quality of day-time environment.* This item rates any problems that may occur with involvement in work and leisure activities and how cooperative the older person is with participation.

There are a few inpatient/community studies that have reported on the use of the HoNOS 65+. McKay and McDonald (2008) described the experience of using the HoNOS 65+ in a small integrated OPMHS in Sydney, Australia. The HoNOS 65+ data had been collected for many years, but they were not being utilised at a local level. A service review recommended integrating outcome measures into routine clinical practice to enhance individual care, team and service operations. At the individual care level, a 'key item' score is derived by clinical team consensus regarding the older person's overall functioning and the main clinical issue that involves the OPMHS. The 'key item' is the most prominent HoNOS 65+ item (e.g. if the admission is for aggressive behaviour it will be item 1).

The advantages of using the HoNOS 65+ were identified as focused care planning, comprehensive data collection and analysis on a regular schedule (admission, review and discharge), evaluation of progress and measuring change in mental health status. At the clinical team level, improvements were noted as improved understanding of the clinical issues faced by the team, factors that influenced outcomes with the team and how effectively the team was performing. In regard to service management, the HoNOS 65+ data were utilised to better characterise the service users, reasons for admission, length of stay and benchmarking activities with other OPMHS.

In another Australian study, Spear et al (2002) found the HoNOS 65+ is sensitive to change and that the community-based OPMHS was having a positive impact on treatment for mental health problems. A study conducted in the United Kingdom (MacDonald 2002) established that the HoNOS 65+ can determine:

- if a service is having an impact on recovery from illness
- different outcomes for similar consumer groups in contact with different services
- changes in outcome over time and relate these to changes in resources and management, and
- significant differences between areas in the patterns of morbidity of otherwise indistinguishable consumer groups.

Life Skills Profile 16 (LSP–16)

The Life Skills Profile 16 (LSP–16) is a shortened version of the LSP–39 (Rosen et al 1989). It measures the level of disability experienced by people with a mental health problem, particularly those living in the community. It is a 16-item scale administered by a mental health worker. The LSP–16 has four subscales, examining the domains of withdrawal, self-care, compliance and antisocial behaviour. The reference period is the previous 3 months. Information is obtained by direct observation or from other people who are in contact with the older person. It can be completed in 5 minutes. The scale has been rated well for clinical utility and feasibility (Pirkis et al 2005). Although recommended for use with older people in the NOCC (Pirkis et al 2005), it does not appear to have been tested specifically with OPMHS users.

Resource Utilisation Groups–Activities of Daily Living (RUG–ADL)

The Resource Utilisation Groups–Activities of Daily Living (RUG–ADL) is a component of the casemix tool RUG–III developed for use in North American RACFs (Fries et al 1994). It was conceptualised from the point of view that diagnosis is a poor predictor of resource use. Factors like objectives of care, functional deficits, rehabilitation problems and behavioural problems are better predictors. The RUG–ADL focuses on basic activities of daily living, such as toileting, bathing, eating and mobility. These four items are rated by a mental health worker and the reference period is 'current status'. Psychometric testing has centred around the RUG–III as a casemix tool, rather than the RUG–ADL as an outcome measure. With that in mind, its content validity has been criticised for not being adequate for mental health problems such as dementia. It has good interrater reliability, but there has been limited or no other standard psychometric testing (Pirkis et al 2005).

Mental Health Inventory (MHI)

The Mental Health Inventory (MHI) (Veit & Ware 1983) is a self-report instrument that measures psychological distress and psychological wellbeing in the general population. It has 38 items, with the majority of items rated from 1 to 6 based on frequency and intensity. A higher score represents more favourable mental health outcomes. The MHI has been used in studies involving older people. Extensive psychometric testing determined adequate to good ratings for content, construct, concurrent and predictive validity, test–retest and interrater reliability. It is sensitive to change and has good clinical utility and feasibility (Pirkis et al 2005).

Kessler–10 Plus (K–10+)

The Kessler–10 (K–10) (Kessler et al 2002) is a 10-item, self-report instrument that measures non-specific psychological distress. It has been incorporated into the United States National Health Interview Survey and Australia's National Health Survey (Australian Bureau of Statistics 2006). Although primarily an epidemiological instrument, it has utility in clinical settings. The Kessler–10 Plus (K–10+) has four additional items that measure distress-specific global impairment, distress-specific service use and self-reported physical health contribution to distress. The reference period is the previous 4 weeks. The items are rated from few or minimal symptoms to extreme levels of distress indicated by the amount of time during the 4-week period the particular problem had been experienced. Clinical utility and feasibility are well regarded. Content, construct and concurrent validity and test–retest reliability are adequate to good. Predictive validity and sensitivity to change could do with further examination (Pirkis et al 2005).

Behaviour and Symptom Identification Scale 32 (BASIS–32)

The Behaviour and Symptom Identification Scale 32 (BASIS–32) (Eisen et al 1986) is a self-report measure of symptoms and behavioural distress. The information can also be obtained via an interview by the mental health worker. Although developed for inpatients, it has subsequently been validated for community and residential settings. It has 32 items based on five subscales, which cover the domains of relation to self and others, depression and anxiety, daily living and role functioning, impulsive and addictive behaviour, and psychosis. Items 3 and 4 relate to work and school activities, which may not be applicable to older people. The BASIS–24 was developed to counteract the problems identified with the BASIS–32, and it is more suitable for older people (Eisen et al 2004). The reference period is the preceding week and it takes 5–10 minutes to complete. The majority of psychometric testing has taken place on the BASIS–32. Despite variation in the psychometric reports, the general consensus is that it has adequate reliability and validity, it is sensitive to change during treatment, and has clinical utility and feasibility. This scale requires a licence and fee payment (Pirkis et al 2005).

SYMPTOM REDUCTION

Instruments such as the BASIS–32 or BASIS–24 may not be specific enough as an outcome measure of treatment effectiveness. There are some very specific instruments available for such purposes with the Hamilton Rating Scale for Depression (HRSD) (Hamilton 1960) being one example. The HRSD has 17 items to measure the severity of depression, which are mainly focused on somatic symptoms. Items cover depressed mood, guilt, suicide, insomnia, work and interests, retardation, agitation, somatic anxiety, gastrointestinal symptoms, general somatic symptoms, loss of libido, hypochondriasis, lack of insight and loss of weight. There are an additional four items that do not measure the intensity of depression, but can be used for diagnostic purposes. It is rated via a semistructured interview with an experienced mental health worker. The reference period is the last week and it takes 20–30 minutes to administer. The majority of items are scored on a 5-point scale from 0 (absent) to 4 (severe). The HRSD assesses change based on the difference in the score from one assessment to another. Although not specifically developed for older people, it has been used extensively with this group.

Other scales such as the Clinical Global Impressions scales (CGI) (Guy 1976) are used to measure symptom severity, treatment response and the efficacy of pharmacological treatment over time. These scales require the older person to be compared with what occurs typically for older people with the same diagnosis. There is a severity scale (CGI–S) that measures severity at the time of assessment on a 7-point scale (normal to extremely ill). The improvement scale (CGI–I) measures how much the older person has improved or worsened to the baseline taken at the beginning of the intervention. This is also a 7-point scale from 'very much improved' to 'very much worse'. The Efficacy Index is a 4-point by 4-point index that measures the therapeutic effect of treatment by side effects. The reference period is the previous week. An interview format is used by the mental health worker, but information can also be obtained from clinical files, other staff and significant others.

QUALITY OF LIFE

Quality of life (QOL) is a ubiquitous concept that has many dimensions. The dimensions generally cover physical, psychological, social and spiritual wellbeing. It is difficult to define because QOL means many different things to many different people. Despite this paradox, QOL is deemed an outcome measure for the evaluation of care provided, and many tools and methods have been devised for measurement (Selai & Trimble 1999). Some tools are global QOL measures, some focus on objective measurement (how a person is doing), others focus on subjective measurement (how a person feels) and others may specifically examine health-related QOL from the perspective of a specific disease (e.g. dementia). The gold standard for QOL measurements is self-report. However, there are some circumstances, such as severe cognitive impairment, where the report may have to be given by another person. There are numerous QOL instruments available and a great variety in the parameters that are measured; therefore, it is paramount that the scale chosen suits the purpose of the activity as judiciously as possible. Reviews of QOL measures can assist greatly with this process (Haywood et al 2005).

The World Health Organization (WHO) has recently developed a QOL measure specifically for older people (Power et al 2005). This instrument measures the older person's perceptions in the context of their cultural and value systems. It also encompasses their personal goals, standards and concerns. It is a six-facet module, with each module containing four items for a total of 24 items. The facets include sensory abilities, autonomy, past, present and future activities, social participation and death, dying and intimacy. Peel et al (2007) established good reliability and validity for the WHOQOL–OLD. It had good face validity, but the researchers suggested it still be administered with either the WHOQOL–100 or the WHOQOL–BREF for a more comprehensive coverage (Power et al 2005). Furthermore, reliability and validity of the WHOQOL–OLD has been examined with a group of Norwegian older people. Internal consistency was reliable except for past, present and future activities; construct validity was only partially supported, but its external validity was rated as good (Halvorsrud et al 2008).

An example of a QOL scale completed by an older person with dementia and also their caregiver is the Quality of Life in Alzheimer's Disease: Patient and Caregiver Report (QOL–AD) (Logsdon et al 2000). It has 13 items which are rated on a 4-point scale, with 1 being poor and 4 being excellent. There is a formula to give a composite score that will give more weight to the older person's rating than the caregiver's rating. It has sound psychometric properties, and moderate levels of cognitive impairment did not have any effect on the reliability or the validity (Burns et al 2004).

CONSUMER AND CARER SATISFACTION

Consumer and carer experience and satisfaction with an OPMHS is a valuable and valid outcome indicator of the quality of the service that has been provided. Satisfaction is determined by undertaking an evaluation of whether or not the older person and their carer's psychological, physical, social and spiritual needs have been met by the service. Such evaluations can provide information that can potentially impact on treatment outcomes (e.g. a clinical intervention may be adapted, enabling easier compliance for the consumer) (Fletcher et al 2008). The feedback received can determine the strengths and weaknesses of the services, and inform priorities and strategies on redeveloping or refining current services or the development of new services. Of note is the importance of consumer opinions because, due to ageist attitudes, older people are sometimes overlooked, particularly if they have a mental health problem, with the assumption they cannot articulate their opinions clearly or accurately. Mozley et al (1999) established that a high proportion of older people can answer questions about such issues as quality of life, even in the presence of cognitive deficits.

There are many areas that can be assessed when undertaking a satisfaction survey. The focus can be on the consumer and carer experience, it can be on the staff, it can be on the physical environment, other consumers and carers, or it can be on broader service delivery issues. In the box below is a snapshot of the many elements that can be examined in relation to consumer and carer satisfaction.

ELEMENTS OF CONSUMER AND CARER SATISFACTION

The elements listed below can be examined in relation to carer and consumer satisfaction.

Perceptions of staff
Elements include:
- source of information
- friendliness
- sensitivity
- attentiveness
- listening and comprehension skills
- courteousness
- respectfulness
- expertise
- generosity with time
- accessibility and availability
- maintenance of privacy and confidentiality
- ability to provide compassion and care, and
- trustworthiness.

Perceptions of the service

Elements include:

- overall satisfaction
- everything done in a timely manner
- user-friendly
- physical environmental qualities (comfortable, safe, clean, private)
- recommendation to others
- expectations have been met
- any gaps in the service, and
- culturally and spiritually congruent.

Perceptions of the treatment plan

Elements include:

- satisfaction with the different components (e.g. psychotherapy, psychoeducation, medication, support groups)
- offered different treatment options
- involved in decision making
- easy to understand and follow
- needs-focused
- advice on how to self-help, and
- follow-up care.

The most common method of gaining the information is through a written survey, which can be mailed, handed out or placed on a website. The questions are usually answered as a 'yes' or 'no', by a Likert scale, short answer/comment or various combinations of these methods. Although these are mainly self-report surveys, they can also be administered via face-to-face or telephone interview format. There are many advantages and disadvantages for whichever method is chosen, and there are many references available on how to construct survey tools.

Similarly, there are many already constructed satisfaction survey tools, some with established validity and reliability. One such scale is the 32-item Verona Service Satisfaction Scale (VSSS–32) (Ruggeri et al 1996). This instrument is a consumer report and was specifically designed for community-based mental health services. It examines the areas of overall satisfaction with professionals' skills and behaviours, information, access, efficacy, type of intervention and the involvement of relatives. It has good test–retest reliability, acceptability, sensitivity and content validity (Ruggeri 2001). Another effective way to measure consumer and carer satisfaction with an OPMHS is by the use of qualitative methods (e.g. focus groups, semistructured interviews and in-depth interviews).

The majority of survey tools and qualitative question guides to evaluate consumer and carer satisfaction have been developed with items generated by the service provider themselves, introducing a certain bias albeit unwittingly in most cases. Qualitative studies are very useful in capturing the aspects that would be relevant to the consumers and carers, and thereby determining quality indicators from their perspective (Willis et al 2009).

There are limitations to conducting satisfaction surveys and qualitative groups and interviews. The participants could be biased, meaning those who are most satisfied are more likely to participate than those people who are not satisfied. Therefore, it is important to contact non-participants to find out why they did not respond or wish to participate. Positive ratings and comments are also influenced by other factors, such as people's reluctance to express negative opinions and the wording and structure of the survey or question guide (Press 2002).

After the data have been collected and analysed, it is important that this is fed back to the actual participants and to the broader group of consumers and carers. They also need to know if any changes are going to be made in relation to the information gained. Sometimes, consumer and carer expectations cannot be met due to lack of willingness, ability and resources. The reasons expectations cannot be met need to be explained to consumers. The loop is vital if the health service wants to continue to gain representative and quality feedback from consumers and carers.

SUMMARY

Outcome evaluation is an important method to ensure continual quality improvement. This chapter has given an overview of some of the methods that can be used to gain the information required for evaluative processes. Being responsive to recommendations or the expressed needs of consumers and their carers enhances engagement with the OPMHS.

FURTHER READING

Press I 2002 Patient satisfaction: defining, measuring and improving the experience of care. Health Administration Press, Chicago

Tansella M, Thornicroft G 2001 Mental health outcome measures. Gaskell, London

USEFUL WEBSITES

Mental Health Outcome and Assessment Tools (MHOAT): www.sswahs.nsw.gov.au/mhealt/mhoat/mhoatsupport.html

National Outcomes and Casemix Collection (NOCC): www.health.gov.au/inter/main/publishing.nsf/Content/mental-nocc

Royal College of Psychiatrists: www.rcpsych.ac.uk/clinicalservicestandards/honos/olderadults.aspx

REFERENCES

Andrews G, Page AC 2005 Outcome measurement, outcome management and monitoring. Australian and New Zealand Journal of Psychiatry 39:649–651

Australian Bureau of Statistics (ABS) 2006 National health survey. ABS, Canberra

Burns A, Beevor A, Lelliott P et al 1999 Health of the Nation Outcome Scales for elderly people (HoNOS 65+). British Journal of Psychiatry 174:424–427

Burns A, Lawlor B, Craig S 2004 Assessment scales in old age psychiatry. Martin Dunitz, London

Cheung G, Strachan J 2007 Routine 'Health of the Nation Outcome Scales for elderly people' (HoNOS 65+) collection in an acute psychogeriatric inpatient unit in New Zealand. Journal of the New Zealand Medical Association 120:1259

Eisen SV, Grob MC, Klein AA 1986 The development of a self-report measure for psychiatric inpatient evaluation. Psychiatric Hospital 17(4):165–171

Eisen SV, Normand SL, Belanger AJ et al 2004 The revised behavior and symptom identification scale (BASIS–R). Medical Care 42:1230–1241

Fletcher K, Parker G, Tully L 2008 Patient satisfaction with the Black Dog Institute Depression Clinic. Australasian Psychiatry 16(1):27–32

Fries BE, Schneider DP, Foley WJ et al 1994 Refining a case-mix measure for nursing homes: Resource Utilization Groups (RUG–III). Medical Care 32(7):668–685

Guthrie D, McIntosh M, Callaly T et al 2008 Consumer attitudes towards the use of routine outcome measures in a public mental health service: a consumer-driven study. International Journal of Mental Health Nursing 17:92–97

Guy W 1976 ECDEU Assessment manual for psychopharmacology. US Department of Health, Education, and Welfare, Public Health Service, Alcohol, Drug Abuse, and Mental Health Administration, Rockville, MD

Halvorsrud L, Kalfoss M, Diseth A 2008 Reliability and validity of the Norwegian WHOQOL–OLD module. Scandinavian Journal of Caring Science 22:292–305

Hamilton M 1960 A rating scale for depression. Journal of Neurology, Neurosurgery and Psychiatry 23:56–62

Haywood KL, Garratt AM, Fitzpatrick R 2005 Quality of life in older people: a structured review of generic self-assessment health instruments. Quality of Life Research 13:1651–1668

HoNOS 65+ Implementation Group 2002 HoNOS 65+ glossary: changes, April. Royal College of Psychiatrists. Research Unit, London

HoNOS 65+ Implementation Group 2004 HoNOS 65+ A tabulated glossary for use with HoNOS 65+ (version 3g: corrected June 2004). Royal College of Psychiatrists, Research Unit, London

Kessler RC, Andrews G, Colpe LJ et al 2002 Short screening scales to monitor population prevalences and trends in non-specific psychological distress. Psychological Medicine 32(6): 959–976

Logsdon RG, Gibbons LE, McCurry SM, Teri L 2000 Quality of Life in Alzheimer's Disease: Patient and Caregiver Reports. In Albert SM, Logsdon RG (eds) Assessing quality of life in Alzheimer's disease. Springer Publishing, New York

MacDonald A 2002 The usefulness of aggregate routine clinical outcomes data: the example of HoNOS 65+. Journal of Mental Health 11(6):645–656

McKay R, McDonald R 2008 Expensive detour or a way forward? The experience of routine outcome measurement in an aged care psychiatry service. Australasian Psychiatry 16(6):428–432

Mozley CG, Huxley P, Sutcliff C et al 1999 'Not knowing where I am doesn't mean I don't know what I like': cognitive impairment and quality of life responses in elderly people. International Journal of Geriatric Psychiatry 14:776–783

Peel N, Bartlett H, Marshall A 2007 Measuring quality of life in older people: reliability and validity of WHOQOL–OLD. Australasian Journal on Ageing 26(4):162–167

Pirkis J, Burgess P, Kirk P et al 2005 Review of standardised measures used in the National Outcomes and Casemix Collection (NOCC). Australian Mental Health Outcomes and Classification Network, Canberra

Power M, Quinn K, Schmidt S 2005 Development of the WHOQOL–OLD module. Quality of Life 14:2187–2214

Press I 2002 Patient satisfaction: defining, measuring and improving the experience of care. Health Administration Press, Chicago

Rosen A, Hadzi-Pavlovic D, Parker G 1989 The Life Skills Profile: a measure assessing function and disability in schizophrenia. Schizophrenia Bulletin 15(2):325–337

Ruggeri M 2001 Satisfaction with psychiatric services. In Thornicroft G, Tansella M (eds) Mental health outcome measures. Springer, Berlin

Ruggeri M, Dall'Agnola R, Bisoffi G 1996 Factor analysis of the Verona Service Satisfaction Scale–32 and development of reduced versions. International Journal of Methods in Psychiatric Research 6:23–38

Selai C, Trimble MR 1999 Assessing quality of life in dementia. Aging and Mental Health 3(2):101–111

Spear J, Chawla S, O'Reilly M, Rock D 2002 Does the HoNOS 65+ meet the criteria for a clinical outcome indicator for mental health services for older people? International Journal of Geriatric Psychiatry 17:226–230

Turner S 2004 Are the Health of the Nation Outcome Scales (HoNOS) useful for measuring outcomes in older people's mental health services? Aging and Mental Health 8(5):387–396

Veit CT, Ware JE 1983 The structure of psychological distress and well-being in general populations. Journal of Consulting and Clinical Psychology 51(5):730–742

Willis R, Chan J, Murray J et al 2009 People with dementia and their family carers' satisfaction with a memory service: a qualitative evaluation generating quality indicators for dementia care. Journal of Mental Health 18(1):26–37

Wing JK, Curits RH, Beevor A 1996 HoNOS Health of the Nation Outcome Scales: report on research and development, July 1993 to December 1995. Royal College of Psychiatrists, London

INDEX

f denotes figures, t denotes tables